From Placebo to Panacea

Putting Psychiatric Drugs to the Test

Edited by

Seymour Fisher

Roger P. Greenberg

John Wiley & Sons, Inc.

New York • Chichester • Weinheim • Brisbane • Singapore • Toronto

Library of Congress Cataloging-in-Publication Data:

From Placebo to Panacea : putting psychiatric drugs to the test / edited
    by Seymour Fisher and Roger P. Greenberg.
        p.   cm.
    Includes bibliographical references and index.
    ISBN 0-471-14848-2 (cloth : alk. paper)
    1. Psychotropic drugs—Effectiveness.   2. Psychiatry—Differential
therapeutics.   3. Mental illness—Chemotherapy—Evaluation.
4. Placebo (Medicine) I. Fisher, Seymour. II. Greenberg, Roger P.
    [DNLM: 1. Mental Disorders—drug therapy.   2. Placebos—
    therapeutic use.   3. Psychotropic Drugs—therapeutic use.   WM 402
    P697 1997]
    RC483.P63   1997
    616.89'18—dc21
    DNLM/DLC
    for Library of Congress   97-1074

Printed in the United States of America

10 9 8 7 6 5 4 3 2 1

Contributors

David O. Antonuccio, Ph.D.
University of Nevada School
of Medicine and Veterans
Affairs Medical Center
Reno, Nevada

Robert F. Bornstein, Ph.D.
Gettysburg College
Gettysburg, Pennsylvania

Robert C. Carson, Ph.D.
Duke University
Durham, North Carolina

David Cohen, Ph.D.
University of Montreal
Montreal, Canada

William G. Danton, Ph.D.
University of Nevada School
of Medicine and Veterans
Affairs Medical Center
Reno, Nevada

Rhoda L. Fisher, Ph.D.
Private Practice
Manlius, New York

Seymour Fisher, Ph.D.
State University of New York
Health Science Center
Syracuse, New York

Michael D. Greenberg, Ph.D.
Duke University and Harvard
Law School (J.D. class of 1999)
Durham, North Carolina, and
Cambridge, Massachusettes

Roger P. Greenberg, Ph.D.
State University of New York
Health Science Center
Syracuse, New York

Barbara Henker, Ph.D.
University of California,
Los Angeles
Los Angeles, California

Carol K. Whalen, Ph.D.
University of California, Irvine
Irvine, California

Preface

MULTIPLE BOOKS CONTINUE to appear with analyses of the therapeutic powers of various psychoactive drugs. What are we offering in this book that is different or special? In answering this question, we will focus first on an issue that we discussed in an earlier edited volume *The Limits of Biological Treatments for Psychological Distress: Comparisons with Psychotherapy and Placebo* (Fisher & Greenberg, 1989). At that time we noted:

> An almost startling complexity faces anyone who seeks to judge the efficacy of the various somatic treatments. The complexity is in part due to the multiple variables influencing any therapeutic outcome and is partially the result of specific troubling inadequacies in current methods for appraising the somatic approaches. We have learned from past literature reviews and discussions with current proponents and opponents of the therapies that the very same set of apparently scientific findings concerning efficacy can be interpreted in quite divergent ways as a function of whichever "theoretical" positions preexist. We have personally been startled to read research reports that seemed ostensibly to indicate a quite limited advantage for a particular drug as compared to a placebo, but then to find such reports hailed in another context as proof the drug is highly effective. The impact of bias is bad enough when one is trying to clarify theoretical issues, but takes on a more immediate seriousness when it influences the treatments of large numbers of distressed humans. (pp. 309–310)

In essence, the sheer complexity and ambiguity of findings bearing on psychoactive drug efficacy often permit wide evaluative latitude when interpreting such findings. The majority of published appraisals of psychoactive drugs are authored by individuals who directly or indirectly are identified with a biological approach to treatment. They have a stake in visualizing psychoactive drugs as potent and beneficial and, therefore, are inclined to introduce a positive twist into their analyses of the pertinent literature. We feel it is important to balance this bias by adopting a counterattitude based on a determined skepticism. All the contributors to this book were chosen because they do not have a significant stake in biological therapies looking good and, indeed, are typified by a questioning posture vis-à-vis biological claims. This is also a form of selectivity or bias, but we regard it as a valuable contrast to other widely prevalent favorably slanted perspectives. In the long run, we think it is good for the psychoactive drug treatment enterprise to be exposed to a probing critique that highlights potential weaknesses and also possible areas that require further thought and analysis. Such aggressive skepticism is encouraged by an awareness of past disappointments typical of the history of treatments for psychological disturbance. The long list of past treatment failures, ranging from insulin coma to lobotomy, speaks for itself. Actually, skepticism should prevail in all evaluations of research, particularly if they involve the welfare of large numbers of persons who are in a state of discomfort.

In our 1989 edited book, we assembled critiques of widely used psychoactive drugs. Systematic analyses were provided concerning the effectiveness of such drugs in relation to depression, anxiety syndromes, schizophrenia, and attention deficit disorders in children. We also appraised in some detail the logic and assumptions underlying the double-blind methodology employed to test the therapeutic powers of psychoactive agents. The picture that emerged was not reassuring about the drug treatment enterprise that anchors the biological approach to managing psychological distress. Numerous problems were uncovered that we will shortly consider.

We learned that the therapeutic efficacies of the antidepressants, anxiolytics, and antipsychotics have been exaggerated. But a more serious problem is that the so-called double-blind design for evaluating drugs, which presumably guarantees that outcome data will not be appreciably contaminated by experimenter bias, is probably vulnerable to such bias. This vulnerability derives particularly from the placebos in drug studies typically being inactive substances that fail to arouse body experiences comparable to those stimulated by active drugs. This contrast in body experience provides solid cues for identifying whether the participant has taken a placebo or an active agent. Inactive placebos are simply not genuine controls, and this leaves a rent in the typical psychoactive drug study design. To a significant but still unknown degree, psychoactive drug trials lack scientific rigor. Further documentation of this point will be provided. Overall, we were left with an impression of uncertainty. It appeared to us that because of the defects in the double-blind design, a good deal of past research dealing with the psychoactive drugs would need to be repeated in better controlled contexts before one could, with any scientific confidence, accept claims concerning their efficacy.

Quite in contrast to the sobering scientific data, the news media and popular persiflage have attributed wondrous qualities to the psychoactive drugs. The florid excitement stirred up by the introduction of the antidepressant Prozac (fluoxetine) illustrates this point only too well. There is widespread belief, in both scholarly and popular circles, that the effects of psychoactive agents are sui generis and that it is unethical to treat psychological disturbance with nondrug approaches. A good deal of published research, however, documents that nondrug agents (e.g., psychotherapy) are equally and sometimes more therapeutically potent. In a related vein, those practitioners who actually prescribe psychoactive drugs in their clinical practices often seem to be only hazily aware of the pertinent scientific literature. They individually compile their own clinical lore and reach idiosyncratic conclusions about optimal dose levels, cookbook combinations of drugs that presumably have augmented effectiveness, and so forth. Anyone familiar with the current clinical scene knows that drug-prescribing concepts and practices are often surprisingly confused (e.g., Dewan & Koss, 1995). Practitioners simply do not have the technical skills to interpret and integrate the up-to-date drug research literature into their work. Therefore, they perseverate on drug treatment modes they learned early in their training or improvise new modes based on their own limited sampling of patients. There is obviously a need to reintegrate into clinical practice the really solid current scientific information available concerning the psychoactive studies.

Another intent of this book is to introduce a wider range of psychological concepts into analyses of psychoactive drug phenomena. Most examinations of such phenomena are anchored in a biological paradigm almost totally bereft of psychological imagery. However, the psychological literature abounds with ideas that offer promise in clarifying various psychoactive drug effects. For example, social psychological notions about expectation, stereotyping, and suggestion are applicable to decoding the link between drug and placebo responses. Similarly, the accumulated body image literature (e.g., Fisher, 1986) would seem to be pertinent to the experiences of taking a psychoactive drug and interpreting its side effects. Personality formulations relating to activity-passivity (independence-dependence, acquiescence) have already shown promise (Cleveland, 1989) in clarifying responses to excitatory versus inhibitory drug effects and differential reactions to placebo versus active drug. There is a need to tap into the true complexity of psychoactive drug effects as mediated by the psychological domain.

The material presented here is organized into four Parts. The first consists of conceptual analysis of ideas that explicitly or implicitly enfold the whole psychoactive drug treatment enterprise. Thus, questions are raised about the usual distinctions between placebo and active drug, and the basic psychosocial nature of drug effects is highlighted. The central point is made that the contrast between psychological and biological is forced and encourages false, oversimplified notions about how psychoactive drugs achieve results.

Another broad conceptual issue considered in Part One relates to the logic of the classificatory system in successive editions of the *Diagnostic and Statistical Manual of Mental Disorders (DSM)* (e.g., American Psychiatric Association, 1994), which serves as a pervasive frame of reference for those who prescribe presumably specific medications for specific forms of psychopathology. The deficiencies of the *DSM* schema are explored not only with reference to its definitional forms and inconsistencies but also in terms of data demonstrating that comorbidity is so widespread as to virtually obliterate the formal boundaries of the *DSM* categories.

Part Two comprises four chapters that scrutinize the research concerned with the efficacy of psychoactive drugs for treating adults with depression, bipolar disorder, various anxiety syndromes, schizophrenic disturbance, and the pathology of the so-called borderline.

Part Three includes a review and evaluation of the existing research bearing on the efficacy and side effects of psychoactive drugs for treating children and adolescents for various forms of psychological disturbance (e.g., depression, ADHD).

Finally, in Part Four we integrate the data provided by the preceding chapters and offer new, often challenging perspectives on the problems of evaluating psychoactive agents.

SEYMOUR FISHER
ROGER P. GREENBERG

REFERENCES

American Psychiatric Association. (1994). *Diagnostic and statistical manual of mental disorders: DSM-IV* (4th ed.). Washington, DC: Author.

Cleveland, S. E. (1989). Personality factors in the mediation of drug response. In S. Fisher & R. P. Greenberg (Eds.), *The limits of biological treatments for psychological distress: Comparisons with psychotherapy and placebo* (pp. 235–262). Hillsdale, NJ: Erlbaum.

Dewan, M. J., & Koss, M. (1995). The clinical impact of reported variance in potency of antipsychotic agents. *Acta Psychiatrica Scandinavica, 91,* 229–232.

Fisher, S. (1986). *Development and structure of the body image* (Vols. 1 & 2). Hillsdale, NJ: Erlbaum.

Fisher, S., & Greenberg, R. P. (1989). *The limits of biological treatments for psychological distress: Comparisons with psychotherapy and placebo.* Hillsdale, NJ: Erlbaum.

Contents

PART ONE

CONCEPTUAL ISSUES

CHAPTER 1

The Curse of the Placebo: Fanciful Pursuit of a Pure Biological Therapy

SEYMOUR FISHER and ROGER P. GREENBERG

T HE TESTING OF psychotropic (and most other) therapeutic drugs is dominated by the aim to demonstrate that a so-called active agent can be distinguished from an inactive one (placebo). The central question posed is whether the active drug produces a discernibly greater therapeutic impact than the placebo. Presumably, if the drug is more curative than the placebo, this proves that the drug is effective because of an active biological constituent that cannot be matched by the placebo, which is defined as lacking biological potency. Active drugs are said to cure largely because they are biologically potent, whereas any curative powers of a placebo are attributed to such nonbiological psychological variables as suggestibility and expectancy.

At one level, the distinction between psychotropic drug and placebo represents a long-term polarity in medicine and biology concerning specific versus nonspecific causes. Shepherd (1993) reviews this polarity in some detail. He points out that the issue of specificity has been a preoccupation in medicine since the time of ancient Greece. He indicates:

> It is bound up with a fundamental dichotomy contrasting the Platonic or "ontological" with the Hippocratic . . . view of disease. . . . The ontological notion of disease postulates an independent, self-sufficient entity (e.g., a

diagnostic category) with its own natural history; the Hippocratic emphasizes the individual biography of the patient. (p. 569)

The ontological perspective, notes Shepherd, "accepted the Cartesian model of the human body as a machine" (Shepherd, 1993, p. 569) and sought to reduce explanations in medicine to specific mechanistic concepts. The opposed perspective considers disease broadly in relation to the overall life circumstances of the individual. In the past 200 years, the pendulum has swung back and forth within this polarity. Explanatory disputes diversely phrased in terms of "bacteriological specificity" at one extreme and "psychosomatic" metaphors at the other have ebbed and flowed.

The need to establish that psychotropic drugs work because they are basically potent biological agents stirred strong interest in the placebo, which represented a control for all the nonbiological therapeutic variance that might contaminate the results of a drug efficacy trial. A considerable literature concerned with placebo controls accumulated. Many observers have probed and analyzed this array of observations (e.g., Beecher, 1955; Brody, 1977; Dinnerstein, Lowenthal, & Blitz, 1966–1967; Evans, 1974; J. D. Frank, 1973; Grunbaum, 1981, 1985; Jospe, 1978; S. Ross & Buckalew, 1983; A. K. Shapiro, 1968; White, Tursky, & Schwartz, 1985). Over and over, the researcher can find discussions about the nature of the placebo and the variables that magnify or minimize its powers. However, the underlying intent of almost all inquiries in psychiatric research concerning placebos has been to muster an experimental design capable of banishing any doubts that psychotropic drugs cure by virtue of a specific biological mechanism. In poring over this literature, however, one is struck with how often it turns out to be difficult to differentiate drug and placebo effects. Most of the studies (e.g., S. Fisher & Greenberg, 1989; White et al., 1985) have shown the therapeutic potential of placebos to be impressive and in many instances (e.g., when treating depression) not markedly less than the level attained by active drugs (e.g., antidepressants). Furthermore, one finds a welter of confused debate about how to differentiate active drug from placebo at a broad theoretical level. Grunbaum (1981, 1985), A. P. Shapiro and Morris (1978), Brody (1977, 1985), and others have argued and disagreed about whether the differentiation relates to being specific versus nonspecific in action or causality; whether it must be linked to physicians' conceptual models of how the agents they administer "work"; whether it is tied to being "intentional" or "nonintentional"; and so forth. Details of these arguments are available in the references just cited.

We are, for reasons soon to be detailed, impressed that theorists have not found it easy to arrive at a sharp logically based frame of reference for rationalizing the long-standing, by now stereotyped, separation of "active psychotropic drug" from "placebo." Actually, we consider the separation to be a Cartesian hangover that is rapidly becoming irrelevant.[1] Such separation derives primarily from the notion that the active drug affects the individual by initiating definable biological (biochemical) processes, whereas the placebo presumably acts through psychological mechanisms. This way of thinking has persisted despite research suggesting that placebo effects are physiologically mediated (e.g., by changes in endorphin levels; Evans, 1985). If the researcher adopts a simple biological monism, the effects produced by placebos are just as biologically mediated as those initiated by so-called active agents. *All* these effects occur in tissue and one is no more biologically real than the other. A response to a placebo is just as biological as a response to an antipsychotic drug. Although this may be obvious, it has somehow not penetrated into most of the functional thinking in this area. It is apropos to cite research (Baxter et al., 1992) showing that successful psychotherapeutic treatment of obsessive-compulsive symptoms produces brain imagery changes parallel to those resulting from successful drug treatment. The talking (psychological) and drug-based therapies are both equally biological as defined by brain imagery measures. Placebos influence behavior because they initiate brain changes; and this is likewise true of active psychotropic drugs. The hazy boundary between placebo and active drug is even more fluid because of the likelihood that psychological variables (when translated into brain changes) also contribute to the "biological" impact of the active drug.

The fluidity of the demarcation between psychotropic drug and placebo cannot be fully grasped until one probes the considerable research literature concerning the role of context in the effects each can produce. When reviewing this literature, we will be alert to the following issues:

- What situational variables mediate response to psychotropic drugs as defined by (a) therapeutic potency; (b) patterns of physiological arousal; (c) modes of coping?
- Analogously, what variables mediate placebo response in relation to (a) therapeutic potency; (b) patterns of physiological arousal; (c) modes of coping?

---

[1] Relatedly, McClelland (1985) asserted: "Above all, they (psychologists) should insist that the term 'placebo'—a term that is a product of the mechanical model of disease, according to which any cure not attributable to the drug is somehow due to mysterious psychological factors—should be abandoned. It is precisely these factors that need to be defined and measured—not covered up with a term like placebo" (p. 455).

In a similar vein, Roberts (1994) concluded: "To invoke the notion of placebo, placebo effect, or placebo response to explain a phenomenon that is not understood is to substitute one ghost in the box for another" (p. 210).

RELATIVITY OF PSYCHOTROPIC DRUG EFFECTS

The contemporary scientific literature concerned with psychotropic drugs, often projects an exaggerated assurance as to what these drugs do. Drug effects and therapeutic powers are typically depicted as if they were inherent in the chemical structure of the drugs in question. There is a widespread amnesia for a large literature published in the 1950s and 1960s documenting how easily state and situational variables actually mediate the impact of any chemical agent on a living system. We will review this earlier literature and also more recent publications highlighting the multiple (often psychosocial) variables that can modify response to the entire range of psychotropic agents. In so doing, we wish to clarify that the input represented by any psychotropic drug is quite ambiguous and capable of almost infinite restructuring. There is no such thing as a fixed biochemically determined effect linked to each drug. There is a final common pathway representing a complex integration of multiple variables that influence the brain. The therapeutic response to a drug may be modified by such diversities as who administers it, the familiarity of the locale in which it is introduced, the verbal label attached to it, the socioeconomic and ethnic identity of the individual who ingests it, and so forth.

Already in the 1950s, as psychotropic drugs were gaining access to treatment programs for psychologically disturbed persons, observers were publishing papers that impressionistically described a range of psychosocial factors that apparently modify drug responses (e.g., Leveton, 1958; Linn, 1959; Sabshin & Ramot, 1956). It was suggested that the impact of various drugs could vary as a function of such variables as the atmosphere of the psychiatric ward on which the patient resides, the attitudes of physicians, nurses, and attendants who supervise the patient, the patient's previous experiences with drugs, and the patient's personality. In these early days of the introduction of psychotropic drugs, much skepticism prevailed concerning their therapeutic power; and therapists who were psychodynamically oriented took an especially resistive, skeptical attitude, which motivated them to look sharply at the nondrug conditions mediating drug effects. This skepticism was spurred in part by the fact that the Old Psychodynamic Guard had to defend itself ardently against a threatening new treatment development. Some of this skepticism is well conveyed by the following statement by Leveton (1958):

> The study of mood-changing drugs and their effect on humans, embraces, in its complexity, all that is known about man—in health and sickness, as an individual, a species, and a social being. He is not a preparation suspended in isotonic saline that awaits the careful variation of a single determinant, and then responds in simple fashion to drugs introduced into the

system. A group of chronic mental patients from a relatively isolated ward with little professional supervision who are brought to a research ward staffed by interested, enthusiastic, and hopeful investigators and given a mood-changing drug, will be influenced by many factors in addition to the specific pharmacodynamic effects of the medication. (p. 232)

Currently, such an outlook is discouraged by the widespread largely unquestioning devotion to psychotropic medications. In any case, it will be useful to systematically review the relativities that researchers have explored pertaining to drug effects. Drug effects are influenced by a surprising range of psychosocial variables. Not only can therapeutic outcome be affected but also physiological response patterns, motor behavior, mood, and so forth. These variables will be examined as they roughly fall on continua of complexity and specificity.

THE BROAD SETTING

Repeatedly, investigators can find observations in the literature indicating that drugs may vary in their impact as a function of gross differences in the locales in which they are administered. First, in drug trials involving multiple clinical centers, it is not unusual to find that the therapeutic results obtained at such centers may differ from each other significantly. One center finds the target drug to be impressively successful but another reports that it does not exceed a placebo control. Greenblatt, Grosser, and Wechsler (1964) compared improvement rates for trials involving three different antidepressants and a placebo at three different hospitals. It was found that imipramine resulted in marked improvement 67% of the time at the most effective site but only 31% of the time at the least effective site. In another study (Feighner, Aden, Fabre, Rickels, & Smith, 1983) that compared imipramine, alprazolam and placebo for treatment of depression at five different locales, variability in outcomes was striking. Thus, after 6 weeks of treatment, some centers found imipramine and placebo to be equivalent; others found imipramine to be superior; and there were numerous other forms of variability among the centers linked to which of various criteria of improvement were adopted. Uhlenhuth et al. (1966) studied the effectiveness of meprobamate for relieving symptoms in "psychoneurotic outpatients" in three clinical locales. Significant differences in outcome emerged as a function of site. Uhlenhuth et al. commented: "It is important to recognize that variations in results among the three clinics in this study came about in spite of painstaking effort to assure uniform experimental conditions" (p. 413). Numerous other studies could be cited in which the therapeutic results varied significantly among the clinical centers involved.

Rarely can one really specify why the results from different psychotropic drug treatment sites are not in agreement. Researchers speculate about possible contributory differences (e.g., sample selectivity, training deficiencies, biased attitudes by personnel), but usually lack the data necessary for a pinpointed formulation. What is relevant from our perspective is that the very same drug given at the same dosage is often differentially therapeutic simply because of the gross fact of having been administered in different places. Presumably, each therapeutic site creates unique attitudinal and interactive conditions that somehow increase or decrease drug potency.

Analogous gross differences in drug effectiveness have been described as a function of "ward atmosphere," "social settings," "situational familiarity," and so forth. Kellam, Goldberg, Schooler, Berman, and Shmelzer (1967) demonstrated that therapeutic improvement of hospitalized schizophrenic patients treated with phenothiazines in 12 different wards (distributed over four hospitals) varied significantly in relation to measures of ward attributes (e.g., amount of social contact, patient-to-staff ratio). In some instances, therapeutic differences between types of wards were of a 30% magnitude. Honigfeld (1964) too reviewed a spectrum of studies exemplifying similar ward differences in drug effects. Also, he presented information indicating that drug potency may vary in relation to whether the drug is administered in a research versus clinical setting.[2] Further, he cited data demonstrating that drug effects may be contingent on whether the drugs in question are administered individually or in groups.[3] Freedman, Engelhardt, Mann, Margolis, and London (1965) found that phenothiazine treatment of schizophrenic patients was differentially successful as a function of whether such patients were given the opportunity to communicate body complaints initiated by the drugs they ingested.

Parenthetically, drugs like alcohol, LSD, and cocaine have been shown to vary in their impact depending on the context in which ingested. Thus, McClelland (1985) noted that "alcohol has no effect on male sexual fantasies if taken in a classroom setting . . . or administered in a styrofoam cup in a laboratory. . . . But if alcohol is taken voluntarily in a party atmosphere it is associated with increases in male sexual fantasies" (p. 454). Pliner and Cappell (1974) reported a difference in response between subjects who drank alcohol while working on a task alone versus in a group. The isolated

---

[2] Beecher (1960) also cites data indicating that morphine more effectively controls pain in naturalistic than research settings.
[3] Barrett (1987) summarized a considerable literature illustrating that drug effects in animals may vary as a function of "reinforcement schedules," "environmental context," and numerous other aspects of the immediate situation in which the effects are being measured.

subjects said the alcohol made them feel dizzy and sleepy, whereas the grouped ones felt happy. Relatedly, cocaine (Van Dyke, Ungerer, Jatlow, Barash, & Byck, 1982) and LSD (Goldstein, Searle, & Schmike, 1960) are experienced more dramatically in a social setting than in the laboratory.

The prior observations represent correlations at a gross, nonspecific level. They do little more than establish that drug effects are at least partially tied to psychosocial conditions.[4] In the following studies, however, greater specificity of explanation is possible.

THE ATTITUDE OF THE DRUG ADMINISTRANT

Some investigations have, more specifically, tested the hypothesis that psychotropic drug effects are shaped to some degree by the attitudes of the drug administrant. Studies in this pool differ a good deal in their designs and their respect for the double-blind. This discussion will be confined to those observing double-blind controls.

Most pertinent studies have concentrated on whether the administrant's degree of positive versus negative feeling toward the patient and the treatment process influence the therapeutic power of the psychotropic drug in question. The two major designs predominating in this literature are as follows: (a) Measure the administrant's personal attitude toward the patient's treatment and relate this to an assessment of the drug's effectiveness; (b) train administrants to role-play favorable or unfavorable attitudes toward the treatment and determine whether differing therapeutic outcomes can thereby be produced.

In the first design, several studies have demonstrated significant differences in therapeutic outcome in relation to the administrant's attitude. Downing, Rickels, and Dreesmann (1973) reported that "neurotic outpatients" who were treated with either diazepam or phenobarbital exhibited significantly greater symptomatic improvement as a function of how favorable and invested their treating physicians were. Baker and Thorpe (1957) found a significant trend for patients to improve more on placebos than tranquilizers when the administrants were nurses who felt negatively about drug therapy for these patients.

Wheatley (1967) described a study involving antianxiety agents prescribed for patients with "chronic anxiety" and two studies in which antidepressants were prescribed for patients with "neurotic depression."

---

[4] Analogous gross differences in drug response have also been documented with reference to geographic locale (e.g., Europe vs. United States) (Denber & Bente, 1966); cultural settings (Keltner & Folks, 1992; Lin, Poland, & Anderson, 1995); and medical vs. psychiatric clinics (Rickels, Ward, & Schut, 1964).

Therapists were classified as optimistic, indifferent, or pessimistic toward the outcome of the treatment. In the anxious sample, a significant positive relationship was detected between how favorable the physician felt and how favorable the treatment outcome was. However, this did not hold true in the depressive samples.

Uhlenhuth, Canter, Neustadt, and Payson (1957) selected two psychiatrists with markedly different attitudes toward drug treatment and monitored the results they obtained when treating "psychoneurotic outpatients with anxiety symptoms" with antianxiety agents. Only in the sample treated by the psychiatrist with a favorable drug attitude did the active drugs prove to be superior to placebo.

Only a few studies are available to be cited for the design based on training administrants to role-play a specific attitude. S. Fisher, Cole, Rickels, and Uhlenhuth (1964) asked physicians to behave either enthusiastically or with scientific skepticism when an antianxiety drug was administered to anxious patients. The enthusiastic condition resulted in such patients improving significantly more on active drug than on placebo. However, the skeptical condition was marked by an absence of difference between active drug and placebo.

Uhlenhuth et al. (1966) conducted a complex experiment that involved 12 different treatment conditions for "psychoneurotic outpatients manifesting anxiety." Three different psychiatric centers participated. One of the experimental variables called for training a set of physicians to express enthusiasm toward the medication and another set to adopt a skeptical attitude. In one of the clinical centers, it was found that the enthusiastic condition resulted in the active drug exceeding placebo in effectiveness, whereas the skeptical condition was marked by a tendency for placebo to exceed drug. In the other two clinical centers, however, this pattern was not duplicated. In fact, some of the results were reversed. Uhlenhuth et al. speculated that the differences in results among the centers might be due in part to differences in socioeconomic status.

Downing and Rickels (1978) were impressed with the variability of the findings just considered; and in reviewing other studies concerned with the relationships between administrant attitudes and drug-placebo differences emphasized that while such attitudes often had a discernible impact, the stability and direction of outcomes were rather unpredictable. Extremely complex interactions occurred that involved not only the administrant's orientation but also patients' attributes, the character of the clinical setting, and so forth.

Another example of the complexity of demonstrating links between administrants' attitudes and the therapeutic power of psychotropic drugs is highlighted in studies (e.g., Downing & Rickels, 1978; Haefner, Sacks, & Mason, 1960) that have found that administrants' attitudes may also influence the dosages prescribed for patients. The greater enthusiasm for a drug may translate into giving larger amounts. Thus, in some instances where dosage levels have not been controlled, the apparent correlation between administrant attitude and therapeutic outcome may reflect dosage differences rather than the direct impact of enthusiasm.[5]

In any case, the intent in this section is to document that drug administrant attitudes can affect therapeutic outcome.[6] One can reasonably say there is a trend for enthusiasm to boost therapeutic efficacy. However, this is not always so and enthusiasm may even result in apparently diminished efficacy, as occurred in the Uhlenhuth et al. (1966) study cited earlier.

Fundamentally, though, the idea that the administrant's attitude can mediate drug effects carries the notion that the drug's impact is influenced by the personal relationship between the drug recipient and the drug administrant. Documentation of this point has been convincingly provided by Krupnick et al. (1996). They asked raters (who viewed videotapes of interactions between patients and therapists) to evaluate the degree to which a favorable "therapeutic alliance" exists. Thus, they judged such variables as whether "Patient and therapist work in joint effort," "Patient experiences therapist as understanding and supportive," and "Therapist acknowledges validity of patient's thoughts, feelings." The patients were all participants in a large-scale study of various treatments of depression (National Institute of Mental Health Treatment of Depression Collaborative Research Program). Four treatment conditions prevailed: interpersonal psychotherapy, cognitive-behavior therapy, imipramine with clinical management, placebo. Measures of the degree to which the patient's behavior (but not the therapist's) indicated the "therapeutic alliance" to be favorable played a significant role in the amount of therapeutic success attained. Surprisingly, the alliance measure was the source of as much variance in the outcomes of the drug (imipramine) and also placebo conditions as it was in the two psychotherapy conditions. It should be emphasized that the measure of psychological relationship (alliance) between patient and therapist contributed substantially to the therapeutic effectiveness of the imipramine treatment. The more positive the relationship, the more therapeutic the drug proved to be. This striking finding reinforces the implications of the more speculative material cited earlier in this section.

---

[5] To complicate matters even further, von Kerekjarto (1966) reported that the sex of the examiner who administers tests for evaluating drug effects can be a significant mediating variable.

[6] A. P. Shapiro, Myers, Reiser, and Ferris (1954) described how the initial apparent success of a new oral hypotensive agent suddenly shifted in the direction of failure as a function of the physician-researcher's change from enthusiasm to pessimism about the drug's basic efficacy.

TESTS OF MORE SPECIFIC HYPOTHESES

Several research studies have focused on whether particular psychological conditions (attitudinal, expectancy) can significantly modify responses to drugs (especially of the psychotropic variety). It is a bit surprising to find that a fair number of older studies have looked into this matter. Current psychotropic drug literature rarely acknowledges what has been learned in this area. Actually, researchers, who in the past were free of many of the current informed consent restraints, conducted diverse imaginative experiments to explore how drug effects vary in relation to such variables as special instructions, the induction of unusual expectations, and even the concealment from patients that a drug has been administered to them.

DISGUISING OR MANAGING THE IDENTITY OF THE DRUG

Particularly striking are the results of experiments in which an active drug is presented to the patient or subject in such a fashion that its identity is concealed, mislabeled, or managed in some way. In 1950, Wolf had already anecdotally reported that when he gave ipecac (a drug that produces nausea) to a female patient who had been continually nauseous for days and he told her that the ipecac was a medicine that would relieve her nausea, "Within 20 minutes the nausea had subsided completely and did not recur until the following morning" (p. 104). This same phenomenon was reported for a second woman. Presumably, simply portraying the ipecac as a cure for nausea was sufficient not only to nullify its nausea-inducing qualities but also to convert it to an antinausea agent. If true, this portrayed a remarkable state of affairs.

More controlled data pertinent to this matter were presented by Luparello, Leist, Lourie, and Sweet (1970). They were interested in whether a bronchodilator (isoproterenol aerosol) and a bronchoconstrictor (carbachol aerosol) could, by means of verbal labeling, be so camouflaged as to reverse their usual physiological effects. The subjects were asthmatics referred from a hospital emergency service. Patients were tested four times (double-blind) with at least 24 hours between sessions. On each occasion they were first evaluated with a body plethysmograph to ascertain their baseline airway resistance levels. After baselines were ascertained, one of the following four conditions was introduced: (a) The patients were told they would be inhaling a bronchodilator (and indeed were given isoproterenol); (b) the patients were informed they would be inhaling a bronchoconstrictor (and instead given the bronchodilator); (c) the patients were told they would be inhaling a bronchoconstrictor (and indeed were given a bronchoconstrictor); (d) the patients were told they would be inhaling a bronchodilator but were actually given a bronchoconstrictor. Following each condition, measures of airway resistance were repeated.

Analysis of the data revealed:

> When instructions to subjects are consonant with the pharmacologic action of the inhalant, the airway reaction to that substance is greater than when instructions are dissonant. In a few instances, instructions to a subject exerted an influence of sufficient magnitude to completely reverse the airway response so that it was opposite in direction from that expected on the basis of the pharmacologic action of the drug alone. (p. 512)

The basic bronchodilating or bronchoconstricting properties of the drugs could be altered and even reversed by presenting subjects with dissimulating images of what they were inhaling.

Penick and Fisher (1965) experimented with whether the impact of epinephrine could be manipulated by inducing special psychological sets in normal subjects. Each subject participated in two sessions, 1 week apart. Eight received an injection of epinephrine at each session and 6 received an injection of saline (placebo). For one of the sessions, subjects were informed they were receiving a stimulant drug that might produce alertness, anxiety, palpitation, and tremor. For the other session, subjects were told they would receive a sedative drug that might produce sleepiness and "washed-out" or slowed-down sensations. Blood samples were drawn before and after the injections; and pulse rate was monitored. Further, subjective response was measured with a symptom checklist. The blood samples were analyzed for glucose and plasma free fatty acids (FFA). The design was single-blind. Only the patient was unaware as to whether adrenaline or saline had been injected.

The data obtained indicated that subjects felt more stimulated during the stimulant than sedative set. But what was most impressive were the findings that the stimulant condition produced significantly more signs of physiological arousal (as measured by heart rate and glucose level and FFA indices) than the presumed sedative condition. Such a pattern of results was not obtained in the placebo controls. Only in the presence of the injected epinephrine did the stimulant versus sedative response difference emerge. The same dose of epinephrine had opposing impacts (defined subjectively and physiologically) in response to opposing expectancies.

Schachter and Singer (1962) had earlier demonstrated that the subjective effects of a dose of epinephrine could be manipulated by situational cues suggesting anger or euphoria.

Frankenhaueser, Post, Hagdahl, and Wrangsjoe (1964) present further evidence that a focused set can modify the effects of a drug. Normal individuals participated in three experimental conditions. One of the conditions called for ingestion of 200 mg of Pentobarbitone (ordinarily a sedative) accompanied by suggestions that this would make one feel "sleepy" and "slow." A second condition involved simply ingesting Pentobarbitone; and a third required ingestion of an inactive placebo, accompanied by the "sleepy" instructions used in the first Pentobarbitone condition. Baseline and posttreatment responses to the experimental conditions were measured by means of self-ratings of mood, pulse rate, blood pressure, and scores on a reaction-time task. A complex pattern of results emerged. Of central importance, however, is that Pentobarbitone plus a depressant set produced significantly more change in a depressant direction, as defined by reaction time (but not pulse rate or blood pressure) and mood scores, than did the Pentobarbitone alone. It also exceeded the placebo (plus depressant set) with reference to mood and reaction time measures of depressant response. The Pentobarbitone condition alone did not differ in its effects from the placebo condition. Thus, the Pentobarbitone plus depressant suggestion affects individuals differently than does Pentobarbitone alone.

Penick and Hinkle (1964) examined the influence of expectation on an appetite-depressing drug (Phenmetrazine). Fifty experiments were carried out on four normal individuals of average weight. In all these experiments, the subjects were given either the active drug or a placebo 30 minutes prior to a test meal. In 28 experiments in which the subjects were not given a description of the drug or the placebo, there was no overall difference in the number of calories consumed for drug versus placebo. However, in 22 subsequent experiments when subjects were told the substance they were ingesting induced "appetite depression," the drug condition resulted in significantly lower caloric intake than was true for the placebo. It was concluded that "the effect of phenmetrazine on food intake was greatly enhanced when subjects knew that they might receive an appetite-depressing drug" (p. 369). The appetite-depressing suggestion was effective only in the context of taking the active drug. It is impressive that the active drug was not more effective than an inert placebo when it was administered in an ambiguous form; whereas it became more effective as soon as it acquired a specific "appetite-depressing" label.

In an interesting bit of deception described by Guy (1967), normal subjects were assigned to either drug or placebo groups. The active drug was Thorazine. However, a unique feature of this elaborate design was that the placebo was actually an equivalent dose of Thorazine labeled as being a less potent agent. This study appeared in an unpublished doctoral dissertation and only an abstract of the findings was available. From the summary that was available, it can be said that the effects (as defined by a battery of measures such as critical flicker frequency, auditory reaction time, and dynamometer strength) of the presumably potent drug differed significantly in a number of respects from those involving the disguised Thorazine. Such differences were in the direction one would expect if the disguised Thorazine was regarded as being of lower potency. It was specifically noted that the response curve for the dynamometer obtained by subjects who received the disguised Thorazine was significantly lower than that for subjects who ingested the Thorazine designated as the potent agent. Also, autonomic responsivity (as defined by heart rate and blood pressure) was lower in the disguised Thorazine condition.

Further forms of disguise were employed in studies by S. Ross, Krugman, Lyerly, and Clyde (1962) and Lyerly, Ross, Krugman, and Clyde (1964). Both of these studies took place in the setting of an elderly male population residing in a Veterans Administration Domiciliary. In the Ross et al. (1962) study, the effects of appropriate and inappropriate instructions on response to amphetamine were measured in terms of motor performance and mood. The appropriate-inappropriate categories refer to whether the properties of the drug were described so as to be either congruent or incongruent with its usual effect (e.g., alerting versus sedative). The Lyerly et al. (1964) study had a similar design, except that two drugs were included (amphetamine and chloral hydrate). What was special about the designs was that a fourfold experimental arrangement was introduced: drug group, drug-disguised group, placebo group, and untreated group. The disguised group received the active drug (concealed in orange juice) and was not aware of having ingested it. Multiple findings emerged from the two studies, but for our purposes it is sufficient to indicate that there were clear trends for the disguised version of the drug to produce different effects than the undisguised version. In the Lyerly et al. (1964) experiment, chloral hydrate and amphetamine initiated different effects when presented to subjects as two distinct identifiable drugs, but, in disguised versions did not elicit distinguishable effects.[7] Lacking differential labels, they were no longer perceived as having unlike properties.[8]

---

[7] When the Lyerly et al. (1964) study was repeated in a sample of young men employed in a veterans center, the results obtained with the elderly sample were not replicated. It was speculated that the marked differences in age and social status between the samples probably explained the contrasting outcomes.

[8] Hughes, Gulliver, Amori, Mireault, and Fenwick (1989) appraised the effects of nicotine gum (under varying instructional conditions) on ability to abstain from smoking. Among the various results to emerge, was the interesting observation that drug-placebo differences under blind conditions disappeared when subjects were explicitly told they were receiving drug or placebo.

MISCELLANEOUS CONTEXT VARIABLES

Several other investigations provide further specialized illustrations of how mediating conditions transform drug response. Hill, Belleville, and Wikler (1957) appraised the effects of morphine and pentobarbital on reaction time (in a sample of imprisoned drug addicts). They set up various conditions in which rewards for good performance on the reaction time task were offered. The rewards (providing cocaine to the addicts) differed in their magnitude and their presumed motivational power. It was found that whether the drugs facilitated or slowed reaction times fluctuated as a function of low versus high incentive conditions. During low incentive, one drug might facilitate reaction time but slow it when higher incentives were provided. Another drug might show quite a reversed pattern. Thus, Hill et al. noted: "The effect of pentobarbital changed from 'depressant' (of reaction time performance) to 'stimulant' when conditions changed from 'Low Incentive' to 'High Incentive,' while the action of morphine changed from 'stimulant' to 'depressant' when identical changes in incentive were made" (p. 35). Even the comparative power of morphine versus pentobarbital to speed up reaction time changed significantly in relation to the level of incentive provided.

To digress for a moment, several studies have demonstrated that the therapeutic power of a drug may vary in relation to the individual's baseline level of anxiety (DiMascio & Barrett, 1965; Janke, 1983; Schneider and also Stifler, cited by Dinnerstein et al., 1966–1967). Thus, DiMascio and Barrett report: "Oxazepam reduced anxiety . . . in the 'high' anxiety subjects. However, in the 'low' anxiety subjects the same dose of oxazepam induced a statistically significant *increase* in level of anxiety" (p. 300). In a related vein, Dinnerstein et al., (1966–1967) observed:

> Employing a self-rating scale measure of anxiety, Stifler reported that subjects showing high anxiety were made less anxious by tranquilizers than by inert material. Under the same testing conditions and instructions, however, subjects who were initially low in anxiety were made more anxious by the tranquilizers than by the inert material. The "active" drugs were active in both groups of subjects, but had opposite directions of effect on the two groups. (p. 109)[9]

It is also striking to learn that the therapeutic power of a psychotropic drug may be influenced by the physical appearance of the pill in which

---

[9] There is some parallel in the fact that schizophrenic patients who live in a family context likely to maintain a high level of anxious emotionality are significantly more likely to relapse when receiving antipsychotic drug therapy than patients living in a family context low in this respect (Kavanagh, 1992).

it is presented. Thus, Schapira, McClelland, Griffiths, and Newell (1970) observed that phobic patients treated with oxazepam showed relatively more improvement when the pills were green and least when red. As will be described later, analogous findings have turned up with respect to the therapeutic effectiveness of placebos.

The ambiguity of the situation in which a drug is presented to an individual may mediate how that drug is experienced. Consider the following. C. W. M. Wilson and Huby (1960) evaluated the responses of normal individuals to caffeine, secobarbital, thiopropazate, and placebo. However, these individuals were not specifically informed as to which drug they were receiving, as the various drugs were randomly administered. Each time a drug was administered, the subjects were asked to describe its effects and to guess its identity. One of the principal findings was, "When they guessed correctly, they responded . . . vigorously; when they guessed incorrectly, the effects of the drug were partially or completely inhibited" (p. 587). C. W. M. Wilson and Huby concluded: "If a drug is administered and a description of its effect is given to the recipient, it can be anticipated that the effect will be more pronounced than if the description is not given. Similarly, some degree of inhibition or variation in the drug's action can be anticipated if a false description of its action is given" (p. 596). Apparently, if the ambiguity of the context makes it difficult for subjects to know specifically the properties of the drug they have ingested, they are less likely to experience that drug in the usual modal fashion. This was interestingly further illustrated in a study by Gammer and Allen (1966) in which normal individuals were asked to report their perceptions of how two different capsules (one containing phenobarbital, another a placebo) affected them. Both were described as having no effects. Interviews with the subjects revealed that they came to believe that the experiment was deceptive and that they were to receive only placebos. Apparently, with this set they could not discern that the phenobarbital was in any way an active agent.

Cumulatively, the studies just reviewed indicate that active drug effects can be manipulated fairly significantly by either camouflaging the drugs or attaching verbal labels to them. It is impressive that simply concealing the identity of a drug or hiding that it has been administered can alter responses, not only subjectively but also in terms of motor performance. Further, the labeling of drugs as possessing or not possessing certain properties can alter their physiological impact (e.g., Luparello et al., 1970). The total pool of studies pertinent to such issues is exiguous, and so it is not really possible at this point to judge the potential limits of manipulated attitudes and expectations for modifying the impact of drugs. However, some of the results described are quite dramatic and it is not a large leap to anticipate the possibility for strong effects. The ability to shape so-called active drug effects with verbal labels parallels an analogous pliability with reference to placebos; and raise questions about the boundaries between categories like "active drug" and "placebo." The overlap between these categories is becoming clearer and clearer. We will shortly devote considerable attention to this matter.

PERSONALITY MEDIATORS

Finally, in our scrutiny of factors mediating responses to active drugs, we should consider personality variables. There have been several major attempts to devise models of how personality traits shape reactions to drugs. Cleveland (1989) summarized them well. He notes three major models. First, a psychoanalytic approach conceptualizes individuals as dedicated to maintaining ego-defense systems and as responding to drugs in terms of how threatening they are to the defense mode. For example, Sarwer-Foner and Ogle (1956) suggested that men with strong passive inclinations who compensatorily mobilize a great deal of masculine energy might find a drug with sedative properties disruptive and disturbing because it interrupted their vigor.

A related model spelled out a Type A versus Type B differentiation. A's were said to be behaviorally assertive, action-oriented, athletic, and not much interested in intellectual or artistic matters. B's were depicted as passive and invested in intellectual pursuits (Klerman, DiMascio, Greenblatt, & Rinkel, 1959). MMPI scores were utilized, in part, to classify individuals as A's or B's. For example, B's were described as low on the MMPI Manic and Ego Strength scales and high on Introversion, Depression, and Anxiety. Presumably, A's would, because of their investment in activity, find sedative drugs particularly disturbing; whereas B's would be especially threatened by a drug like reserpine because its "visceral effects" would impinge on their presumed introspective hypochondriacal sensitivity.

Eysenck (1983) presented a third primary model. It was derived from his theory of personality (Eysenck, 1947), which reduces personality to three axes: Extroversion versus Introversion, Psychoticism versus Impulse control, Neuroticism versus Emotional stability. Eysenck hypothesized that as individuals differed with respect to these categories they would respond differentially to drugs that produced effects specifically pertinent to such categories. Extroverts were conceptualized as being unusually susceptible to inhibitory and introverts to stimulant states. Therefore, stimulant drugs should increase introversive and depressants augment extroversive inclinations.

Janke (1983), Cleveland (1989), and Zubin and Katz (1964) have appraised the large research literature concerned with testing Eysenck's model of drug response. The findings generate mixed impressions. There seems to be a basic solidity to the formulation but so many other factors impinge on drug effect (e.g., dose, time of day) that the Eysenck paradigm holds its own only within a narrow territory.

As for the validity of the psychoanalytic model (e.g., Sarwer-Foner & Ogle, 1956) and that proposed by Klerman et al. (1959), there are early promising findings based on small samples, but little subsequent data that would provide a confident anlage. They represent potentially fertile areas for future research.

We have searched the world literature for other research data bearing on the role of personality variables in drug responses. From the late 1950s to the present, we located about 50 pertinent publications based on experimental designs. Aside from the Eysenck-inspired studies, this work has been largely nontheoretical. It also fails to evidence any broad consistencies with respect to specific personality traits predicting particular patterns of drug response. The major generalization we derived was that the more psychologically unstable persons are, the more likely they are to respond strongly or in atypical ways (as defined by subjective sensations and physiological measures) to various drugs (e.g., depressant, stimulating). Multiple studies, including the following ones, have demonstrated this point:

- Kornetsky and Humphries (1957) found that normal subjects high in Depression and Psychasthenia (as defined by the MMPI) showed maximum subjective reactions to drugs like chlorpromazine and LSD.
- Bartholomew and Marley (1959) reported that individuals high in neuroticism were particularly susceptible to the effects of methylpentynol and more likely to develop toxic symptoms.
- Idestrom and Schilling (1970) found that normal subjects high on Psychasthenia (MMPI) were unusually sensitive to amobarbital.
- Naditch, Alker, and Joffe (1975) noted that in a sample of "drug users" adverse reactions to psychoactive drugs were more likely in those whose MMPI scores indicated higher levels of maladjustment.
- Multiple findings delineating positive correlations (in normal subjects) between neuroticism and deviant or intense responses to various psychoactive drugs are described in a volume by Janke (1983).
- Interestingly, Nakano, Ogawa, and Kawazu (1980) even found that the rate of oral absorption of diazepam in normal individuals was positively correlated with degree of neuroticism.

Numerous other findings similar in tenor to the preceding illustrative studies could be cited (e.g., Faravelli & Sacchetti (1984); E. Frank, Kupfer, Jacob, & Jarrett, 1987; Levinson, Malen, Hogben, & Smith, 1978; Lindemann

& von Felsinger, 1961; Shawcross & Tyrer, 1985; von Felsinger, Lasagna, & Beecher, 1955).

In short, those persons who are most uncertain and troubled about their modes of adaptation seem to respond most idiosyncratically to psychoactive drugs. Whether it is reasonable to label this as a personality phenomenon is debatable. However, a persistent maladaptive stance may represent an inability to maintain an integrated, functioning personality structure.

The problem in demonstrating that drug effects are linked to personality variables is intensified by the enormous range of factors that influence such effects. Many of these factors have already been described. A vivid example of the complexity and paradox involved is provided by repeated observations that a psychoactive drug may reduce anxiety in anxious individuals but increase anxiety in those who are low anxious (e.g., DiMascio, 1968; Gardos, DiMascio, Saltzman, & Shader, 1968; Janke, 1983; Parrott & Kentridge, 1982). When one begins to consider, on the one hand, such drug response complexities as circadian rhythms, group versus individual contexts, previous drug experiences, dose level variations, relationship with the drug administrant and, on the other hand, the uncertainties of personality measurements, it is obvious that the odds are against clearly and consistently demonstrating personality-drug action connections.

THE PLACEBO EXPLANATION: THE POWER OF THE "INERT" SUBSTANCE

"The Placebo" image has become central in discussions of drug therapies. At one extreme, the placebo represents control, assurance that the unruly semichaotic nature of drug testing will be contained and scientifically disciplined. At the other extreme, the placebo is redolent with meanings pertaining to all those subjective "psychological" variables that mess up biological paradigms.

Because placebos are so often perceived as ephemeral and somehow unreal, expositions of the placebo often start out with graphic accounts of how powerful it can be. This is an instructive thing to do; and so we will begin by rounding up some pertinent illustrations. First, there is no scientifically supported statement that can be made about modal placebo effects across multiple conditions. The literature includes a remarkable range of placebo effectiveness. The spectrum of power extends from practically 0% to 90% (Brody, 1977). S. Ross and Buckalew (1983) reviewed 20 years of placebo research (more than 50 research papers) and found reasonable experimental evidence that placebos can diversely influence psychomotor behavior, physiological variables, short-term memory, self-perception, recovery from illness, and so forth. Ross and

Buckalew concluded: "It seems apparent that placebos can be as efficacious in effecting change in physiological and mental conditions as many 'active' preparations with which they are compared" (p. 466).

Brody (1977) cites the following litany of instances in which placebos have produced significant relief for "cough, mood changes, angina pectoris, headache, seasickness, anxiety, hypertension, status asthmaticus, depression, and the common cold . . ." (p. 11). Significant placebo effects have been traced also to surgical procedures (e.g., Johnson, 1994; Turner, Deyo, Loesser, Von Korff, & Fordyce, 1994) and the use of impressive medical devices and gadgets (White et al., 1985).

The power of placebos to cure what are typically regarded as medical illnesses has been widely documented (e.g., Jospe, 1978; Leavitt, 1995; White et al., 1985). A paper describing the success of placebos in treating ulcerative colitis provides a convincing illustration. Meyers and Janowitz (1989) reviewed 11 controlled trials in which there were placebo controls. Most of the colitis patients were mildly to moderately ill. They were appraised by endoscopic, pathological, and/or clinical criteria. The results indicated that in the placebo samples "up to 52% improved clinically and 50% sigmoidoscopically" (p. 33). Similar rates of placebo healing have been depicted with reference to patients with gastric ulcers, rheumatoid arthritis, and urinary incontinence (Lundh, 1987). Placebos have turned out to be about 50% to 60 % as effective as analgesics for reducing pain (Evans, 1974).

Particularly impressive with regard to the physiological translation of placebos are multiple reports of "toxic effects" directly traceable to ingesting specific placebos. As early as 1954, Wolf and Pinsky described instances in which patients on a medical ward who were receiving placebos (in the course of a research protocol) developed such symptoms as "diffuse itchy erythematous maculopapular rash," "overwhelming weakness, palpitation, and nausea," and "epigastric pain . . . followed by watery diarrhea, urticaria, and angioneurotic edema of the lips" (p. 340). They also cited studies by other investigators in which dramatic toxic reactions occurred. They described an investigation of streptomycin as follows: "Of the patients given only placebo, 61% showed one or more of the 'evidences' of 'streptomycin' toxicity. The disturbances included high-tone and low-tone hearing loss, eosinophilia, and impairment of urea clearance" (p. 340).[10]

---

[10] Turner et al. (1994) highlight some similarities between the "pharmacokinetics" of placebo and active drugs: "Placebos have demonstrated time-effect curves and peak, cumulative (greater effects with repeated administrations), and carryover effects after cessation of treatment, which mimic those of active medications" (p. 1610).

Apropos of toxic effects, a number of studies (e.g., Honigfeld, 1964; Reed & Witt, 1965) have reported dramatic instances in which persons involved in LSD studies have responded to LSD placebos by becoming disorganized and grossly disturbed. Relatedly, Levy and Jankovic (1983) described a patient whose hysterical conversion symptoms (e.g., pseudoseizures, "profound unresponsiveness") could be triggered by an intravenous placebo.

This brief sampler of the potency of placebos would be incomplete without an account of the work of Roberts (1994, 1995), who assumed that the usual double-blind, placebo-controlled design for testing drugs might actually conceal the real power of the placebo. That is, since patients and therapists participating in such a design are explicitly aware that an inert substance might be introduced, they would probably entertain relatively modest expectations of consistent therapeutic success. However, in the typical clinical context where both patients and therapists have a relatively straightforward (uncomplicated by the expectation of a placebo) anticipation of successful treatment, the placebo effect might be maximized. Roberts solicited from various sources examples of earlier medical treatments that had apparently achieved high levels of success, but then had eventually been shown to have no real therapeutic power. Examples of such treatments are "glomectomy" for asthma and "gastric freezing" for duodenal ulcers. A detailed objective analysis of the early success rates of such treatments (as available in published studies) indicated that they were originally reported to be of the order of 40% "excellent," 30% "good," and 30% "poor." That is, the overall success rates were of the order of 70%. However, when better controlled investigations were initiated, the actual subsequent effectiveness of such treatments was no greater than placebo improvement rates. It was only when bathed in the early exuberant enthusiasm of the initial introduction of these treatments that the true maximum placebo effect could break through. Over time, as formal controls were applied, the apparent 70% therapeutic triumph dwindled to insignificance. Roberts' work provides a glimpse of the amazing therapeutic potential of the unrestrained placebo.

That the double-blind tends to constrain placebo effects is affirmed by the work of Kirsch and Weixel (1988) and Kirsch and Rosadino (1993). In both instances, the effects of placebos (represented as caffeine) were appraised under double-blind versus conditions in which subjects were deceptively convinced that they would receive only caffeine (with no possibility of a placebo). In these studies, the results were significantly different for the two sets of conditions. Generally, the effects of the placebo were greater in the context in which subjects were persuaded there was no likelihood of a placebo being introduced.

There is no question but that presumably inert substances can, when managed or disguised in various ways, instigate therapeutic and somatic responses largely comparable to those associated with what are labeled as active drugs. No body system seems immune to registering placebo power. Although a few scattered papers (e.g., Quitkin et al., 1987; Rothchild & Quitkin, 1992) have claimed that a therapeutic response to a placebo can be distinguished from the response to an active drug, they are not impressive with regard to the magnitude or consistency of the distinction. We can only point out again how vague is the boundary between the realms of the placebo and the "real" drug.

ACTIVE VERSUS INERT PLACEBOS

With rare exceptions, an inert placebo arouses fewer body sensations than an active drug. The problems associated with this sensory disparity are touched on in Chapter 4, which deals with depression. Quite simply, the muted sensory quality of the typical placebo is obviously different from the sensorily brighter experience of the active drug, and this (among other variables such as side effects) enables both patients and researchers participating in drug trials to break the double-blind. We (S. Fisher & Greenberg, 1993) have actually shown that participants in double-blind studies can guess significantly better than chance which patients are receiving active drug versus placebo. This means that those who conduct drug trials and who are typically highly motivated to demonstrate that the active drug is "better," more effective than the placebo, have the opportunity to exercise their bias. The objectivity presumably guaranteed by the double-blind is largely fictitious and so the biases aimed at differentiating drug and placebo are relatively unrestrained. Exploratory data indicate that when placebos are used that induce clear body sensations the difference between active drug and placebo wanes. Thomson (1982) reported that when he examined studies in which antidepressants were compared with an active placebo (atropine) the former proved not to be significantly more therapeutically effective than the latter. This contrasts with the often observed therapeutic advantage of antidepressant over placebo, when the placebo is an inert substance that arouses few body sensations.[11] However, it is apropos

---

[11] The difference between active and inactive placebos is here depicted as revolving around the simple distinction that one arouses body sensations and the other, largely, does not. However, there are studies suggesting that the matter is actually more complex. Such studies (Kast, 1961; Lipman, Park, Rickels, & Chase, 1966) have shown that highlighting specific body sensations (e.g., dry mouth) produced by a substance like atropine may have favorable or unfavorable therapeutic effects as a function of positive or negative attitudes induced by the "drug" administrant toward the body sensations. What is particularly noteworthy is that a body experience like dry mouth may have therapeutic implications in some contexts but antitherapeutic in others. This suggests that the matter of creating an effective active placebo involves not simply instilling body sensations but

to add that in our own analyses (S. Fisher & Greenberg, 1989) of the average reported therapeutic advantage of antidepressant over "inert" placebo, the difference was only of the order of 19%. Others (e.g., Depression Guideline Panel [DGP], 1995; Foulds, 1958; E. Frank, Karp, & Rush, 1993) have come up with similar estimates. Thus, even under conditions in which biases in favor of distinguishing active drug and placebo are rampant, the magnitude of the distinction is not impressive. Some would argue, on the basis of the Thomson findings just cited, that the real difference between antidepressant and placebo probably does not amount to much. Relatedly, R. L. Fisher and Fisher (1996) report that in the case of children and adolescents no one has been able to demonstrate differences between the therapeutic effects of antidepressants and placebos. Chapter 4 in this book, by Greenberg and Fisher, spells out the relatively small therapeutic advantage lithium demonstrates over placebo, when treating bipolars. Chapter 5, by Cohen, describes the difficulties in establishing that antipsychotics are more therapeutic than placebos.

MANIPULATION OF PLACEBO PHENOMENA

The psychosocial relativity that is characteristic of active drug effects also applies to placebos. Numerous situational variables influence the direction and intensity of placebo potency. An amazing fluidity characterizes the interactions of such variables.

ADMINISTRANT ATTITUDES

First of all, serious evidence affirms that positive placebo effects are likely to be increased as a function of what may be loosely referred to as the enthusiasm and perceived therapeutic conviction of the placebo administrant. A. K. Shapiro (1964) summarizes several pertinent findings in the literature as follows: "Placebo effectiveness may decrease from 70 to 25 percent when attitudes toward treatment changed from positive to negative . . ." (p. 78). Relatedly, Gryll and Katahn (1978), after describing their study of the effects of dentists' variations in the ways they delivered a placebo disguised as a pain-alleviating drug, stated: "The results agree with and extend previous findings . . . that a physician's warm, supportive attitude can potentiate the occurrence of placebo effects" (p. 259). While a number of the studies in this area are not well controlled, there is a detectable trend in the direction defined by Gryll and Katahn. It is also

---

perhaps a pattern of sensations that can be perceived as having positive or encouraging significance. Knowledge in this area is minimal, and a good deal of further exploration is needed.

pertinent that, as earlier noted, Krupnick et al. (1966) reported that degree of therapeutic improvement of depressed individuals receiving a placebo is positively and significantly correlated with a measure of how favorable the "therapeutic alliance" is between patient and placebo administrant.

PLACEBO LABELING

A spectrum of studies documents that inert placebos may be shifted to and fro in their effects as their labels are manipulated. Butler and Steptoe (1986) measured the effects of placebo medication on pulmonary responses in adult asthmatics who were recruited to participate in a laboratory study of the "effectiveness of a new bronchodilator." Distilled nebulized water was inhaled by the subjects on three separate occasions. They were told at Session 1 that they were inhaling water; at Sessions 2 and 3 they were informed they were inhaling a substance likely to cause chest tightness and wheezing. Just prior to inhaling the water in Sessions 2 and 3, subjects inhaled from an aerosol that presumably contained either a powerful new drug (placebo) capable of blocking the irritant or a nonactive substance (neutral). Pulmonary function, autonomic reactivity (e.g., heart rate) and psychological parameters (e.g., anxiety level) were measured. It was found that "the asthmatic participants produced a bronchoconstrictive response to the suggestion that they were inhaling an irritant chemical but this effect was blocked by the 'placebo therapy'" (p. 180). The belief that the placebo one had received was a drug capable of neutralizing an irritant was sufficient to block the effect of another placebo which, in a different context, was lung-irritating.

In an experiment by Frankenhaueser, Jarpe, Svan, and Wrangsjo (1963) to test the reversal of placebo effects, normal female subjects came to the laboratory for three sessions. The first was for purposes of general orientation and training in a reaction-speed test. In one of the remaining two sessions, the subjects were given two inert white pills said to contain a sleep-producing drug; whereas in the other session, they received inert pink pills described as stimulants. Pulse rate and blood pressure were measured once before and three times after ingestion of the placebos. Also, reaction-speed to an auditory signal was measured before and after each placebo. In addition, subjects rated their subjective mood states after each placebo. Analysis of the data indicated distinctly opposed patterns of response in relation to whether the placebos had been labeled as depressant or stimulant. This was demonstrated in terms of pulse rate, blood pressure, reaction-speed, and self-rated mood.

Brodeur (1965) examined the impact, in one normal sample, of being told that the inert placebo ingested was an amphetamine-like stimulant; and in a second sample the effect of being told the placebo was a tranquilizer. Control subjects were simply told they were controls and were to receive a placebo. Pulse rate and both self-ratings and self-written descriptions of mood were obtained at a baseline point and after ingestion of the placebos. The overall findings were phrased as follows: "The effects of both stimulation and tranquilization can be induced in healthy subjects . . . by means of a pill and a bit of knowledge suggesting the specific effects of taking such a pill . . ." (p. 450).[12]

A similar "tranquilizer versus energizer" dimension was explored by Loranger, Prout, and White (1961). They told psychiatric inpatients (and also the participating psychiatrists and nurses) that they were testing a new "tranquilizer" and a new "energizer." Different samples were given either a tranquilizer or energizer that was, in actuality, an inactive placebo pill. A control group received no pills at all. Treatment lasted for 6 weeks and weekly ratings were made of various aspects of the patients' behaviors (e.g., depression, energy, sociability). The tranquilized sample improved significantly more than the control group on overall behavior and with reference to depression and restlessness. This difference dissipated in a subsequent 2-week follow-up. The energized sample's ratings proved not to be significantly different from those of the controls. Thus, only the tranquilizing placebo had a detectable impact.

The widely cited work of Storms and Nisbett (1970) illustrates how attributing contrasting qualities to identical inert placebos can eventuate in behavioral differences. They recruited insomniac subjects who were told they were participating in a study of the effects of bodily activity on dreams. The members of one sample were, shortly before going to bed, given a pill portrayed as likely to increase their arousal. Another sample was told the pill would be relaxing. It had been hypothesized that some degree of insomnia is due to excess emotionality at bedtime. Therefore, if the insomniacs could attribute their emotionality to an "arousing" pill, they would, overall, be less upset and fall asleep faster. On the other hand, those taking the "relaxing" pill, who expected to feel relaxed, would find their insomnia-linked disturbance, by way of contrast, magnified, and consequently be delayed in falling asleep. The hypothesis was significantly supported by the findings. Subsequent studies (e.g., Bootzin, Herman, & Nicassio, 1976), however, raised serious questions about these results. A later review (M. Ross & Olson, 1981) of the literature concerned with the

---

[12] Brodeur (1965) refers to a previous study by Lyerly et al. (1964) that he describes as not having successfully manipulated placebos to produce tranquilizing versus stimulant effects. The design of that study, however, was not only much more complex but also less specific in its instructions to subjects with reference to the sedative versus stimulant variable.

effectiveness of divergent attributions to placebos revealed other studies with results analogous to those of Nisbett and Storm, but there was a good deal of complex inconsistency.

The divergent results that follow from divergent labeling of placebos is particularly well illustrated in an experiment reported by Sternbach (1964). Subjects were tested on three different occasions. In each instance, they swallowed a gelatin capsule containing a magnet that permitted measurement of stomach movements. In one condition, the capsule was described as likely to produce strong churning sensations; in a second condition, the capsule was depicted as likely to make the stomach feel full and heavy; and a third condition represented the capsule as having only control purposes. The magnetic tracings of stomach movements conformed significantly to the expected opposing patterns of placebo instructions in 4 of the 6 subjects who were studied.

The preceding examples show how labeling of the placebo can influence its impact on various aspects of behavior. Many other illustrations can be found in Jospe (1978) and White et al. (1985). The implications of such material are, in certain respects, quite striking. It is also apparent that the results described are sometimes tenuous and inconsistent. Caution is in order when interpreting the findings.

The literature dealing with placebos is vast. Because of space limitations, a full-fledged review is not possible here. It has been shown that the power of placebos is linked to an amazing array of variables and conditions. The potency of placebos has been variously correlated with the appearance of the pill (e.g., size, color), method of delivery (e.g., orally vs. by injection), stress level, previous experience with drugs, quantity of pills, circadian rhythms, potency of the active drug with which the placebo is being compared, and so forth (Jospe, 1978; Pollmann & Hildebrandt, 1981; White et al., 1985). It is doubtful that any behavioral phenomenon has ever been demonstrated to be more complex.[13,14]

PLACEBO AS DEFENSE

A collection of experiments directly or indirectly highlight the individual's use of placebos for ego-defensive purposes. An endless literature

---

[13] There are also complex phenomena involving contexts in which placebos reinforce or detract from the effectiveness of designated active drugs (e.g., Casey et al., 1985; White et al., 1985).

[14] A curious example of the devious processes involved in placebo effects is provided by reports (Epstein & Cluss, 1983; Horowitz et al., 1990) that not only did the consistency with which samples of patients took their medications (respectively for fever and myocardial infarction) foster recovery but also the consistency with which placebo samples did so!

documents that when psychologically distressed persons find themselves caught up in a paradigm in which a placebo substance, defined as possessing the power to relieve distress is made available, they often manage to derive therapeutic advantage. They utilize this paradigm to attain various degrees of relief from their distress. They extract an advantage, feel "better off."[15]

It is well established that persons employ a broad repertoire of strategies to enhance themselves, to manage and buffer that which is threatening. Numerous studies have shown that they strive at both conscious and unconscious levels to bolster self-esteem, to minimize feelings of threat, to allay sensations of pain and discomfort, to deny vulnerability, and, whenever possible, to cast the world in optimistic tones (Breznitz, 1983; S. Fisher & Fisher, 1993; Ihilevich & Gleser, 1986; Taylor, 1989). The following experiments illustrate with focal specificity the larger proposition just stated. They capture individuals in action when they seize on the placebo as an opportunity to comfort and bolster self.

Gibbons and Wright (1981) are social psychologists who were interested in maneuvers motivated by ego defensiveness. Previous research indicated that individuals may hide information from themselves that might cast them in a negative light. Gibbons and Wright state: "People sometimes seek ambiguity rather than clarity as to their behavior and the motives behind it. They do this to avoid learning something about themselves that they may not wish to know, in other words, because of ego defensiveness" (p. 588). The Gibbons and Wright project is of special interest because it provided subjects with the opportunity to incorporate a placebo into defensive strategies. In one experiment, the researchers selected (by means of a well-validated questionnaire) a sample of men with high sex guilt and a sample with low sex guilt. These men were exposed on different occasions to an erotic film (containing explicit scenes of nudity and sexual intercourse) and a control nonerotic film. Prior to viewing each of the films, they were asked to swallow a placebo capsule said to contain a stimulant drug that might produce some side effects (e.g., increases in heart rate, breathing rate, sweaty palms). The "side effects" cited were chosen because they are associated with sexual arousal. After reviewing the film, the subjects were asked to rate how sexually aroused they felt, how arousing the drug and the film were, what affects were experienced, and miscellaneous other reactions. It had been hypothesized that the individuals with high sex guilt would find the arousal created by the erotic film to be particularly threatening and so would be more motivated than the low sex guilt subjects "in taking advantage of the causal

---

[15] Obviously, placebos can also produce negative and even toxic effects, the focus here is on positive therapeutic outcomes.

ambiguity surrounding the source of their arousal." Presumably, this would result in "an increase in the amount of arousal they choose to attribute to the 'drug' and a corresponding decrease in the amount they attribute to the erotic film. No differences in attributions were expected in the nonarousing film condition" (p. 590).

Analysis of the data significantly supported the hypothesis. Those who had need to allay their sex guilt perceived the placebo as having heightened physiological intensity.[16]

Analogous findings were reported by Briddell et al. (1978). In their experimental design, they randomly assigned males ("social drinkers") whose level of sex guilt was measured with the same questionnaire used in the Gibbons and Wright (1981) study, to one of two expectancy conditions; in which they were informed that the beverage they consumed contained alcohol or no alcohol. For half of the subjects in each expectancy category, the beverage was alcoholic liquor; for the other half it was nonalcoholic. After the subjects had consumed the beverages pertinent to their assignment, they were exposed to three tape recordings: one depicting "mutually enjoyable heterosexual intercourse"; a second, "forcible rape"; and a third, "sadistic aggression" (but no sexual advances) toward a woman. During exposure to these tapes, physiological recordings were obtained of heart rate, finger temperature, and penile tumescence. Also subjective ratings of arousal were secured.

One of the principal findings was that men who believed they had ingested alcohol evidenced greater penile tumescence than those who believed they had not consumed alcohol. This pattern was not found for heart rate or temperature. The fact that subjects had or had not actually consumed alcohol did not significantly influence tumescence level. The expectancy effect on tumescence of believing one had consumed alcohol attained statistical significance only in the rape and sadistic aggression conditions. It is important to point out that the alcohol expectancy (but no alcohol actually ingested) condition is equivalent to a placebo. Further, the subjective ratings of arousal the men made following each rape recording were significantly higher as a function of the expectancy that alcohol had been consumed. The sex guilt scores were significantly and negatively correlated with subjective sexual arousal for the heterosexual intercourse condition and the forcible rape condition, but were not correlated with penile tumescence.

---

[16] Gibbons and Wright (1981) also performed a second experiment (involving women rather than men) with a design that duplicated the first except that the subjects were arbitrarily made to feel sexually aroused by giving them false physiological feedback while looking at erotic pictures. The results supported those of the first experiment, "although they were clearly weaker" (p. 597).

What is of prime interest here is that the placebo alcohol condition (belief one has consumed alcohol when this is not so) enhances tumescence, whereas actual consumption of alcohol does not. But what is even more noteworthy is that the effect of the placebo condition turns out to be greater during the deviant theme conditions (rape, sadistic aggression) than during the normal heterosexual intercourse story. If one presumes that it is more forbidden for a man to feel sexually excited by rape or sadistic aggressive themes than by willing heterosexual intercourse themes, it would appear that the disinhibiting effects of the men's belief they had ingested alcohol occurred particularly in the context of higher levels of sexual inhibition. Thus, one could conceptualize the alcohol placebo as having enabled the men to enjoy the forbidden themes by defining the situations as involving forces (being intoxicated) beyond their control. The alcohol placebos could be said to have relieved them of responsibility for the unworthy fantasies that had been aroused by the rape and sadistic tapes.

This interpretation is favored by the data from a similar type of study (G. T. Wilson & Lawson, 1976) involving alcohol that demonstrated that the belief one had consumed alcohol had a greater effect in increasing penile tumescence in reaction to a deviant (homosexual) film than to a conventional heterosexually oriented film. Once again, the alcohol placebo provided a strategy for rationalizing or excusing sexual arousal in a context where it is normally not acceptable.

Further, Hull and Bond (1986), employing a meta-analysis of nine studies involving comparisons of alcohol placebos with actual alcohol consumption, found that the assumption one had ingested alcohol had a sizable impact on sexual arousal, whereas consumption of alcohol, as such, had only minimal effect. This pattern held up both in terms of physiological (e.g., tumescence) and subjective measures. It was striking that the expectancy effects were greatest for individuals high in sex guilt. Hull and Bond noted: "Such results provide additional support for the view that for some individuals alcohol expectancy (alcohol placebo) functions as an excuse to become sexually aroused" (p. 354).

Multiple additional studies have looked at the ego-defensive functions of placebos in relation to other drives and motives. Nisbett and Schachter (1966) showed that if individuals could attribute their discomfort, during exposure to electric shocks, to a placebo (whose side effects were said to be similar to the discomfort produced by shock), they judged the shock to be less painful and could tolerate more of it. Davison and Valins (1969), Loftis and Ross (1974) and M. J. Weiner (1971) also demonstrated that the impact of electric shocks could be buffered by providing a placebo to which the shock effects could be attributed. Analogous buffering effects by placebos have been documented with respect to anxiety generated by a film

(Girodo, 1973); tension induced by dissonance (Zanna & Cooper, 1974); disappointment aroused by failure experiences (B. Weiner & Secord, 1975); and guilt engendered by cheating (Dienstbier & Munter, 1971).

In brief, the literature reveals that individuals may utilize placebos to cope with and buffer such diverse unacceptable experiences as guilty sexual imagery, pain, anxiety, fear of failure, and sensations of dissonance. This opens the door to conceptualizing placebo response as one more manifestation of those broad forms of adaptation referred to as "defense mechanisms." The placebo response is not some unique, specialized construct. Rather, it is as commonplace as all the popular forms of self-defense (e.g., projection, denial, rationalization) that sustain people 24 hours a day. Many explanations for placebo phenomena have been offered. Theories have been formulated that variously highlight expectancy (e.g., Kirsch, 1985; M. Ross & Olson, 1981), conditioning (e.g., Archer, 1995; White et al., 1985), and suggestion (e.g., J. D. Frank, 1973; A. P. Shapiro & Morris, 1978) as causal variables. Research support for such theories (White et al., 1985) is promising. However, these theories refer primarily to specialized mechanisms for placebo action. They do not, by and large, perceive placebo phenomena within the wider perspective that they basically represent ways of defending the self. As will be discussed later in more detail, the placebo response is part of a general capacity to adapt, to capitalize on the potential provided by pretense and illusion, and to mobilize one's creative (self-healing) powers; the placebo response does not derive primarily from passivity but rather from active intentions.

PERSONALITY PREDICTORS

The zeal to find the Holy Grail does not exceed the investment that has, over the years, been dedicated to uncovering the personality correlates of being a placebo responder. This was especially true in the 1950s and 1960s. However, after a series of early reports that seemed promising, the view gradually prevailed that, in the first place, there probably is no such thing as a consistent placebo reactor. Whereas some studies (e.g., Batterman, 1957; Joyce, 1959; Lasagna, Mosteller, von Felsinger, & Beecher, 1954) did report consistencies in individuals' responses to placebos across situations, many have not (e.g., Honigfeld, 1964; Liberman, 1964, 1966; Shapiro, 1971). It is now fashionable to dismiss as illusory the whole concept of a personality type "susceptible" to placebos.

S. Fisher (1967) pointed out that although it has been difficult to demonstrate consistency in placebo response one should not dismiss data that periodically describe significant correlations between personality variables and particular forms of placebo reactivity. He also suggests:

> If one is interested in studying placebo consistency . . . then one must avoid placebo situations which either are too potent or too ineffectual. In studying placebo consistency, the various placebo situations must be closely matched for overall placebo effect so that each situation contributes the same weight to the composite response. (p. 512)

One can simply write off correlations of personality variables with placebo response as chance findings, methodological defects, and so forth; but there is always the possibility one is dealing with an elusive phenomenon hard to pin down.

The obstacles in finding individual consistencies across multiple placebo contexts have largely shut off thinking about the "placebo reactor" issue. Research in this area has mobilized a bewildering array of placebo test situations. Subjects are exposed to pills, capsules, injections, sounds, invisible magnetic fields—all defined as potent agents. Further, such "potent agents" have been presented as variously able to alleviate pain, sleeplessness, psychological distress, memory difficulties, motor deficiencies, tension, shyness, too great an appetite for food, guilt about forbidden impulses (e.g., sexual), hypertension, and so forth. Even further, these presumably potent agents have been taken by subjects under conditions varying sharply in degree of stress, after being primed by figures differing dramatically in their authority and prestige, after the target symptoms have been experienced for very brief versus extended periods, and so forth. This is a chaotic level of diversity.

If one is looking for consistency in placebo response, what is a fair paradigm for examining the issue? If there are such animals as placebo reactors, should they be equivalently responsive to a placebo delivered by an authority figure, one delivered by self, and one delivered by a low prestige figure? Should they be equally responsive to a placebo offered by someone they trust versus one they do not trust? Should they be equivalently responsive to placebo agents that are cast as having strong versus weak powers?

Basically, the question is whether consistency can meaningfully be defined in terms of whether individuals respond to any series of disparate placebo situations presented to them. Consistency may perhaps better be conceptualized in terms of what is meaningful to the individuals involved. Thus, certain persons, with special hypochondriacal anxieties, might respond consistently only to those placebos that target salient somatic symptoms. Others might respond consistently only to placebos presented in a context where response signals pleasing authority figures. The consistency would represent a need to be submissive and thereby to win favor. If the presenters of the placebo provided cues that they did not believe in the placebo (as often occurs in clinical trials), those who wish to please authorities might express their consistency by *not* responding to the placebo. Still others might respond consistently only to those placebos that provide them with excuses for denying responsibility for certain classes of impulses. Thus, placebos that were defined as having the power to arouse sensations of emotional excitement might be responded to consistently whenever individuals were struggling with unacceptable urges (e.g., sexual, hostile) and needed to attribute them to outside sources. The matter of consistency can be decoded only within the context of a potentially infinite number of individual scripts.

In surveying the entire research literature for attempts to correlate personality variables with measures of placebo response, we have found about 50 studies based on formal research designs. The detailed findings are largely striking for their contradictions and the failure to obtain solid cross-validations. However, two trends deserve description.

Sociability

First, and with considerable uncertainty, we will mention a trend for placebo response to occur more often in persons who can be described as sociable or interested in relating to others than in those who are characterized as self-sufficient and inclined toward being distant from others. A number of studies provide data supporting this view (viz., Black, 1966; Gelfand, Ullman, & Krasner, 1963; Gowdy, 1983; Joyce, 1959; Lasagna et al., 1954; Muller, 1965; Sharp, 1965; Trouton, 1957; Vrhovac, 1977). There are also a number of studies that explicitly failed to discern such a difference. However, the sociability variable has surfaced sufficiently often in various guises that it should be considered as a potential lead.[17]

If further confirmation of the sociability findings could be achieved, what would be a reasonable explanation? It is possible that the placebo is a construction that acquires potency from a social encounter and that the placebo responder is especially tuned to opportunities for bolstering self on the basis of interactions with others. By way of contrast, the non-placebo responder would look more to self, as a separate power or entity, to generate opportunities. Thus, presumably, the placebo would, for the placebo reactor, be a carrier of meaning. It condenses a vision of opportunity leveraged by the symbolism or energy or revised perspective triggered by a social encounter. Openness to such meaning would probably

---

[17] Rawlinson (1985) came to a similar conclusion after examining a number of pertinent studies: "Those patients who benefit from placebo therapy tend to be more communicative, more socially responsive, . . ." (p. 410).

be greatest in these who are sociable, who are enthusiastic about harvesting profits from social paradigms.

ACQUIESCENCE

While we have only hesitantly put forward the concept of sociability as a personality dimension pertinent to placebo responding, we can more confidently do so with reference to a variable identified as acquiescence. The idea that acquiescence might be an important personality mediator in this respect was first formally enunciated by S. Fisher and Fisher (1963). They set up a design in which normal (33 male and 39 female) college students were asked to respond to the Bass (1956) measure of social acquiescence, which is based on the number of times agreement is registered with a series of sayings or proverbs (e.g., "seeing is believing;" or "still water runs deep"). The students were then asked to swallow a placebo capsule that was presented as a harmless drug that could initiate a variety of feelings or sensations. The situation was dramatized by attaching each subject to an apparent apparatus for measuring physiological arousal. After swallowing the capsule, the subjects reported both spontaneously and by responses to a questionnaire what sensations and feelings the capsule had aroused. Analysis of the data demonstrated a significant positive correlation between the number of sayings with which individuals agreed and the number of presumed drug effects reported. In terms of the attributes Bass ascribed at that time to agreement with the sayings (proverbs), this meant that the greater the inclination to please others the larger were the number of effects initiated by the capsule.

While Bass (1956) originally presented data suggesting that the acquiescence score was a measure of the degree to which one "resembles Sinclair Lewis' 'Babbitt'—an unquestioning conformer to social demands" (p. 299), subsequent research came up with more complex information. Thus, McGee (1962), after reviewing a series of pertinent studies in this area concluded: "Acquiescers are stimulus accepting, uninhibited, conformers; nonacquiescers are stimulus rejecting, inhibited, independents" (p. 291). The concept of being stimulus accepting versus rejecting is not clearly defined but refers generally to being open to the influence of environmental inputs versus carefully controlling their entry into self. McGee also summarizes work by Couch and Keniston (1960) who probed in depth the personal attributes of persons varying in their tendencies to agree with statements. He portrays their findings as follows:

> Yeasayers are impulsive, emotionally reactive, extraverted, externally oriented, low in psychological inertia, and possess passive egos; naysayers are guarded, defensive, constricted, inhibited, introverted, withdrawing,

introspective, high in psychological inertia, slow and critical reactors, and possess active egos. (p. 290)

These descriptors are obviously not completely consistent, but broadly speaking, they depict individuals with higher acquiescence scores as more socially involved, more likely to interact spontaneously with others, than are those with lower acquiescence scores. Apparently, the less acquiescent are more wary of others, more self-oriented. This is particularly interesting relative to the tentative observation that several studies suggest placebo responders are inclined to be "sociable." It should be cautioned, however, that while the Bass acquiescence measure is significantly positively correlated with the Couch and Keniston measure, the degree of relationship is fairly low.

The meaning of the acquiescence dimension takes on importance because further studies that confirmed a relationship between acquiescence and placebo responding expressed some puzzlement about the underlying implications of this relationship.

The first study that sought to test the original S. Fisher and Fisher (1963) findings was carried out by McNair, Kahn, Droppleman, and Fisher (1968). The subjects were 40 men and 20 women who were being treated either with diazepam or placebo (double-blind) for "functional psychoneurotic complaints and manifest anxiety" in a psychiatric outpatient facility. The Bass Social Acquiescence Scale was administered prior to beginning treatment. Response to treatment was measured with both self-ratings and scales filled out by interviewers. The results were supportive of the Fisher and Fisher report. McNair et al. (1968) stated: "Considered in conjunction with the Fishers' report on acquiescence and placebo response, this is the first time to our knowledge that a predictor of placebo reactivity has passed the test of an independent replication" (p. 542). Another interesting trend was that the nonacquiescent seemed to respond more favorably to the drug (diazepam) than did the acquiescent. Indeed, the high acquiescent patients on drug were the only group that did not improve significantly from their pretreatment baseline.

A follow-up investigation of the sample just described was published by McNair, Fisher, Sussman, Droppleman, and Kahn (1970). It embraced 73% of that original sample. Each patient was reevaluated roughly 18 weeks after the completion of the first study. Various self-ratings and ratings by a research social worker (blind to medication and acquiescence type) were obtained with respect to symptoms, mood, and distress levels. The same significant pattern of relationships between acquiescence and placebo and active drug effects was affirmed after a 4-month period. Incidentally, high acquiescers significantly more often refused to participate in the follow-up than the low acquiescers, which was interpreted to mean that high acquiescence may not be an indicator of conformity.

The next attempt at cross-validation was launched by McNair, Fisher, Kahn, and Droppleman (1970). The design involved a double-blind comparison of chlordiazepoxide and placebo in female psychiatric patients who differed in their Bass (1956) Social Acquiescence scores. The design was unusual because it involved comparing a high and a low acquiescent scorer within each of four sets of pairs. Each patient completed five cycles of crossovers during which they switched back and forth between placebo and active drug. It should also be mentioned that all patients were simultaneously participating in weekly psychotherapy sessions. Evaluations of improvement were based on daily self-ratings. The results were once again supportive of the S. Fisher and Fisher (1963) reported positive relationship between acquiescence and placebo response. They also supported the previous McNair et al. (1968) observations concerning the negative relationship of acquiescence to therapeutic response to an active antianxiety drug. McNair, Fisher, Kahn, and Droppleman (1970) reported as follows:

> Low Acquiescent patients reported less anxiety on drug days than on placebo days. For Low Acquiescers, Tension-Anxiety decreased the longer they remained on drug (up to seven days), and their level of anxiety increased the longer they remained on placebo . . . . High Acquiescers reported no anti-anxiety effects of the drug. (pp. 134–135)

Next in this chain of inquiry was an investigation by McNair, Gardos, Haskell, and Fisher (1979). Three samples of psychiatric patients (consisting of men and women) with anxiety symptoms were evaluated. Two of the samples received one week of placebo treatment and were then randomly assigned to an anxiolytic or antidepressant drug. A quasi-control group received no medication while waiting a week before beginning psychotherapy. The Bass Social Acquiescence Scale was administered at baseline to all patients. Degree of improvement was measured with self-ratings and ratings by observers. Only the improvement data pertinent to the placebo were reported. In one group, a clear significant trend emerged for patients with high acquiescent scores to obtain greater relief during placebo treatment than did the low acquiescent. In a second group, several measures of improvement during placebo treatment (based on observer ratings) correlated positively and significantly with acquiescence, but, measures of improvement based on self-ratings did not show the same relationship. McNair et al. (1979) concluded: "The pattern of findings (in one sample) and on physician ratings (in the second) is consistent with the inference that . . . the Social Acquiescence Scale is a replicated predictor of placebo response" (p. 249). Note that acquiescence was not predictive of improvement in the control group that was just waiting for a week before beginning psychotherapy. This supports the idea that acquiescence is specifically predictive of placebo improvement rather than that arising spontaneously.[18]

Pichot and Perse (1968) independently hypothesized that a measure of acquiescent set would predict placebo response. They used two different measures of acquiescence derived from the MMPI. In one experiment, they studied 111 male medical students who "at the end of the morning . . . took a placebo which was presented to them as an experimental therapeutic product . . . The next morning all subjects completed a nine item questionnaire concerning the effects they had experienced" (p. 54). The data significantly demonstrated that degree of placebo response was positively and significantly linked to the acquiescence scores.

A second experiment was also undertaken. It involved 53 physicians who had taken the MMPI (from which acquiescence scores were derived). They were asked to determine "the value of a new drug" by taking, over a 4-week period, a capsule a day (half of the capsules containing an inert substance and half chlordiazepoxide). Self-ratings provided data concerning the character of each individual's responses to the capsules. Once again, a significant trend was found for acquiescence to be positively predictive of favorable response to the placebo. Only minimal details were provided by Pichot and Perse concerning their procedures and analyses. Incidentally, their experiments were not undertaken to test the original S. Fisher and Fisher (1963) findings, but rather evolved from their own speculations.

Two studies were carried out primarily to ascertain how well body image parameters predict responses to placebo and various active drugs. However, these studies also secondarily sought to determine if the Bass Social Acquiescence Scale could predict such responses. In one investigation (Fast & Fisher, 1971), a series of body image evaluations was obtained from 15 normal males and 15 normal females. After baseline measures, a placebo substance was injected and subjects asked to report their body sensations and degree of anxiety. This same procedure was then repeated with an injection of epinephrine. Seven days later, the subjects again responded to a second (larger) dose of epinephrine and subsequently to another placebo injection. The Bass scale was administered just prior to the second epinephrine injection. Analysis of the data indicated that acquiescence was not significantly correlated with the number of subjective bodily effects produced by either of the placebos. However, as predicted, the greater were individuals' acquiescence levels, the more anxiety they

---

[18] Incidentally, a measure of autonomic awareness was included in this study. The results indicated that high somatizers showed less symptom reduction during both placebo treatment and in the control group.

experienced during epinephrine as compared with placebo. This prediction obviously grew out of the McNair et al. (1968; McNair, Fisher, Kahn, et al., 1970) demonstration that effects produced by active drugs are more disturbing for (viewed more negatively by) acquiescent individuals than are those resulting from placebo.

In a second body image investigation, Clausen and Fisher (1973) appraised the body image effects of amphetamine, pentobarbital, and placebo on 75 normal females. The drugs were taken at high and low dose levels. Along with a battery of body image tests, The Bass Social Acquiescence Scale was administered at baseline. Further, mood self-ratings were secured at baseline and following ingestion of the drug and placebo capsules. Few definitive findings emerged for the acquiescence scores. There was a significant trend for anxiety during a high pentobarbital dose to be positively and significantly correlated with acquiescence. This is congruent with one aspect of the McNair et al. (1968; McNair, Fisher, Kahn, et al., 1970) data. However, level of anxiety during the placebo condition was, contrary to expectation, not correlated with acquiescence.

Halm (1967) probed the effects of asking male college students to ingest either a placebo presented as an energizing drug or one labeled as a tranquilizer. Twenty were given the "energizer" and 20 the "tranquilizer." At baseline, the Bass Social Acquiescence Scale and self-rated mood questionnaires were administered. Other measures were also administered that are not pertinent to our present purpose. The mood measures were reported after the placebos had been ingested. In analyzing the results, a composite index was first constructed that combined the subjects in both the energized and tranquilized groups by simply transforming their mood scores to indicate the degree to which they had been affected in the direction expected on the basis of the instructions given. The mood scale used to measure the impact of the placebos contained five dimensions (sleepy, friendly, aggressive, unhappy, clear thinking, dizzy). The "sleepy" dimension was most pertinent to the major intent of the instructions given with each placebo, which focus primarily on manipulating the subject's degree of alertness or arousal. Congruent with this point, it was found that acquiescence was positively and significantly correlated with the degree to which subjects reported the placebos had altered the "sleepy mood factor." Acquiescence was not significantly correlated with changes in any of the other mood factors.[19,20]

---

[19] A Galvanic Skin Reaction (GSR) measure that was included in the study simply could not differentiate the energized and tranquilized groups.

[20] A. K. Shapiro, Struening, Barten, and Shapiro (1975) describe a Placebo Test they devised that calls for individuals to take a placebo (labeled as a drug) at home and to record

We have reviewed the literature pertaining to acquiescence studies in some detail to demonstrate how substantial the accumulated data actually are. With minor exceptions, there have been repeated confirmatory cross-validations that acquiescence predicts largely positive therapeutic response to placebos and largely negative therapeutic reactions to active drug agents. This statement needs to be modified in the sense that acquiescence has not only predicted positive therapeutic effects of placebos but also the intensity of somatic experiences (some of which have negative connotations) evoked by placebos (S. Fisher & Fisher, 1963; A. K. Shapiro, Struening, Barten, & Shapiro, 1975). A respectable body of research exists that documents the importance of an acquiescent orientation in mediating both placebo responses and certain classes of drug reactions. This stands in direct contradiction to repeated declarations in the literature (A. P. Shapiro & Morris, 1978) that no personality variables have consistently shown promise in predicting placebo phenomena.

That acquiescence simultaneously predicts reactions to placebos and active drugs deserves comment. It highlights the point made earlier that the boundary between "active" drug and placebo is ambiguous. To find that a variable, which can be conceptualized as being of personality-level significance, is linked with what are usually regarded as two different response systems dramatizes the fact of overlap. The usual separation of placebo response as a psychological species and drug response as a biological species is difficult to maintain because acquiescence predicts for both realms. At this point, there is no satisfactory explanation of the reversal in relationship of acquiescence to placebo compared with active drug.

One of the prime questions that remains is what basic meaning to assign to the acquiescence dimension. It will be recalled that Bass (1956) originally equated acquiescence with a "Babbit-like" conformance, a nonintellectual style of yielding to social demands. In Bass's original paper, however, he also reported positive correlations between acquiescence and sociability, effectiveness as a salesman, and being "outwardly-oriented," "socially uncritical," and "ethnocentric." In a second paper (1961), he also described positive correlations between acquiescence and being nonskeptical, not doing well as a supervisor, being dissatisfied with self, and being inclined to overgeneralize.

In later reports, McNair, Fisher, Sussman, et al. (1970; McNair et al., 1979) underscored the possibility that acquiescence reflects a style of

---

their reactions to it. In a population of patients in a psychiatric outpatient facility, they found a measure of acquiescence (derived from the MMPI) not to be correlated with the patients' ratings of how therapeutic the "drug" was but significantly positively correlated with the number of reported somatic effects (side effects) it apparently aroused.

"glib" careless thinking. They also reported that they could not accept the notion that high acquiescence is synonymous with being conforming. As previously noted, this view evolved from one of their projects in which they tried to persuade individuals who had participated in one study to return for a follow-up. They discovered that the highly acquiescent were the most resistive. In another study, however, McNair and Barrett (1979), after factor analyzing the Bass scale, concluded that one of the factors extracted should be labeled "traditionalism," which they defined as endorsing conventional, simplistic values and respect. The basic theme of this "traditional" orientation was described as follows: "You get the rewards or solve human problems by playing it safe, by acting cautiously, by obeying the rules, by following but not leading. Finally there are touches of grace and gentleness . . ." (p. 168).

Other studies of the acquiescent or related sets abound (e.g., Couch & Keniston, 1960; Gage & Chatterjee, 1960; Schutz & Foster, 1963). The earlier cited analysis of this literature by McGee (1962) reviewed the twistings and turnings that had already emerged by that time. It did affirm, though, that there was "general agreement in the literature that there is a trait of response acquiescence and that it is probably closely related to some personality variable" (p. 291). As already noted, McGee felt the underlying nature of the variable could be conceptualized as indicating that "acquiescers are stimulus accepting, uninhibited, conformers; nonacquiescers are stimulus rejecting, inhibited, independents" (p. 291).

The general impression from this matrix of data is that the best supported distinction between the high and low acquiescer relates to the need to cultivate ties or forms of closeness with others versus holding to a self-articulated ("I am an independent person") position. The high acquiescer's strategies for maintaining ties may vary (e.g., being submissive, being resistive), but the underlying motivation seems to be to mix it up with people. Generally, the acquiescer wants to evoke responses from others and to transmit a willingness to be part of the social structure. As earlier proposed, the placebo seems to be a selective catalyst for triggering, in acquiescers, expectations concerning potential advantages to be gained from placebo dialogues. The low acquiescer stands off in a more reserved stance and is less trusting of any possible advantages to investing in the socially energized potentialities conjured up by the placebo.

THE NATURE OF THE PLACEBO RESPONSE

Placebo responses not only are powerful and ubiquitous but also can be pumped up or reduced by an array of such variables as personality, degree of enthusiasm of the placebo administrant, and the texture of the illusory attributions mobilized. The psychopharmacology literature is populated with theories concerning the underlying nature of the placebo response. These theories are anchored in concepts like expectancy, suggestibility, conditioning, and attribution (e.g., Jospe, 1978; White et al., 1985). No one of these mechanisms is explanatorily satisfactory. Respectable data exist indicating that each probably applies to different degrees in different contexts. Another potentially interesting explanatory perspective, however, is to conceptualize the placebo paradigm in terms of defense mechanisms.[21]

Thus, we reviewed a number of studies indicating that placebos may be empowered as a means of denying, concealing, or justifying certain feelings or fantasies. Illustratively, placebo experiences may be constructed that permit individuals with high sex guilt to enjoy certain forbidden sexual images by attributing the associated body arousal to the placebo; or persons who are tempted to cheat may indulge the temptation by projecting the anxiety thereby triggered on to placebo-attributed arousal. Such observations suggest that motivation may be an important player in determining placebo response. The intensity with which individuals seize upon a potential placebo opportunity or attribution may depend on how much they are in need of the type of experience the placebo appears to provide.

Jensen and Karoly (1991) conducted a pertinent study in which they examined the role of motivation in determining how strongly individuals responded to a placebo pill that was supposed to have sedating properties. They had structured the experiment so that one sample was assigned to a high motivated condition and another to a low motivated one. The high motivated state was created by telling the subjects that persons who respond to the "drug" to be offered had previously been found to possess a cluster of positive personality traits, whereas those who do not so respond have been identified with a negative personality type. The low motivated sample was essentially told that any relationship between responding to the "drug" and one's personality was negligible. The results showed a significantly greater sedation response in the high as compared with the low motivated subjects. Motivation to emulate the good personality type determined the degree of sedation experienced. Other studies (e.g., Aletky & Carlin, 1975; Gibbons & Hormuth, 1981) have also demonstrated the role of motivation in placebo reaction.

The dominant view in the placebo literature is that the placebo response is the result of deception and represents a form of submission to a figure of higher authority (usually a physician). Placebo responding is typically

---

[21] Speculations concerning psychodynamic influences on drug and placebo responses can be found in early papers by Bellak, Hurvich, Silvan, and Jacobs (1968) and Azima and Sarwer-Foner (1961).

conceptualized as a species of passivity, a loss of autonomy, a form of susceptibility to being manipulated. The power of the placebo is regarded as flowing from the administrant to the placebo responder. The psychopharmacology establishment has often cast the placebo responder as a nuisance, a representative of a form of inferiority, someone to get rid of (e.g., by means of a preliminary washout).

However, we would propose that the placebo response is not something bestowed, but rather represents the ability of individuals, when they consciously or unconsciously detect an advantage, to imaginatively mobilize certain feelings, moods, and therapeutic strategies. Impressive creativity is implicit in the ability of persons to view themselves as being in a situation that enables them to revise negative self-destructive attitudes or to court new forms of experience or to magnify and minimize (reframe) various somatic sensations. The context of the placebo encounter can have stimulating meanings that may variously be paraphrased as "You have a chance to change yourself radically—to pull yourself together" or "You can experience new sensations, thoughts, and emotions that you rarely allow yourself" or "You can engage in forms of imaginative play that are usually off-limits." Such ideas and concepts probably play a role in other forms of self-transformation such as encountered in religious conversion experiences, psychotherapy-inspired changes, and encounters with radically new environments or persons (S. Fisher & Fisher, 1993). Plotkin (1985) points out how strongly inclined the health establishment is to attribute cures to the therapist's competency, the therapist's potency; and to minimize the contribution of the patient's resources to any recovery process.[22] The fact that individuals can take advantage of cues and ideas offered by the placebo context is not a sign of passivity but rather of the ability to mobilize oneself imaginatively. What is called passivity may really be a willingness to be receptive to communications.[23] One argument against interpreting placebo response as a form of submission is that despite strenuous efforts, no one has been able to demonstrate convincingly that placebo responding is correlated with measures of suggestibility or hypnotic susceptibility (White et al., 1985). Apropos of interpreting placebo responding as a form of creative fantasy, Fisher and Fisher

---

[22] Plotkin (1985) states: "To whatever extent a therapeutic improvement is attributed to a placebo effect, that improvement . . . is the direct achievement of the patient himself or herself. That is, it is the patient, through the exercise of personal competence, who directly achieves the therapeutic outcome" (p. 245).

[23] Bootzin et al. (1976) suggested that the ability to be "reflective" may be involved in certain forms of placebo response.

(1993) have outlined in some detail the imaginative ability and the talent required to construct self-protective illusions and defenses.

Since little or no data exist concerning the specific ways in which placebos achieve their effectiveness, one can only cautiously speculate. M. Ross and Olson (1981) contributed the following possibilities:

- "Placebos alleviate patient's anxiety about their symptoms and thereby effect an improvement" (p. 427).
- "Individuals accentuate the positive after receiving placebos. They may observe small changes in their conditions that they would have failed to notice in the absence of the placebo, and they may downplay the significance of negative changes that would otherwise have caused them considerable concern . . . ." (p. 427).
- "Recipients of placebos do not truly perceive any changes in their condition but simply comply with the demands of the situation. Subjects in experiments and patients being treated with placebos know the effects that the placebos should have. They may feel that it is important, either for the sake of science or for their own well-being, that the experimenter's or therapist's prognosis be affirmed" (p. 427).
- "A fourth . . . possibility is that expectancies produce actual somatic changes (e.g., in the endorphin system) . . . ." (p. 427).

The following supplementary alternatives are expressed more in the language of self-defense strategies:

- The placebo context may facilitate the use of defense mechanisms that have in the past proven effective for that individual. For example, introducing the concept of a curative substance that is simultaneously "out there" and has special powers meaningful to the self may make it easier to engage in certain forms of projection or displacement that involve spatial distancing.
- The responsibility apparently assumed by the placebo for one's state could conceivably make the individual more comfortable about "letting go" and venting feelings ("I am doing this because the drug is making me") that had been denied or repressed.
- The pretend ambiance associated with placebo dialogues might encourage the individual to reinstitute some of the basic illusory optimistic attitudes that are known to facilitate normal adaptation (S. Fisher & Fisher, 1993; Taylor, 1989).
- A placebo, which is typically presented as a drug, could increase body awareness. Research findings (S. Fisher & Fisher, 1993) suggest that such augmented awareness can increase the accuracy of perceptions

of one's emotional states and this could obviously be beneficial because it would facilitate more realistic interpretation of body cues.

Exploration of the various mechanisms basic to the placebo's power will open novel perspectives on the whole process of how individuals capitalize on opportunities and cues that help them to mobilize their self-saving resources.

CONCLUSION

The obsessive effort to find pure biologically based drug treatments for psychological distress is rooted in false premises. First of all, as indicated, so-called psychological variables that shape behavior are just as biologically mediated as psychotropic drugs. Further, the differences between placebo effects (the presumed epitome of the psychological) and "active drug" effects are often hazy and shifting. If active drugs are regarded as achieving their potency by influencing specific brain centers and synaptic functions, one can just as logically presume that placebos are influential because they activate other brain loci that modulate variables like self-efficacy, anxiety, and ability to try out new roles and new forms of pretense.

The literature reviewed in this chapter illustrates not only the variability in drug and placebo responses as a function of psychosocial context but also the overlapping nature of placebo and drug phenomena. The impact of both placebos and psychotropic drugs is influenced by such a melange as whether administered in group or individual settings, the optimism of the administrant, the nature of the ward or clinic atmosphere, and personality factors. Krupnick et al. (1996) demonstrated rather dramatically that the character of the "alliance" between patient and therapist contributes significantly to the therapeutic efficacy of imipramine (and placebo) for depression. However, most impressive concerning the relativities of drug and placebo responses is that simply altering the verbal label associated with a substance may significantly increase or decrease certain of its apparent therapeutic, subjective, and physiological powers. It is striking that thorazine represented as a placebo differs in its consequences from thorazine presented as an active agent (Guy, 1967). The effects of a drug or placebo may be grossly reversed merely by introducing reversed descriptions of the substance's potentialities. Thus, a bronchodilator can be converted to a bronchoconstrictor by telling individuals the proper deceptive story (Luparello et al., 1970). A disguised drug affects individuals differently than it does when offered in its conventional identity. There are also instances in which placebos neutralize active drugs and placebos neutralize other placebos. In addition, psychotropic drugs and placebos often do not really differ much in their therapeutic powers (e.g., in the case of antidepressants for adults and children). This is especially true when one takes into account the bias in favor of the active drug that pervades drug trials because of the inadequate safeguard against such bias provided by the double-blind.

If one grasps the considerable functional similarities between psychotropic drugs and placebos and if one is not driven by ideological needs for biological purity, it seems quite logical to design treatments for psychological distress that maximize the potential of the placebo element. We are to some unknown degree already taking advantage of the placebo effects that are implicit in the matrix of the active drug as we proffer it to the distressed. The magnitude of this implicit placebo effect is unknown because it is doubtful that it can be accurately measured by the size of the simple placebo control effect. We have already spelled out in some detail how the usual placebo control lacks the drama of the active drug that is not only delivered with greater conviction but also initiates a scenario of active body experiences signaling "This is the real thing." We do not actually know empirically whether the so-called active psychotropic drugs would have much potency left if their full placebo component were to be magically extracted. However, this possibility can be glimpsed in studies cited earlier in which active drugs lose a good deal of their potency when disguised as placebos.

Placebo effects have so impressed some observers that they have proposed giving placebos to the distressed, first, before offering the active drug. Brown (1994) suggested such a possibility apropos of the use of antidepressants. An issue that is immediately raised about such placebos is that they call for deception. Presumably, the placebo can be effective only if the distressed individual is not aware that it is an inert substance. Nevertheless, there is a hint that placebos can sometimes be effective even when individuals are explicitly told that they are not ingesting the real thing. In one study (Park & Covi, 1965), patients responded positively to an undisguised placebo and later revealed that they did so because they did not believe a physician would prescribe an ineffective agent. In any case, with reference to the dishonesty presumably associated with giving individuals an inert substance and pretending it is the active drug, one could logically argue that it is just as dishonest to provide the active drug and not to reveal that a significant fraction of its potency probably derives from placebo elements.

Our own proposal is that placebo effects should be maximized by either using placebo substances that arouse discernible and convincing body experiences or providing active drugs under conditions that will optimize the recipients' conviction that such drugs truly guarantee an opportunity to mobilize and "get better." Optimizing variables would include enthusiastic administrants who sincerely expect positive change, an impressive looking capsule or pill, a clear presentation of the benefits to be expected, comforting rationalization of unpleasant side effects, and the reassurance there is ample scientific proof of efficacy. Interestingly, Plutchik, Platman, and Fieve (1969) proposed that one way to cope with the uncertainty linked to the use of the double-blind when testing drugs would be to set up trials in which a deliberate effort was made to maximize all the biases (e.g., administrant enthusiasm) favoring the drug in question. This would define the highest possible therapeutic power that could be expected from that drug.

No drug can be aloof from the social atmosphere in which it is administered. The goal in treating distressed patients is not to provide some pure form of therapy but rather to embrace every possible curative force. A biologically pure treatment for psychological disturbance has been and remains a mythic hope.

REFERENCES

Aletky, P. J., & Carlin, A. S. (1975). Sex differences and placebo effects: Motivation as an intervening variable. *Journal of Consulting and Clinical Psychology, 43,* 278.

Archer, T. (1995). The role of conditioning in the use of placebo. *Nordic Journal of Psychiatry, 49,* 43–53.

Azima, H., & Sarwer-Foner, G. J. (1961). Psychoanalytic formulations of the effects of drugs in pharmacotherapy. *Revue Canadienne de Biologie, 20,* 603–614.

Baker, A., & Thorpe, J. (1957). Placebo responses. *American Medical Association Archives of Neurology and Psychiatry, 78,* 57–60.

Barrett, J. E. (1987). Nonpharmacological factors determining the behavioral effects of drugs. In H. Y. Meltzer (Ed.), *Psychopharmacology: The third generation of progress* (pp. 1493–1501). New York: Raven Press.

Bartholomew, A. A., & Marley, E. (1959). Susceptibility to methylpentynol: Personality and other variables. *Journal of Mental Science, 105,* 955–970.

Bass, B. (1956). Development and evaluation of a scale for measuring social acquiescence. *Journal of Abnormal and Social Psychology, 53,* 296–299.

Bass, B. M. (1961). Some recent studies in social acquiescence. *Psychological Reports, 9,* 447–448.

Batterman, R. C. (1957). Placebo and nonreactors to analgesics. *Federation Proceedings, 280,* Abstract No. 1197.

Baxter, L. R., Schwartz, J. M., Bergman, K. S., Szuba, M. P., Guze, B. H., Mazziotta, J. C., Akazraju, A., Selin, C. E., Ferng, H. K., Munford, P., & Phelps, M. E. (1992). Caudate glucose metabolic rate changes with both drug and behavior therapy for obsessive-compulsive disorder. *Archives of General Psychiatry, 49,* 681–689.

Beecher, H. K. (1955). The powerful placebo. *Journal of the American Medical Association, 159,* 1602–1606.

Beecher, H. K. (1960). Stress and effectiveness of placebos and "active" drugs. *Science, 132,* 91–92.

Bellak, L., Hurvich, M., Silvan, M., & Jacobs, D. (1968). Toward an ego psychological appraisal of drug effects. *American Journal of Psychiatry, 125,* 593–604.

Black, A. A. (1966). Factors predisposing to a placebo response in new outpatients with anxiety states. *British Journal of Psychiatry, 112,* 557–567.

Bootzin, R. R., Herman, C. P., & Nicassio, P. (1976). The power of suggestion: Another examination of misattribution and insomnia. *Journal of Personality and Social Psychology, 34,* 673–679.

Breznitz, S. (Ed.). (1983). *The denial of stress.* New York: International Universities Press.

Briddell, D. W., Rimm, D. C., Caddy, G. R., Krawitz, G., Sholis, D., & Wunderlin, R. J. (1978). Effects of alcohol and cognitive set on sexual arousal to deviant stimuli. *Journal of Abnormal Psychology, 87,* 418–430.

Brodeur, D. (1965). The effects of stimulant and tranquilizer placebos on healthy subjects in a real-life situation. *Psychopharmacologia, 7,* 444–452.

Brody, H. (1977). *Placebos and the philosophy of medicine.* Chicago: University of Chicago Press.

Brody, H. (1985). Placebo effect: An examination of Grunbaum's definition. In L. White, B. Tursky, & G. E. Schwartz (Eds.), *Placebo: Theory, research, and mechanisms* (pp. 37–57). New York: Guilford Press.

Brown, W. A. (1994). Placebo as a treatment for depression. *Neuropsychopharmacology, 10,* 265–269.

Butler, C., & Steptoe, A. (1986). Placebo responses: An experimental study of psychophysiological processes in asthmatic volunteers. *British Journal of Clinical Psychology, 25,* 173–183.

Casey, J. F., Bennett, I. F., Lindley, C. J., Hollister, L. E., Gordon, M. H., & Springer, N. N. (1985). Drug therapy in schizophrenia. *Archives of General Psychiatry, 42,* 887–896.

Clausen, J., & Fisher, S. (1973). Effects of amphetamine and barbiturate on body experience. *Psychosomatic Medicine, 35,* 390–405.

Cleveland, S. E. (1989). Personality factors in the mediation of drug response. In S. Fisher & R. P. Greenberg (Eds.), *The limits of biological treatments for psychological distress* (pp. 235–262). Hillsdale, NJ: Erlbaum.

Cooper, J., Zanna, M. P., & Taves, P. A. (1978). Arousal as a necessary condition for attitude change following induced compliance. *Journal of Personality and Social Psychology, 36,* 1101–1106.

Couch, A., & Keniston, K. (1960). Yeasayers and naysayers: Agreeing response set as a personality variable. *Journal of Abnormal and Social Psychology, 60,* 151–174.

Davison, G. C., & Valins, S. (1969). Maintenance of self-attributed and drug-attributed behavior change. *Journal of Personality and Social Psychology, 11,* 25–33.

Denber, H. C. B., & Bente, D. (1966). Clinical response to pharmacotherapy in different settings. In H. Brill (Ed.), *Neuropsychopharmacology: Proceedings of* the Fifth International Congress of the Collegium Internationale Neuropsychophar-macologicum (pp. 517–519). New York: Excerpta Medica Foundation.

Depression Guideline Panel (DGP). (1993). *Depression in primary care: Vol. 2. Treatment of major depression* (Clinical Practice Guideline, No. 5, AHCPR Publication No. 93-0551). Rockville, MD: Department of Health and Human Services, Public Health Services, Agency for Health Care Policy and Research.

Dienstbier, R. A., & Munter, P. O. (1971). Cheating as a function of the labeling of natural arousal. *Journal of Personality and Social Psychology, 17*, 208–213.

DiMascio, A. (1968). Personality and variability of response to psychotropic drugs: Relationship to "paradoxical effects." In K. Rickels (Ed.), *Non-specific factors in drug therapy* (pp. 40–58). Springfield, IL: Thomas.

DiMascio, A., & Barrett, J. (1965). Comparative effects of Oxazepam in "high" and "low" anxious college students. *Psychosomatics, 6*, 298–302.

Dinnerstein, A. J., Lowenthal, M., & Blitz, B. (1966–1967). The interaction of drugs with placebos in the control of pain and anxiety. *Perspectives in Biology and Medicine, 10*, 103–117.

Downing, R. W., & Rickels, K. (1978). Nonspecific factors and their interaction with psychological treatment in pharmacotherapy. In M. A. Lipton, A. DiMascio, & K. F. Killam (Eds.), *Psychopharmacology: A generation of progress* (pp. 1419–1428). New York: Raven Press.

Downing, R. W., Rickels, K., & Dreesmann, H. (1973). Orthogonal factors vs. interdependent variables as predictors of drug treatment response in anxious outpatients. *Psychopharmacologia, 32*, 93–111.

Epstein, L. H., & Cluss, P. A. (1983). Bio-behavioral effects of compliance. *Journal of Pediatrics, 103*, 665.

Evans, F. J. (1974). The placebo response in pain reduction. *Advances in Neurology, 4*, 289–296.

Evans, F. J. (1985). Expectancy, therapeutic instructions, and the placebo response. In L. White, B. Tursky, & G. E. Schwartz (Eds.), *Placebo: Theory, research, and mechanisms* (pp. 215–234). New York: Guilford Press.

Eysenck, H. J. (1947). *Dimensions of personality.* London: Keegan, Trench, Trubner.

Eysenck, H. J. (1983). Drugs as research tools: Experiments with drugs in personality research. *Neuropsychology, 10*, 29–43.

Faravelli, C., & Sacchetti, E. (1984). Subjective side effects during treatment with clomipramine: Relationship to symptoms, plasma levels and personality. *Medical Science, 12*, 1111–1112.

Fast, G. J., & Fisher, S. (1971). The role of body attitudes and acquiescence in epinephrine and placebo effects. *Psychosomatic Medicine, 33*, 63–84.

Feighner, J. P., Aden, G. C., Fabre, L. F., Rickels, K., & Smith, W. T. (1983). Comparison of alprazolam, imipramine, and placebo in the treatment of depression. *Journal of the American Medical Association, 249*, 3057–3064.

Fisher, R. L., & Fisher, S. (1996). Antidepressants for children: Is scientific support necessary? *Journal of Nervous and Mental Disease, 184*, 99–108.

Fisher, S. (1967). The placebo reactor: Thesis, antithesis, synthesis, and hypothesis. *Diseases of the Nervous System, 28*, 510–515.

Fisher, S., Cole, J. O., Rickels, K., & Uhlenhuth, E. H. (1964). Drug-set interaction: The effect of expectations on drug response in outpatients. *Neuropsychopharmacology, 3,* 149–156.

Fisher, S., & Fisher, R. L. (1963). Placebo response and acquiescence. *Psychopharmacologia, 4,* 298–301.

Fisher, S., & Fisher, R. L. (1993). *The psychology of adaptation to absurdity: Tactics of make-believe.* Hillsdale, NJ: Erlbaum.

Fisher, S., & Greenberg, R. P. (Eds.). (1989). *The limits of biological treatments for psychological distress: Comparisons with psychotherapy and placebo.* Hillsdale, NJ: Erlbaum.

Fisher, S., & Greenberg, R. P. (1993). How sound is the double-blind design for evaluating psychotropic drugs? *Journal of Nervous and Mental Disease, 181,* 345–350.

Foulds, G. (1958). Clinical research in psychiatry. *Journal of Mental Science, 104,* 259–265.

Frank, E., Karp, J. F., & Rush, A. J. (1993). Efficacy of treatments for major depression. *Psychopharmacology Bulletin, 29,* 457–475.

Frank, E., Kupfer, D. J., Jacob, M., & Jarrett, D. (1987). Personality features and response to acute treatment in recurrent depression. *Journal of Personality Disorders, 1,* 14–26.

Frank, J. D. (1973). *Persuasion and healing.* Baltimore: Johns Hopkins University Press.

Frankenhaueser, M., Jarpe, G., Svan, H., & Wrangsjo, B. (1963). Psychophysiological reactions to two different placebo treatments. *Scandinavian Journal of Psychology, 4,* 245–250.

Frankenhaueser, M., Post, B., Hagdahl, R., & Wrangsjo, B. (1964). Effects of a depressant drug as modified by experimentally-induced expectation. *Perceptual and Motor Skills, 18,* 513–522.

Freedman, N., Engelhardt, D., Mann, D., Margolis, R., & London, S. (1965). Communication of body complaints and paranoid symptom change under conditions of phenothiazine treatment. *Journal of Personality and Social Psychology, 1,* 310–318.

Gage, N. L., & Chatterjee, B. B. (1960). The psychological meaning of acquiescence set: Further evidence. *Journal of Abnormal and Social Psychology, 60,* 280–283.

Gammer, C. E., & Allen, V. L. (1966). Note on the use of drugs in psychological research. *Psychological Reports, 18,* 654.

Gardos, G., DiMascio, A., Saltzman, C., & Shader, R. I. (1968). Differential actions of chlordiazepoxide and oxazepam on hostility. *Archives of General Psychiatry, 18,* 757–760.

Gelfand, S., Ullman, L. P., & Krasner, L. (1963). The placebo response: An experimental approach. *Journal of Nervous and Mental Disease, 136,* 379–387.

Gibbons, F. X., & Gaeddert, W. P. (1984). Focus of attention and placebo utility. *Journal of Experimental Social Psychology, 20,* 159–176.

Gibbons, F. X., & Hormuth, S. E. (1981). Motivational factors in placebo responsivity. *Psychopharmacology Bulletin, 17,* 77–79.

Gibbons, F. X., & Wright, R. A. (1981). Motivational biases in causal attributions of arousal. *Journal of Personality and Social Psychology, 40,* 588–600.

Girodo, M. (1973). Film-induced arousal, information search, and the attribution process. *Journal of Personality and Social Psychology, 25,* 357–360.

Goldstein, A., Searle, B. W., & Schmike, R. T. (1960). Effects of secobarbital and of D-Amphetamine on psychomotor performance of normal subjects. *Journal of Pharmacology and Experimental Therapeutics, 130,* 55–58.

Gowdy, C. W. (1983). A guide to the pharmacology of placebos. *Canadian Medical Association Journal, 128,* 921–925.

Greenblatt, M., Grosser, G. H., & Wechsler, H. (1964). Differential response of hospitalized depressed patients to somatic therapy. *American Journal of Psychiatry, 120,* 935–943.

Grunbaum, A. (1981). The placebo concept. *Behavior Research and Therapy, 19,* 157–167.

Grunbaum, A. (1985). Explication and implications of the placebo concept. In L. White, B. Tursky, & G. E. Schwartz (Eds.), *Placebo: Theory, research and mechanisms* (pp. 9–36). New York: Guilford Press.

Gryll, S. L., & Katahn, M. (1978). Situational factors contributing to the placebo effect. *Psychopharmacology, 57,* 253–261.

Guy, W. H. (1967). Placebo proneness: It's relationship to environmental influences and personality traits. *Dissertation Abstracts, 28*(5-B), 2137–2138.

Haefner, D. P., Sacks, J. M., & Mason, A. S. (1960). Physicians' attitudes toward chemotherapy as a factor in psychiatric patients' responses to medication. *Journal of Nervous and Mental Disease, 131,* 64–69.

Halm, J. (1967). *The relationship of field articulation and affective placebo reaction.* Unpublished doctoral dissertation, Yeshiva University, New York.

Hill, H. E., Belleville, R. E., & Wikler, A. (1957). Motivational determinants in modification of behavior by morphine and pentobarbital. *Archives of Neurology and Psychiatry, 77,* 28–35.

Honigfeld, G. (1964, April). Non-specific factors in treatment. *Diseases of the Nervous System, 25,* 225–239.

Horowitz, R. I., Viscoli, C. M., Berkman, L., Donaldson, R. M., Horowitz, S., Murray, C. J., Ransohoff, D. F., & Sindelar, J. (1990). Treatment adherence and risk of death after a myocardial infarction. *Lancet, 336,* 542–545.

Hughes, J. R., Gulliver, S. B., Amori, G., Mireault, G. C., & Fenwick, J. F. (1989). Effect of instructions and nicotine on smoking cessations, withdrawal symptoms, and self-administration of nicotine gum. *Psychopharmacology, 99,* 486–491.

Hull, J. G., & Bond, C. F., Jr. (1986). Social and behavioral consequences of alcohol consumption and expectancy: A meta-analysis. *Psychological Bulletin, 99,* 347–360.

Idestrom, C. M., & Schilling, D. (1970). Objective effects of dexamphetamine and amobarbital and their relations to psychasthenic personality traits. *Psychopharmacologia, 17,* 399–413.

Ihilevich, D., & Gleser, G. C. (1986). *Defense mechanisms.* Owosso, MI: DMI Associates.

Janke, W. (Ed.). (1983). *Response variability to psychotropic drugs*. New York: Pergamon Press.

Jensen, M. P., & Karoly, P. (1991). Motivation and expectancy factors in symptom perception: A laboratory study of the placebo effect. *Psychosomatic Medicine, 53*, 144–152.

Johnson, A. G. (1994). Surgery as a placebo. *Lancet, 344*, 1140–1142.

Jospe, M. (1978). *The placebo effect in healing*. Lexington, MA: Heath.

Joyce, C. R. B. (1959). Consistent differences in individual reactions to drugs and dummies. *British Journal of Pharmacology, 14*, 512–521.

Kast, E. C. (1961). Methodology in clinical drug evaluation: Phenyramidol in the treatment of hypertrophic arthritis. *Chic Medicine, 63*, 17–21.

Kavanagh, D. J. (1992). Developments in expressed emotion and schizophrenia. *British Journal of Psychiatry, 160*, 601–620.

Kellam, S. G., Goldberg, S. C., Schooler, N. R., Berman, A., & Shmelzer, J. L. (1967). Ward atmosphere and outcome of treatment of acute schizophrenia. *Journal of Psychiatric Research, 5*, 145–163.

Keltner, N. L., & Folks, D. G. (1992). Culture as a variable in drug therapy. *Perspectives in Psychiatric Care, 28*, 33–36.

Kirsch, I. (1985). Response expectancy as a determinant of experience and behavior. *American Psychologist, 40*, 1189–1202.

Kirsch, I., & Rosadino, M. J. (1993). Do double-blind studies with informed consent yield externally valid results? *Psychopharmacology, 110*, 437–442.

Kirsch, I., & Weixel, L. J. (1988). Double-blind versus deceptive administration of a placebo. *Behavioral Neuroscience, 102*, 319–323.

Klerman, G. L., DiMascio, A., Greenblatt, M., & Rinkel, M. (1959). The influence of specific personality patterns on the reactions of psychotropic agents. In J. M. Masserman (Ed.), *Biological psychiatry* (pp. 224–238). New York: Grune & Stratton.

Krugman, A. D., Ross, S., & Lyerly, S. (1964). Drugs and placebos: Effects of instructions upon performance and mood under amphetamine sulphate and chloral hydrate with younger subjects. *Psychological Reports, 15*, 925–926.

Krupnick, J. L., Sotsky, S. M., Simmens, S., Moyer, J., Elkin, I., Watkins, J., & Pilkonis, P. A. (1996). The role of the therapeutic alliance in psychotherapy and pharmacotherapy outcome: Findings in the National Institute of Mental Health Treatment of Depression Collaborative Research Program. *Journal of Consulting and Clinical Psychology, 64*, 532–539.

Lasagna, L., Mosteller, F., von Felsinger, J. M., & Beecher, H. K. (1954). A study of the placebo response. *American Journal of Medicine, 16*, 770–771.

Leavitt, F. (1995). *Drugs and behavior* (3rd ed.). Thousand Oaks, CA: Sage.

Leveton, A. F. (1958). The evaluation and testing of psychopharmaceutic drugs. *American Journal of Psychiatry, 116*, 97–103.

Levinson, P., Malen, R., Hogben, G., & Smith, H. (1978). Psychological factors in susceptibility to drug-induced extrapyramidal symptoms. *American Journal of Psychiatry, 135*, 1375–1376.

Levy, R. S., & Jankovic, J. (1983). Placebo-induced conversion reaction: A neurobehavioral and EEG study of hysterical aphasia, seizure, and coma. *Journal of Abnormal Psychology, 92*, 243–249.

Liberman, R. P. (1964). An experimental study of the placebo response under three different situations of pain. *Journal of Psychiatric Research, 2,* 233–246.

Liberman, R. P. (1966). The elusive placebo reactor. In H. Brill (Ed.), *Neuro-psycho-pharmacology: Proceedings of the Fifth International Congress of the Collegium Internationale Neuro-psycho-pharmacologicum* (pp. 557–566). New York: Excerpta Medica Foundation.

Lin, K., Poland, R. E., & Anderson, D. (1995). Psychopharmacology, ethnicity and culture. *Transcultural Psychiatric Research Review, 32,* 3–40.

Lindemann, E., & von Felsinger, J. M. (1961). Drug effects and personality theory. *Psychopharmacologia, 2,* 89–92.

Linn, E. L. (1959). Sources of uncertainty in studies of drugs affecting mood, mentation, or activity. *American Journal of Psychiatry, 116,* 97–103.

Lipman, R. S., Park, L. C., Rickels, K., & Chase, C. (1966). Paradoxical influence of a therapeutic side-effect interpretation. *Archives of General Psychiatry, 15,* 462–474.

Loftis, J., & Ross, L. (1974). Effects of misattribution of arousal upon the acquisition and extinction of a conditional emotional response. *Journal of Personality and Social Psychology, 30,* 673–682.

Loranger, A. W., Prout, C. T., & White, M. A. (1961). The placebo effect in psychiatric drug research. *Journal of the American Medical Association, 176,* 920–925.

Lundh, L. (1987). Placebo, belief, and health. *Scandinavian Journal of Psychology, 28,* 128–143.

Luparello, T. J., Leist, N., Lourie, C. H., & Sweet, P. (1970). The interaction of psychologic stimuli and pharmacologic agents on airway reactivity in asthmatic subjects. *Psychosomatic Medicine, 32,* 509–513.

Lyerly, S. B., Ross, S., Krugman, A. D., & Clyde, D. (1964). Drugs and placebos: The effects of instructions upon performance and mood under amphetamine sulphate and chloral hydrate. *Journal of Abnormal and Social Psychology, 68,* 321–327.

McClelland, D. C. (1985). The social mandate of health psychology. *American Behavioral Scientist, 28,* 451–467.

McGee, R. K. (1962). Response style as a personality variable: By what criterion? *Psychological Bulletin, 59,* 284–295.

McNair, D. M., & Barrett, J. E. (1979). Two Bass scale factors and response to placebo and anxiolytic drugs. *Psychopharmacology, 65,* 165–170.

McNair, D. M., Fisher, S., Kahn, R. J., & Droppleman, L. F. (1970). Drug-personality interaction in intensive outpatient treatment. *Archives of General Psychiatry, 22,* 128–135.

McNair, D. M., Fisher, S., Sussman, C., Droppleman, L. F., & Kahn, R. J. (1970). Persistence of a drug-personality interaction in psychiatric outpatients. *Journal of Psychiatric Research, 7,* 299–305.

McNair, D. M., Gardos, G., Haskell, D. S., & Fisher, S. (1979). Placebo response, placebo effect, and two attributes. *Psychopharmacology, 63,* 245–250.

McNair, D. M., Kahn, R. J., Droppleman, L. F., & Fisher, S. (1968). Compatibility, acquiescence and drug effects. In H. Brill (Ed.), *Neuro-psycho-pharmacology:*

Proceedings of the Fifth International Congress of the Collegium Internationale Neuro-psycho-pharmacologicum (pp. 536–542). New York: Excerpta Medica Foundation.

Meyers, S., & Janowitz, H. D. (1989). The "natural history" of ulcerative colitis. An analysis of the placebo response. *Journal of Clinical Gastroenterology, 1,* 33–37.

Muller, B. P. (1965). Personality of placebo reactors and nonreactors. *Diseases of the Nervous System, 26,* 58–61.

Naditch, M. P., Alker, P. C., & Joffe, P. (1975). Individual differences and setting as determinants of acute adverse reactions to psychoactive drugs. *Journal of Nervous and Mental Disease, 161,* 326–335.

Nakano, S., Ogawa, N., & Kawazu, Y. (1980, March). Influence of neuroticism on oral absorption of diazepam. *Clinical and Pharmacological Therapy, 27,* 370–374.

Nisbett, R. E., & Schachter, S. (1966). Cognitive manipulation of pain. *Journal of Experimental Social Psychology, 2,* 227–236.

Park, L. C., & Covi, L. (1965). Nonblind placebo trial. *Archives of General Psychiatry, 12,* 336–345.

Parrott, A. C., & Kentridge, R. (1982). Personal constructs of anxiety under the 1,5 benzodiazepine derivative related to trait-anxiety levels of the personality. *Psychopharmacology, 78,* 353–357.

Penick, S. B., & Fisher, S. (1965). Drug-set interaction: Psychological and physiological effects of epinephrine under differential expectations. *Psychosomatic Medicine, 27,* 177–182.

Penick, S. B., & Hinkle, L. E., Jr. (1964). The effect of expectation on response to Phenmetrazine. *Psychosomatic Medicine, 26,* 369–373.

Pichot, P., & Perse, J. (1968). Placebo effects as response set. In K. Rickels (Ed.), *Non-specific factors in drug therapy* (pp. 50–58). Springfield, IL: Thomas.

Pliner, P., & Cappell, H. (1974). Modification of affective consequences of alcohol. *Journal of Abnormal Psychology, 83,* 418–425.

Plotkin, W. B. (1985). A psychological approach to placebo: The role of faith in therapy and treatment. In L. White, B. Tursky, & G. E. Schwartz (Eds.), *Placebo: Theory, research, and mechanisms* (pp. 237–254). New York: Guilford Press.

Plutchik, R., Platman, S. R., & Fieve, R. R. (1969). Three alternatives to the double-blind. *Archives of General Psychiatry, 20,* 428–432.

Pollmann, L., & Hildebrandt, G. (1981). Circadian variations of potency of placebos on pain threshold in healthy teeth. *International Journal of Oral Surgery, 10,* 208–211.

Quitkin, F. M., Rabkin, J. G., Markowitz, J. M., Stewart, J. W., McGrath, P. J., & Harrison, W. (1987). Use of pattern analysis to identify true drug response: A replication. *Archives of General Psychiatry, 44,* 259–264.

Rawlinson, M. C. (1985). Truth-telling and paternalism in the clinic: Philosophical reflections on the use of placebos in medical practice. In L. White, B. Tursky, & G. E. Schwartz (Eds.), *Placebo: Theory, research, and mechanisms* (pp. 403–418). New York: Guilford Press.

Reed, C. F., & Witt, P. N. (1965). Factors contributing to unexpected reactions to two human drug-placebo experiments. *Confina Psychiatrica, 8,* 57–68.

Rickels, K. (Ed.). (1968). *Non-specific factors in drug therapy.* Springfield, IL: Thomas.

Rickels, K., Ward, C. H., & Schut, L. (1964, March). Different populations, different drug responses. *American Journal of the Medical Sciences, 247,* 106–113.

Roberts, A. H. (1994). "The powerful placebo" revisited: Implications for headache treatment and management. *Headache Quarterly, Current Treatment and Research, 5,* 208–213.

Roberts, A. H. (1995). The powerful placebo revisited: Magnitude of nonspecific effects. *Mind Body Medicine, 1,* 35–43.

Ross, M., & Olson, J. M. (1981). An expectancy-attribution model of the effects of placebos. *Psychological Review, 88,* 408–437.

Ross, S., & Buckalew, L. W. (1983). The placebo as an agent in behavioral manipulations: A review of problems, issues, and affected measures. *Clinical Psychology Review, 3,* 457–471.

Ross, S., Krugman, A. D., Lyerly, S. B., & Clyde, D. J. (1962). Drugs and placebos: A model design. *Psychological Reports, 10,* 383–392.

Rothchild, R., & Quitkin, F. M. (1992). Review of the use of pattern analysis to differentiate true drug and placebo responses. *Psychotherapy and Psychosomatics, 58,* 170–177.

Sabshin, M., & Ramot, J. (1956). Pharmacotherapeutic evaluation and the psychiatric setting. *Archives of Neurology and Psychiatry, 75,* 362–370.

Sarwer-Foner, G. J., & Ogle, W. (1956). Psychodynamic aspects of reserpine: Its uses and effects in open psychiatric settings. *Developments in Social Therapy, 1,* 11–17.

Schachter, S., & Singer, J. (1962). Cognitive, social and physiological determinants of emotional state. *Psychological Review, 69,* 379–399.

Schapira, K., McClelland, H., Griffiths, M., & Newell, D. (1970). Study on the effects of tablet colour in the treatment of anxiety states. *British Medical Journal, 2,* 446–449.

Schutz, R. E., & Foster, R. J. (1963). A factor analytic study of acquiescent and extreme response set. *Educational and Psychological Measurement, 23,* 435–447.

Shapiro, A. K. (1964). Factors contributing to the placebo effect. *American Journal of Psychotherapy, 18,* 73–88.

Shapiro, A. K. (1968). Semantics of the placebo. *Psychiatric Quarterly, 42,* 653–695.

Shapiro, A. K. (1971). Placebo effects in medicine, psychotherapy, and psychoanalysis. In S. L. Garfield & A. E. Bergin (Eds.), *Handbook of psychotherapy and behavior change* (pp. 439–475). New York: Wiley.

Shapiro, A. K., Struening, E. L., Barten, H., & Shapiro, E. (1975). Correlates of placebo reaction in an outpatient population. *Psychological Medicine, 5,* 389–396.

Shapiro, A. P., & Morris, L. A. (1978). The placebo effect in medical and psychological therapies. In S. L. Garfield & A. E. Bergin (Eds.), *Handbook of psychotherapy and behavior change* (pp. 369–410). New York: Wiley.

Shapiro, A. P., Myers, T., Reiser, M. F., & Ferris, E. B., Jr. (1954). Comparison of blood pressure response to Veriloid and to the doctor. *Psychosomatic Medicine, 16,* 478–488.

Sharp, H. C. (1965). Identifying placebo reactors. *Journal of Psychology, 60,* 205–212.

Shawcross, C. R., & Tyrer, P. (1985). Influence of personality on response to monamine oxidase inhibitors and tricyclic antidepressants. *Journal of Psychiatric Research, 19,* 557–562.

Shepherd, M. (1993). The placebo: From specificity to the non-specific and back. *Psychological Medicine, 23,* 569–578.

Sternbach, R. A. (1964). The effects of instructional sets on autonomic responsivity. *Psychophysiology, 1,* 67–72.

Storms, M. D., & Nisbett, R. E. (1970). Insomnia and the attribution process. *Journal of Personality and Social Psychology, 16,* 319–328.

Taylor, S. E. (1989). *Positive illusions: Creative self-deception and the healthy mind.* New York: Basic Books.

Thomson, R. (1982). Side effects and placebo amplification. *British Journal of Psychiatry, 140,* 64–68.

Trouton, D. S. (1957). Placebos and their psychological effects. *Journal of Mental Science, 103,* 344–354.

Turner, J. A., Deyo, R. A., Loesser, J. D., Von Korff, M., & Fordyce, W. E. (1994). The importance of placebo effects in pain treatment and research. *Journal of the American Medical Association, 271,* 1609–1614.

Uhlenhuth, E. H., Canter, A., Neustadt, J. D., & Payson, H. E. (1957). The symptomatic relief of anxiety with meprobamate, phenobarbital, and placebo. *American Journal of Psychiatry, 115,* 905–910.

Uhlenhuth, E. H., Rickels, K., Fisher, S., Park, L. C., Lipman, R. S., & Mock, J. (1966). Drug, doctor's verbal attitude and clinic setting in the symptomatic response to pharmacotherapy. *Psychopharmacologia, 9,* 392–418.

Van Dyke, C., Ungerer, J., Jatlow, P., Barash, P., & Byck, R. (1982). Intranasal cocaine: Dose relationships of psychological effects and plasma levels. *International Journal of Psychiatry in Medicine, 12,* 1–13.

von Felsinger, J. M., Lasagna, L., & Beecher, H. K. (1955). Drug induced mood changes in man: Personality and reactions to drugs. *Journal of the American Medical Association, 157,* 1113–1119.

von Kerekjarto, M. (1966). Studies on the influence of examiner's sex on the effects of drugs. In H. Brill (Ed.), *Neuropsychopharmacology: Proceedings of the Fifth International Congress of the Colleguim Internationale Neuropsychopharmacologicum* (pp. 552–556). New York: Excerpta Medica Foundation.

Vrhovac, B. (1977). Placebo and its importance in medicine. *Journal of Clinical Pharmacology, 15,* 161–165.

Weiner, B., & Secord, J. (1975). Misattribution for failure and enhancement of achievement striving. *Journal of Personality and Social Psychology, 31,* 415–421.

Weiner, M. J. (1971). Contiguity of placebo administration and misattribution. *Perceptual and Motor Skills, 33,* 1271–1280.

Wheatley, D. (1967, November). Influence of doctors' and patients' attitudes in the treatment of neurotic illness. *Lancet, 2,* 1133–1135.

White, L., Tursky, B., & Schwartz, G. E. (Eds.). (1985). *Placebo: Theory, research, and mechanisms.* New York: Guilford Press.

Wilkins, W. (1985). Placebo controls and concepts in chemotherapy and psychotherapy research. In L. White, B. Tursky, & G. E. Schwartz (Eds.), *Placebo: Theory, research and mechanisms* (pp. 83–109). New York: Guilford Press.

Wilson, C. W. M., & Huby, P. M. (1960). An assessment of the responses to drugs acting on the central nervous system. *Clinical Pharmacology and Therapeutics, 2,* 587–598.

Wilson, G. T., & Lawson, D. M. (1976). Expectancies, alcohol, and sexual arousal in male social drinkers. *Journal of Abnormal Psychology, 85,* 587–594.

Wolf, S. (1950). Effects of suggestion and conditioning on the action of chemical agents in human subjects—The pharmacology of placebos. *Journal of Clinical Investigation, 29,* 100–109.

Wolf, S., & Pinsky, R. H. (1954). Effects of placebo administration and occurrence of toxic reactions. *Journal of the American Medical Association, 155,* 339–341.

Zanna, M. P., & Cooper, J. (1974). Dissonance and the pill. *Journal of Personality and Social Psychology, 29,* 703–709.

Zubin, J., & Katz, M. M. (1964). Psychopharmacology and personality. In P. Worchel & D. Byrne (Eds.), *Personality and change* (pp. 367–395). New York: Wiley.

CHAPTER 2

Treatment Implications of Psychiatric Comorbidity

MICHAEL D. GREENBERG

C OMORBIDITY OF MENTAL illness has become the focus of increasing scholarly attention in recent years, as psychiatric epidemiologists have documented the alarming trend for "mental illness" to comprise multiple and concurrent *DSM* mental disorders. At the same time, research on treatment outcome is just beginning to examine the prognostic implications of comorbid disorders for many standard psychopharmacological treatments. Preliminary findings, though inconsistent, suggest that medications may exert diminished potency for many individuals who present with multiple psychiatric conditions at the same time. Concurrent with recent empirical investigations of comorbidity, psychiatric theorists have devoted increasingly intense scrutiny to the etiologic pathways that might explain the proliferation of comorbid mental disorders. Insight into comorbidity remains limited, however, except for recognition that the manifestation of mental illness is neither as straightforward nor as readily classifiable as the exclusion criteria of the *Diagnostic and Statistical Manual of Mental Disorders*, fourth edition (*DSM-IV*; American Psychiatric Association [APA], 1994) might otherwise be taken to imply.

The burgeoning psychiatric research literature on comorbidity is an interesting historical phenomenon, in addition to its immediate relevance to psychiatric treatment and clinical practice. A computerized database search (Psychlit) using the keyword "comorbidity" retrieved 1,175 journal articles published during the years 1990 through 1994 . Closer examination revealed that for every year during that interval, the number of published comorbidity articles exceeded the number of articles published in the preceding year (which, by the way, reflects a highly significant linear trend, $r^2 = .935$, $p < .01$).[1] A similar database search for the same period yielded more than 200 book chapters devoted in part or in whole to the same subject. These findings are all the more striking when compared with interest in comorbidity reflected by journal articles published 15 to 20 years ago. Medline database search for the years 1967 to 1980 yielded *no* articles referring to "comorbidity," nor was that term anywhere evident in casual inspection of several textbooks on psychiatric diagnosis published during the 1960s and 1970s (Akiskal & Webb, 1978; Slater & Roth, 1969; Wolman, 1978). All of which serves to raise the question: How has comorbidity so rapidly and recently captured the minds of so many researchers in psychiatry and the behavioral sciences?[2]

The answer may derive partly from an implicit sense of urgency in the field, as large-scale epidemiological studies have suggested that mental disorder is proliferating widely, and in what might almost be deemed an epidemic pattern. The Epidemiologic Catchment Area study (ECA) (Robins & Regier, 1991), a multisite survey of Axis I mental illness in several community and hospital populations, found lifetime prevalence rates for Axis I mental disorders in the United States falling roughly at 30%. Results from the more recent and methodologically superior National Comorbidity Study (NCS) (Kessler et al., 1994) found lifetime prevalence rates approaching 50%. Furthermore, these rates almost certainly underestimate prevalence based on current diagnostic standards, as neither the ECA nor the NCS included an evaluation of Axis II disorders (with the exception of antisocial personality disorder), nor did either of the studies employ the *DSM-IV*, which significantly expands the diagnostic system over earlier *DSM* editions. It remains to be seen whether rising prevalence rates reflect an actual increase in vulnerability to psychiatric disorders over time, as opposed to an artifactual shift due to changing diagnostic methods and systems. Either way, results from these studies suggest that the experience of mental disorder, and particularly of comorbid mental disorder, may no longer meet the statistical anomaly criterion implied by the introduction to the *DSM-III-R* (APA, 1987; see also discussion in Wakefield, 1992).

At the same time that recent epidemiological studies have suggested high prevalence rates for unitary mental disorders, additional results have

---

[1] A similar literature search on the keywords "comorbid" and "comorbidity" was earlier undertaken by Lilienfeld, Waldman, & Israel (1994), with findings akin to those described here.

[2] Double entendre notwithstanding, one might raise a related question: How high would prevalence rates need to rise before researchers begin to question their own independence from the putative object of their study?

suggested that the simultaneous co-occurrence of *multiple* mental disorders may also represent a serious and widespread problem. Results from the NCS (Kessler et al., 1994) suggest that about 30% of the general population suffers from a lifetime prevalence of comorbid mental disorder. In other words, more than half of those individuals who acknowledged the symptoms of one form of illness also endorsed criteria for at least one additional form of illness. Here again, the results do not include prevalence data for the *DSM* Axis II disorders; consider that in a related research literature examining personality disorder and major depression, many studies have estimated rates of comorbidity approaching or exceeding 50% (e.g., see review in Farmer & Nelson-Grey, 1990). The implication of such findings is that large numbers of people suffer from multiple mental disorders at the same time—perhaps even a majority of those individuals who are diagnosable for *any* individual form of disorder. The additional implication is that mental disorder in the "real world" is often more complex and more severe than it appears in the context of diagnostically controlled studies of treatment outcome.

It is probably not by coincidence that research efforts on comorbidity have arisen mainly in the past 10 to 15 years, following the introduction of the *DSM-III* in 1980 (APA). Prior to 1980, the *DSM* diagnostic system was comparatively abstract and psychodynamic, whereas the 1980 revision favored instead a more concrete and behavioral approach. The merits of this change have been frequently extolled and occasionally criticized (e.g., Kirk & Kutchins, 1992, 1994; Klerman, 1990; Spitzer & Williams, 1994; M. Wilson, 1993), with arguments that shall not be recapitulated here. It suffices to say that the introduction of the *DSM-III* culminated an extensive effort to improve diagnostic uniformity and reliability among clinicians, as well as to reconstruct psychiatric taxonomy within a more objective and atheoretical framework. The advent of the *DSM-III* may therefore be directly linked to the recent explosion of interest in comorbidity. By defining mental disorders in behavioral terms and adopting a multiaxial format for personality disorders, the *DSM-III* allowed researchers in 1980 to study "pure" disorders with a previously unrealized degree of rigor and generality. In the 1990s, however, the countervailing trend has been increasing recognition that real-world disorders manifest only rarely in their pure diagnostic forms.

Why is an understanding of comorbidity important, particularly in a textbook about the treatment efficacy of psychiatric medications? There are several reasons for this emphasis ranging from the prosaic to the esoteric. Most prosaically, there is the fundamental epidemiological finding that substantial numbers of individuals in the general population suffer from more than one mental disorder at once. This implies, at best, that the average clinician often faces a more complex set of treatment problems than is typically addressed by outcome research studies. The efficacy of antidepressant treatments, for example, is usually studied in terms of some measure of reduction in symptoms of depression. In the case of comorbid disorders, by contrast, the clinician is confronted with a mixture of many symptoms superimposed, perhaps combining the features from two or three or more separate disorders (e.g., depression, polysubstance abuse, and avoidant personality disorder). In such complicated cases, it may be difficult for a clinician even to decide what "improvement" means, much less to distinguish improvement in depressive symptoms from all the other chronic and acute symptoms with which an individual patient may present. In practice, it is the clinician's task to treat the "whole individual," rather than discrete forms of illness as addressed by studies of outcome. Thus, the clinician may often wind up trying to mix disparate forms of medication treatment (and even psychotherapy) to "match" the particular set of comorbidities for a given patient. This practice necessarily deviates from the results of controlled outcome studies, with consequences that are difficult to quantify idiographically, much less across patients.

If it is difficult for practicing clinicians to apply the findings from outcome research to the treatment of comorbidity, then treatment-outcome researchers themselves struggle with an even more difficult problem due to the prevalence of myriad forms of comorbid illness. The difficulty for outcome researchers is largely methodological, and derives from the inferential limits imposed by the characteristics of an empirical subject pool. Consider the following questions: Should antidepressant medication trials exclude subjects based on secondary diagnosis or history of anxiety disorder, personality disorder, eating disorder, substance-use disorder, psychotic symptoms, obsessive-compulsive disorder, posttraumatic stress disorder, attention-deficit/hyperactivity disorder, or the like? Should medication trials exclude subjects based on prior history of antidepressant medication use, electroconvulsive therapy, or psychiatric hospitalization, or demographic characteristics such as age, gender, race, or ethnicity? Arguments about the preceding can be made in either direction, depending on the philosophy of any particular investigator. Studies at the more inclusive end of the spectrum will accept patients with all sorts of comorbid conditions (and demographic backgrounds), possibly making the results more generally applicable, but also conflating results across many different kinds of people who might actually exhibit systematically different patterns of response to drug treatment.[3] At the more exclusive end of the

---

[3] For example, different forms of comorbidity in depression may actually correspond to the elusive "depressive subtypes" that researchers have labored for so long, and so generally without success, to find.

spectrum, studies may demonstrate relatively specific treatment effects for small groups of precisely diagnosed people . . . with findings that possess only limited applicability to the population at large. Both approaches to treatment outcome studies may be required to make results at once easily interpretable and at the same time generally applicable.

In addition to problems with exclusion criteria, there is a possibility that ignoring comorbidity may lead researchers of treatment outcome to systematically overestimate therapeutic effects in controlled trials. The general estimate of prevalence for comorbid mental illness using NCS data (and excluding Axis II conditions) is about 30% (Kessler et al., 1994). Given that the overall NCS prevalence of mental illness falls around 50%, the implication is that more than half of those people who meet criteria for one psychiatric disorder may also meet criteria for at least one other disorder. This is an important point, partly because it means that superficially comparable outcome studies may actually employ very different research samples, but also because it means that the more exclusive outcome studies may select for a comparatively healthy group of subjects, relative to the population at large. If there is any general trend toward treatment resistance associated with comorbid disorders (as some previous reviews have suggested in part; see Ilardi & Craighead, 1994/1995; Reich & Green, 1991), then it follows that outcome studies excluding comorbid conditions (or focusing on some comorbidities to the exclusion of others) may systematically overestimate the magnitude of treatment effects as they would appear in the general population.

On a more esoteric plane, an understanding of comorbidity is important because of its implications for psychiatric taxonomy and the medical model of mental illness. It has long been the premise of biological psychiatry that discrete forms of psychopathology are driven by physical mechanisms that correspond directly to the specific neuroregulatory effects of the standard psychiatric medications. The reasoning that supports this conclusion is based partly on outcome studies that purport significant therapeutic effects associated with medication treatment (as with the antidepressants; see Greenberg & Fisher, 1989), combined with the results of studies on the pharmacodynamics of the medications themselves (i.e., the effects of the medications on synaptic or cellular processes such as reuptake, neurotransmitter catabolism, or compensatory regulation of postsynaptic receptor density). A full discussion of the logical and empirical shortcomings in this line of reasoning goes beyond the scope of the current chapter (the interested reader is referred to an excellent discussion offered by Wencel, 1995). For current purposes, it suffices to point out that comorbidity may dramatically complicate the task of isolating the physical concomitants of putatively discrete disease processes. Given current empirical techniques, it often remains difficult to distinguish the independence of concurrent mental disorders even on the basis of their behavioral features, much less their underlying substrates (e.g., Frances, Widiger, & Fyer, 1990; Horowitz & Malle, 1993; Hudson & Pope, 1990). In this vein, it seems plausible that concurrent disorders such as depression and substance abuse might interact simultaneously at psychological and biological levels, thus sabotaging a patient's ability to cope with the symptoms of either individual disorder, while undermining responsiveness to treatment interventions and serving to maintain the pathology in the face of disease-specific efforts to treat it. The future prospects for empirically deconfounding such complex interactions appear somewhat less promising than one might infer from recent reviews with an optimistic tenor (e.g., Michels & Marzuk, 1993a, 1993b).

Comorbidity is an important topic for several reasons. On a historical level, comorbidity appears to have gained enormous attention in a very short span of time. On an epidemiological level, comorbidity represents a widespread trend for individuals to suffer from multiple mental disorders concurrently. On a methodological level, comorbidity creates a complicated set of diagnostic and measurement problems for studies examining treatment response for psychiatric medications. On an etiologic level, comorbidity raises the prospect that discrete disorders may interact causally with one another over time, in a pattern that defies efforts at diagnostic deconstruction, much less clinical intervention. On a taxonomic level, comorbidity suggests that mental disorders may be less discrete than the exclusion rules of the *DSM-IV* seem to imply. And on a philosophical level, high comorbidity rates raise questions regarding the putative specificity of the biological bases of mental illness. The study of comorbidity is the study of mental illness as it actually manifests in the world, as well as the difficulties inherent in conducting psychiatric research. An understanding of comorbidity issues is a prerequisite for the clinical examination of studies on psychiatric treatment outcome.

The purpose of this chapter is to describe empirical findings on comorbidity, and briefly to address their relevance to future research in psychiatry and the behavioral sciences. The chapter will begin with a review of results from the ECA and NCS studies, discussing epidemiological findings on comorbidity with particular attention to methodological and clinical implications. The comorbidity of Axis II disorders will also be discussed, by reference to the research literature on major depression, anxiety disorders, and the personality disorders. After a description of the epidemiological approach to comorbidity, the chapter will then turn to studies on comorbidity and somatic treatment outcome, again examining clinical findings as well as measurement and methods issues. Finally, the concluding sections of the chapter will provide a coherent summary of the empirical findings on comorbidity and will present the clinical, philosophical, and taxonomic implications in greater detail.

Comorbidity refers in general to the most complicated, mutually recursive, diagnostically ambiguous forms of psychopathology to which human beings are sometimes vulnerable. The study of comorbidity is therefore interesting, in part because of the insights it offers about general psychopathology, but also because of the insights that it offers into the limits of empirical studies on psychopathology. If the current chapter illuminates some of these insights for the unfamiliar reader, then the purpose of the discourse will have been well served.

EPIDEMIOLOGY AND COMORBIDITY

The Epidemiologic Catchment Area Study

In the years prior to 1980, *DSM*-based psychiatric taxonomy had not yet achieved the degree of acceptance and uniformity it enjoys today. Early versions of the *DSM* (i.e., *DSM-I*, 1952; *DSM-II*, 1968) were much more abstract and psychodynamic systems than were the taxonomic revisions that followed. Because the earlier systems were less concrete and behavioral in their formulation, they reportedly suffered from major deficits in diagnostic reliability. Two clinicians attempting to diagnose the same patient while using the same diagnostic system might often have come to different conclusions regarding the diagnosis. Not surprisingly, this sort of disagreement was widely viewed as a major epistemological problem that undercut efforts to achieve greater uniformity in clinical standards and research methods (Kirk & Kutchins, 1992; M. Wilson, 1993). Pressure had been building, therefore, to develop an improved diagnostic system that might address these flaws. At a minimum, the new system would be aimed toward improving interclinician diagnostic reliability, while providing a standard lexicon for defining psychiatric disorders. Early strides in this direction included the publication of the Feighner criteria (Feighner et al., 1972) and the Research Diagnostic Criteria (Spitzer, Endicott, & Robins, 1978), culminating in the publication of the *DSM-III* in 1980.

At the same time that psychiatric taxonomy was moving toward the *DSM-III*, government interest in the provision of mental health services led to the formulation of a President's Commission on Mental Health in the late 1970s. Basic questions were raised about the prevalence for different psychiatric disorders, and it subsequently became apparent that even psychiatric experts could not provide clear answers. Several early epidemiological studies had been undertaken in the 1950s and 1960s using the *DSM-I* diagnostic system. The findings for lifetime prevalence had varied widely, with results ranging from 11% to 57% (see discussion in Regier & Robins, 1991). Setting aside any reliability problems associated with the *DSM-I*, these early epidemiological studies also suffered from significant methodological deficits, including problems with sampling procedures and ambiguities in the interpretation of the *DSM-I* criteria. These factors, taken together with the need for more rigorous epidemiological data based on the evolving *DSM-III* system, led to a new National Institute of Mental Health (NIMH) mandate for psychiatric epidemiology: the Epidemiologic Catchment Area study (ECA) (Robins & Regier, 1991). At its inception in 1980, the ECA was the first large-scale, multisite study to undertake an epidemiological survey using modern *DSM* criteria.

Starting in 1980, the ECA began its collection of psychiatric data on roughly 20,000 subjects drawn from community and hospital populations. In contrast to earlier epidemiological studies where subjects were obtained from a single, limited geographic region, the ECA was designed as a "multisite collaborative approach" (Robins & Regier, 1991, p. 7). The advantages to the multisite design included improved access to special (i.e., minority) populations, semiindependent replication of findings by researchers working at different locations, and centralized oversight and training for research methodology. Sites for the ECA were selected by competitive application to the NIMH. Five contract proposals were accepted for the study, with participation by researchers at Yale University, Johns Hopkins University, Washington University (of St. Louis), Duke University, and the University of California at Los Angeles. Each site became a "catchment area" for the study, offering a local sample with distinctive variations in demographics, ethnicity, and urbanicity for the target subject pool. The aim of the ECA was to study psychiatric epidemiology in a manner that would permit inferences about prevalence in the American population as a whole.

The methodology of the ECA involved stratified random sampling of community and hospital populations within each catchment area. Data on psychiatric disorders were mostly gathered by psychiatric laypeople trained in the administration of the Diagnostic Interview Schedule (DIS) (Robins, Helzer, Croughan, & Ratcliff, 1981), a structured diagnostic interview for the *DSM-III* Axis I disorders. Interviews for the ECA were conducted in person and by phone, with relatively low rates of noncompliance; validity and reliability of the data-gathering process were addressed by an extensive internal review (see Leaf, Myers, & McEvoy, 1991, for details). Unsurprisingly, full findings from the ECA were quite voluminous, and the results included numerous published journal articles on diagnostic and epidemiological topics. The most comprehensive summary of the ECA findings was released as a textbook in

1991 (Robins & Regier, 1991), with overview chapters on methods and general findings, as well as specific chapters devoted to each of the major classes of disorder (e.g., affective disorders, alcohol disorders, generalized anxiety disorders). Findings from the ECA included prevalence rates for the major disorders (findings presumably representative of prevalence in the general U.S. population), along with extensive secondary analyses regarding the demographic, environmental, and clinical correlates of the disorders.

Based on the results of the full ECA research cohort, the lifetime prevalence rate for *DSM-III* disorders was judged to be 32%, with an annual prevalence rate of 20% and a monthly prevalence rate of 15.4% (Regier et al., 1990; Robins, Locke, & Regier, 1991). Roughly 3 people out of every 10 acknowledged some previous life history consistent with *DSM-III* diagnosis, and more than 1 person in 10 acknowledged the symptoms of an acute disorder within the preceding month.[4] These findings appear to suggest relatively high rates of psychiatric morbidity in the general population of the United States. Moreover, the DIS interview employed by the ECA study omitted a number of *DSM-III* disorders from its evaluation, including PTSD, the eating disorders, and the personality disorders (except for *antisocial* personality disorder). Presumably, a full diagnostic evaluation including these additional syndromes might have led to even higher prevalence rates for psychiatric disorder in general.

Because general prevalence rates for the ECA were fairly high, it should come as little surprise that comorbidity rates were high as well. The ECA rate for *lifetime comorbidity* (i.e., the percentage of individuals who reported suffering from two or more psychiatric disorders over the course of a lifetime) was found to be 18% in the general population (Robins et al., 1991). In other words, more than one person out of every two who reported lifetime prevalence for *one* disorder also reported prevalence for one or more additional disorders. According to the ECA results, those disorders with especially high rates of lifetime comorbidity included alcohol abuse/dependence (52%), simple phobia (63%), drug abuse/dependence (75%), depressive episode (75%), and obsessive-compulsive disorder (79%), with six additional disorders (agoraphobia, dysthymia, schizophrenia, panic, somatization, antisocial personality) all garnering lifetime comorbidity rates in excess of 80%. Interpretation of the preceding must be qualified because the ECA researchers did *not* here employ the *DSM-III* exclusion hierarchy

---

[4] Note that prevalence rates as published in the ECA were based on an elaborate statistical weighting of the data to make the sample representative of the United States as a whole (see Leaf, Myers, & McEvoy, 1991).

(which automatically precludes some diagnoses when observed in the presence of others), nor does "lifetime comorbidity" necessarily imply that two disorders occur together in time. Nevertheless, the findings suggest (minimally) that the diagnosis of one major psychiatric disorder often represents an important risk factor/diagnostic marker for additional forms of mental illness.

Beyond the preceding analysis, the ECA investigators also examined *acute* comorbidity (i.e., co-occurence of two disorders in the span of the preceding year). Findings were reported in terms of *odds ratios*, the increased likelihood for an individual suffering from any one specific disorder also to meet criteria for a second specific disorder. All possible pairwise comparisons were undertaken for the 11 major disorders surveyed in the ECA study, resulting in the examination of 55 different forms of comorbidity. Although the subsequent pattern of results is too complex to summarize fully here, the general finding was for strong comorbidity relationships between 23 pairs of psychiatric disorders,[5] such that diagnosis of one disorder posed a substantial incremental risk for diagnosis of a second disorder. Based on supplementary analyses, the investigators further determined that their findings could be attributed neither to shared symptoms between the disorders, nor to any identified shared risk factors. The conclusion, therefore, was that individuals suffering from one form of disorder were placed at increased risk for developing additional disorders: an etiologic hypothesis.

The ECA study was a watershed event for psychiatric epidemiology, following in the wake of the 1980 publication of the *DSM-III*. Review of the ECA findings is illustrative of the enormous logistical and technical difficulties inherent to addressing basic questions about the prevalence of mental illness in the United States. Elaborate methods were developed by the ECA for use in diagnostic training, interviewing, reliability checking, population sampling, and data analysis, with independent teams of psychiatric investigators at five different catchment sites devoting years to the pursuit of the investigation. The most general finding from the ECA was a lifetime prevalence rate for *DSM-III* disorders of 32%, and a lifetime comorbidity rate of 18%: More than 3 people out of every 10 acknowledged a history of some form of *DSM-III* disorder, and of those so afflicted, more than 1 in 2 reported a history of *multiple* forms of disorder. With the full publication of the ECA findings in 1991, the dramatic scope of psychiatric comorbidity in the U.S. population became fully apparent.

---

[5] Pairs that included various combinations of the affective, anxiety, schizophrenic, somatoform, and substance-use disorders.

THE NATIONAL COMORBIDITY STUDY

Although the ECA represented a major step forward in American psychiatric epidemiology, critics noted that the ECA suffered from numerous methodological problems, some of which may have qualified the generality of its findings (e.g., Kessler, 1994a; Parker 1987; Shrout, 1994). Criticisms against the ECA included *sample size* (which was judged insufficient for detailed examination of low-prevalence disorders), *nonresponse bias* (which might have rendered the ECA results unrepresentative of prevalence in the general population), *inappropriate institutional samples* (which represented only a minuscule proportion of the general population), and *validity and reliability issues surrounding the DIS diagnostic interview* (which might have resulted in underestimates in the ECA lifetime prevalence rates; see Parker, 1987). In addition, the ECA was also criticized for using several local sites for data collection, rather than employing a truly national sample. Kessler noted that the local ECA samples were "an odd collection which in some cases were not even representative of their own [geographic] areas" (Kessler, 1994a, p. 83); in consequence, Kessler suggested that a national sampling procedure might at once have proven more cost-effective than the ECA, while also offering improved access to underrepresented populations (e.g., rural Americans, Native Americans).

Apart from these method issues, substantial taxonomic progress had occurred in the interval between the inception of the ECA in 1980, and its full publication of results in 1991. In 1987, the *DSM-III* diagnostic system was superseded by the *DSM-III-R* (American Psychiatric Association, 1987), a revision that involved significant changes in the classification rules for mental disorders (see H. S. Wilson & Skodol, 1988). The drawbacks to rapid turnover in *DSM* diagnostic revisions have been discussed elsewhere in detail (e.g., Carson, 1991; Zimmerman, 1988, 1990; Zimmerman, Jampala, Sierles, & Taylor, 1991); it was an unintended consequence of the *DSM-III-R* that by the time the full ECA results were published in 1991, those results were already, in some practical sense, out of date. Researchers had been busy for several years in developing new structured interviews and outcome studies using the revised criteria of the *DSM-III-R*. Meanwhile, at least one group of investigators noted the difficulty in generalizing the results of earlier studies to a new diagnostic format in which the defining parameters had been changed, occasionally with unforeseen results (e.g., Blashfield, Blum, & Pfohl, 1992). The ECA findings, although retaining their probative value, possessed somewhat diminished applicability to ongoing *DSM*-based clinical practice and research.

The National Comorbidity Survey (NCS) (Kessler, 1994a, 1994b) was the second, large-scale, psychiatric epidemiological study of the United

States, designed in part to remedy some of the method drawbacks to the earlier ECA. The mandate for the NCS was "to study the prevalence, causes, and consequences of comorbidity between substance-use disorders and non-substance psychiatric disorders in the U.S." (Kessler, 1994a, pp. 86–87). The study obtained its diagnostic interview data on a nationally representative sample of 8,098 individuals, using psychiatric laypeople as interviewers and employing a modified version of the CIDI (Composite International Diagnostic Interview) (World Health Organization, 1990) to obtain *DSM-III-R* diagnoses. Subjects for the NCS were limited to individuals ranging in age from 15 to 54,[6] and the response rate among those asked to participate was 82%. All statistical analyses were adjusted according to the results of a secondary survey of nonresponders to the initial interview (see Kessler, 1994a, for details). Preliminary findings from the NCS have appeared in a series of papers published over the past few years (e.g., Blazer, Kessler, McGonagle, & Swartz, 1994; Kessler 1994a, 1994b; Kessler et al., 1994; Kessler, Sonnega, Bromet, Hughes, & Nelson, 1995; Magee, Eaton, Wittchen, McGonagle, & Kessler, 1996). The definitive compilation of NCS findings (by analogy to the Robins & Regier, 1991, textbook on the ECA) remains forthcoming.

Based on the results from the full NCS dataset, the lifetime prevalence rate for *DSM-III-R* disorders was judged at 48%, with an annual prevalence rate of 29% (Kessler, 1994b; Kessler et al., 1994). Interestingly, these rates appear substantially higher than those found for the ECA study; this difference was attributed in part to the use of different diagnostic systems (i.e., *DSM-III* vs. *DSM-III-R*), in part to the use of different diagnostic interviews (DIS vs. modified CIDI), in part to the recruitment of a younger research sample (limited to ages 15–54 in the NCS), and in part to the correction of NCS data for nonresponse bias (see Kessler, 1994b for discussion). Setting aside the differences between the ECA and NCS figures, the NCS suggests even more strongly than the ECA that mental disorder is widely prevalent in the general population of the United States. The NCS, like the ECA, omitted a number of *DSM* disorders from its clinical interviews, including the personality disorders (except for antisocial personality disorder) and the eating disorders. Presumably, an evaluation that included these categories might have led to even higher general prevalence rates.

Turning to the NCS data on comorbidity, the lifetime prevalence rate for comorbid psychiatric disorders in the United States was found to be 29%, or somewhat more than half of all the individuals who acknowledged a

---

[6] The age range in which comorbidity was most commonly found in the ECA (see Kessler, 1994a).

prior history of at least one disorder. Findings in regard to more acute (e.g., 1-year) comorbidity were not presented in either of the overview articles on the NCS (Kessler, 1994b; Kessler et al., 1994), although the available preliminary data seem to reinforce the ECA finding that diagnosis of one mental disorder is a strong predictor for diagnostic history of a second disorder. As yet, NCS findings on prevalence for specific forms of comorbidity remain very limited. One recent NCS study (Kessler et al., 1995) found that the lifetime comorbidity rate associated with PTSD diagnosis was in excess of 80%. Likewise, a second NCS study (Magee et al., 1996) found lifetime comorbidity rates in excess of 80% for the conditions of simple phobia, social phobia, and agoraphobia. More detailed comorbidity data regarding other forms of psychiatric disorder remain to be published for the NCS.

By contrast with the results from the earlier ECA study, results from the NCS are still in the process of preliminary analysis. The NCS was designed specifically to address some of the method deficits in the earlier ECA, and was also structured to employ a more recent diagnostic system, the *DSM-III-R*. Initial results from the NCS confirm the earlier ECA findings of widespread prevalence and comorbidity of mental disorders in the United States, although the difference between ECA and NCS results raises questions regarding methods and diagnostic systems in the two studies. Then too, there has been another diagnostic shift since the NCS data were gathered, with the introduction of the *DSM-IV* (APA, 1994). It remains to be seen whether the revisions of the *DSM-IV* may impair the precision of NCS prevalence estimates, at least as relating to the new diagnostic standard. Nevertheless, the cumulative findings of the ECA and NCS suggest, at minimum, that morbidity and comorbidity of mental disorders are fairly common in the population of the United States.

AXIS II AND EVERYTHING AFTER

The foregoing discussion illuminates the complexity involved in addressing a deceptively simple question: "How common is mental illness in the United States?" The conduct of a successful epidemiological survey rests on the conjunction of many elements, including (but not limited to) sampling procedure, interview procedure, diagnostic procedure, and statistical procedure. Each of these can become problematic in an undertaking as large as a national survey. Suspending questions about the validity of the methods in such surveys, it can be supremely challenging for investigators even to describe what was done in sufficient detail to permit replication. Fairly small details (such as the standards for training psychiatric interviewers, or the protocol for contacting research subjects) can potentially exert a significant impact on the results of a survey. Multiply these effects by the number of small details involved in conducting such a survey, and one begins to sense the magnitude of effort invested in a study like the NCS. The point here is not simply that the results of the ECA and NCS are imperfect (although they are), but rather that it is only by Herculean effort that such studies can be undertaken at all.

It is perhaps for this reason that neither the ECA nor the NCS included an evaluation of the Axis II personality disorders[7] in their epidemiological surveys. The *DSM personality disorders* correspond to constellations of enduring and inflexible behavioral traits that are maladaptive or subjectively distressful (APA, 1980, 1987, 1994); whereas there exists some consensus that assessment for the disorders on Axis I has improved in reliability since 1980 (see discussion in Kirk & Kutchins, 1992), assessment for the more complicated and abstract disorders on Axis II has remained problematic (Zimmerman, 1994). And though reliability for personality disorder diagnosis can be improved through semistructured assessment techniques and clinically skilled interviewers, the cost in time and money is substantial, particularly when added to the already substantial expense of structured Axis I interviewing (such as undertaken in the ECA and NCS). Thus, the personality disorders have not yet been included in any of the major attempts to survey prevalence and comorbidity of the Axis I disorders, despite findings of 10% to 13% prevalence for Axis II disorders in more limited epidemiological studies (see review in Weissman, 1993). What follows is a brief review of comorbidity findings in regard to the Axis II personality disorders, major depression, and the anxiety disorders.

The research literature on the comorbidity of personality disorder and major depression includes studies that fall into several categories, based on the methods used for gathering the data. At least five studies have employed retrospective chart reviews to gather diagnostic data (Charney, Nelson, & Quinlan, 1981; Fogel & Westlake, 1990; Goethe, Szarek, & Cook, 1988; Koenigsberg, Kaplan, Gilmore, & Cooper, 1985; Mezzich, Fabrega, & Coffman, 1987), while two other studies used self-report questionnaires (Joffe & Regan, 1988; Libb et al., 1990), eight studies used diagnostic interviews (Alnaes & Torgersen, 1988; Davidson, Miller, & Strickland, 1985; Friedman, Aronoff, Clarkin, Corn, & Hurt, 1983; Marton et al., 1989; Pfohl, Stangl, & Zimmerman, 1984; Pilkonis & Frank, 1988; Sanderson, Wetzler, Beck, & Betz, 1992; Shea, Glass, Pilkonis, Watkins, & Docherty, 1987); and

---

[7] As defined by the *DSM-III* (APA, 1980), Axis II is composed of 11 different categories of personality disorder, as well as several categories of *developmental* disorder. For purposes of this chapter, the term "Axis II" will be employed as a synonym for personality disorder, and not in the more inclusive sense described by the *DSM*.

two studies used some combination of diagnostic techniques (Reich & Noyes, 1987; Zimmerman, Pfohl, Coryell, Corenthal, & Stangl, 1991). The object of interest in all these studies was the prevalence of Axis II disorder in clinical samples of patients meeting criteria for major depression. The range of comorbidity rates derived from these studies has been broad, varying from 15% (Mezzich et al., 1987) to 100% (Joffe & Regan, 1988). By eliminating studies that used retrospective chart reviews or self-report assessment instruments, attention can be focused solely on the more rigorous investigations, with a slight reduction in the range of prevalence estimates: from 35% (Shea et al., 1987) to 85% (Alnaes & Torgersen, 1988). Part of the disparity among these studies may derive from nonequivalent samples, with some studies drawing subjects from outpatient populations, and other studies drawing from institutional samples. Still, the general findings suggest that comorbid diagnosis of acute personality disorder is fairly common in clinical samples of depressed patients, with comorbidity rates often approaching or exceeding 50% (e.g., Pfohl et al., 1984; Reich & Noyes, 1987; Zimmerman, Pfohl, et al., 1991).

Similarly suggestive findings were described in a review article on the anxiety disorders by Brown & Barlow (1992). According to the reviewers, comorbid personality disorder manifests commonly in samples of patients suffering from anxiety disorders such as panic, agoraphobia, generalized anxiety disorder, and obsessive-compulsive disorder, with reported comorbidity rates ranging from 27% to 65% across seven different studies. A detailed examination of these studies goes beyond the bounds of the current chapter (as it also did for Brown & Barlow, 1992), but the fairly broad range in comorbidity rates is again presumably attributable to some combination of differences in research samples, methods, and assessments across studies. Although the "true" rate of comorbidity remains uncertain, the aggregate findings indicate that between ¼ and ⅔ of individuals suffering from anxiety disorders are also likely to meet criteria for an Axis II personality disorder. This reflects a substantial percentage of anxiety-disordered individuals, even if the true comorbidity rate falls toward the bottom of the specified range.

A caveat here is in order. If findings from the ECA and NCS require careful scrutiny for complete understanding, then the findings on Axis II comorbidity are nearly Byzantine by comparison. Results represent the accumulated wisdom of about two dozen studies, mostly small-scale surveys on samples from psychiatric inpatient and outpatient populations. The generality of these findings has often been held suspect, in part because of the idiosyncratic samples and exclusion criteria employed, but also because of dramatic variation among Axis II assessment procedures. Some studies have used semistructured interviews (e.g., the

Structured Interview for Disorders of Personality [SIDP]; the Personality Diagnostic Examination [PDE]) to generate Axis II diagnoses, whereas other studies have used questionnaire assessments (e.g., the Millon Clinical Multiaxial Inventory [MCMI]; the Personality Disorders Questionaire [PDQ]). These different techniques are well known to produce widely discrepant results (Zimmerman, 1994), nor has any diagnostic "gold standard" ever been identified. Furthermore, the majority of studies in this literature are based on *DSM-III* criteria: The subsequent introduction of *DSM-III-R* and *DSM-IV* has served to lend additional ambiguity to an already chaotic subject matter. And although the Axis II comorbidity literature has been previously surveyed by several reviewers (e.g., Brown & Barlow, 1992; Farmer & Nelson-Grey, 1990; Shea, Widiger, & Klein, 1992), the full extent of this methodological morass has never been made fully explicit. The current review has focused mainly on general comorbidity findings rather than methodological conundrums, but readers should not be deceived regarding the turbidity of the findings.

Large-scale studies such as the ECA and NCS possess no analogs in the domain of Axis I/Axis II comorbidity. Whereas the large-scale epidemiological studies have suggested substantial Axis I comorbidity rates in the general population, similar findings can only be inferred regarding Axis I/Axis II comorbidity, because (to date) the relevant empirical literature has drawn exclusively on relatively small, clinical samples. The method issues involved in interpreting these smaller studies are, in some ways, even more convoluted than those involved in interpreting the ECA and NCS: Caution must be employed accordingly. Nevertheless, studies on Axis I/Axis II comorbidity have consistently revealed substantial rates of co-occurrence. Some reviewers have consequently suggested that the Axis I and Axis II disorders may be etiologically related (e.g., see discussion in Akiskal, Hirschfeld, & Yerevanian, 1983), while other reviewers have noted that the two Axes may be less orthogonal than the *DSM* nosology asserts (e.g., Widiger & Shea, 1991). Most important, however, is the simple recognition that *DSM*-based comorbidity is, in practice, even more common than the ECA and NCS appear to suggest.

COMORBIDITY AND SOMATIC
TREATMENT OUTCOME

Until now, this chapter has focused on comorbidity primarily as an epidemiological phenomenon. Studies like the NCS, as well as many smaller-scale studies such as those on the Axis II disorders, have demonstrated that psychiatric illnesses often occur together, and that a presenting history for one illness often poses an incremental risk for life history of additional forms of illness. Attaching specific numbers to this trend is difficult, in part because of a host of methodological reasons previously described, and also in part because of an evolving diagnostic system that has already distanced much of the available research base from the de facto clinical standard of the *DSM-IV*. Despite the ambiguous meanings of specific numbers, the general trend is important to treatment providers for two reasons. First, the trend suggests that mental disorder is relatively common, with large numbers of people in the population suffering from "disorder" at some point during their lives. Second, the trend suggests that clinical practice may frequently involve treatment for more than one psychiatric disorder at a time. Whereas in controlled research trials the "problem" may be defined, for example, simply as depression, in practice other psychiatric problems often present concurrently. At a minimum, therefore, comorbidity research implies that clinical practice often involves more complicated cases or problems than those typically addressed in studies of treatment outcome.

In addition to this general implication, a more specific set of research findings bears on the relationship between comorbidity and treatment outcome. As empirical interest in comorbid disorders has expanded, investigators have begun to target comorbidity as a potential moderator for treatment effects. Some of the relevant studies have been naturalistic and retrospective, examining the records of large numbers of former hospital patients to identify predictors of outcome/relapse (e.g., Charney, Nelson, & Quinlan, 1981; Rounsaville, Dolinsky, Babor, & Meyer, 1987). Other studies have been efficacy trials for various forms of somatic treatment: trials that either included an assessment for comorbidity as a potential moderator of outcome, or else focused on the comparison between outcome in comorbid versus "pure" diagnostic cases. These studies focus directly on the impact of comorbid diagnosis on outcome for specific forms of psychopharmacological treatment (e.g., study might examine the impact of comorbid substance use disorder on outcome for tricyclic medication treatment of unipolar major depression). The question of interest here is no longer simply "Does the medication work?" but rather, "For whom does the medication work with greatest comparative efficacy?" Comorbidity outcome research seeks to determine whether individuals suffering from multiple disorders may be less amenable to standard forms of treatment. The research also raises the prospect of identifying specific diagnostic subgroups that might exhibit differential patterns of treatment response.

Before examining some of the empirical studies that have addressed these issues, several methodological precursors demand attention. First, a question: How do researchers select which variations of comorbidity will be made the focus for a particular study? The *DSM-IV* contains in excess of

300 diagnostic categories (APA, 1994); thus there are on the order of 45,000 possible pairwise combinations of disorders (not accounting, of course, for exclusion hierarchy rules). Even granting that many of the possible combinations are foreclosed by exclusion, there likely remain thousands of valid combinations of disorders. No psychiatric research study can examine the relationship between thousands (or tens of thousands) of variables simultaneously. In consequence, the method for most comorbidity studies has either been to select a specific pair of disorders of interest, or else (retrospectively) to compare a "pure" disorder to the same disorder in the presence of generic comorbidity. Both strategies present problems. The former poses ancillary difficulty in terms of handling *tertiary* comorbidities. Should individuals with a third disorder be excluded from study? Or simply documented for their participation? Or matched between treatment groups, to unbias any comparison between outcome in the two focal conditions? The alternate research strategy of treating comorbidity as a blanket, all-encompassing category suffers from conflating diagnostic groupings that may exert qualitatively different effects on treatment response. The upshot is that the conduct of comorbidity outcome studies involves more subtle method issues than might be evident at first glance, and no one method can resolve all the dilemmas.

A related problem in comorbidity studies involves the measurement of treatment "outcome." Even in the most diagnostically unambiguous of research trials, "outcome" is ordinarily measured by some standardized assessment instrument (such as the Beck Depression Inventory or the Hamilton Rating Scale for Depression). Typically, improvement is defined in terms of posttreatment scores on such instruments, or else by change in such scores from pretreatment to posttreatment, or by percentage of change in posttreatment scores from a pretreatment baseline, or by comparison of posttreatment scores with an arbitrary threshold of "recovery," or by any of several other analogous techniques. The equivalence of these measures is, at best, debatable (e.g., see discussions in M. D. Greenberg, Craighead, Evans, & Craighead, 1995; Murray, 1989), nor is it clear the extent to which any of the measures provides an unambiguous index of improvement in real-world functioning. But these problems, endemic to the literature on treatment outcome, become magnified in the domain of comorbidity research. If an individual is suffering from two disorders at once, how should posttreatment improvement be measured? Can symptom variance for one disorder be ignored in favor of symptom variance in the other? Can outcome be measured independently for both disorders, with the implicit assumption that no significant interaction takes place? Should symptomatology for the comorbid disorder be employed as a statistical covariate, rather than a dependent measure in statistical analysis? Most of the studies discussed in the following make use of simple comparisons between pure versus comorbid cases in examining outcome for a primary disorder. The superficial clarity of this approach begs the question of what kind of outcome should be measured, and in what manner.

Having acknowledged some of the method problems intrinsic to comorbidity outcome research, what follows is a brief review of comorbidity treatment studies that focus, in some manner, on somatic forms of intervention. These studies compose something of a diagnostic grab bag, with attention scattered across various forms of comorbidity and treatment, and only relatively few studies devoted to any particular combination of disorders and type of treatment. As described earlier, there are potentially thousands of kinds of comorbidity from which to choose, and the controlled investigation of comorbidity remains a relatively recent innovation in treatment outcome research. For current purposes, available findings will be summarized for several combinations of the following sorts of disorder: unipolar major depression, the anxiety disorders, the personality disorders, and the substance use disorders.

DEPRESSION AND PERSONALITY DISORDER

Undocumented clinical wisdom has long held that individuals suffering from major depression and concurrent personality disorder represent a particularly difficult population to treat (e.g., Akiskal, Hirschfeld, & Yerevanian, 1983). This wisdom derives some empirical support from the research literature on depression and personality traits, which includes several studies in which "pathological" scores on personality trait inventories (e.g., the neuroticism index on the Maudsley Personality Inventory) have generally been found to predict poor treatment response or propensity to relapse for major depression (e.g., Duggan, Lee, & Murray, 1990; Faravelli, Ambonetti, Pallanti, & Pazzagli, 1986; Weissman, Prusoff, & Klerman, 1978). The preceding studies either involved retrospective samples of patients treated naturalistically, or else formal treatment trials of antidepressants such as amitriptyline or clomipramine; it is noteworthy, however, that at least one other comparable study yielded more equivocal results in regard to the prognostic significance of personality trait measures (Zuckerman, Prusoff, Weissman, & Padian, 1980).

Other relevant research on personality and depression includes at least two studies on "treatment resistant" depression, with findings suggestive of a link between personality pathology and poor antidepressant treatment response. Frank and Kupfer (1990) examined Axis II personality disorder as a concomitant to poor response for a combination treatment consisting of imipramine and interpersonal therapy, whereas MacEwan and Remick (1988) undertook a retrospective examination of personality factors (and other clinical correlates) associated with poor response to somatic interventions (including trials with tricyclics, MAOIs, and ECT). Although neither of these studies reported significant statistical findings, both reported clinical observations of "suggestive correlation" between Axis II history and poor treatment response for depression.

In addition to these more generic studies on personality pathology and treatment resistance for depression, a series of investigations has been undertaken to examine the prognostic relationship between the *DSM* Axis II disorders and somatic treatment outcome for depression. These studies have included both naturalistic retrospective investigations, as well as controlled clinical medication trials, and the literature has previously been a focus for several reviews on the relationship between depression and personality (e.g., Farmer & Nelson-Grey, 1990; Ilardi & Craighead, 1994/1995; Reich & Green, 1991; Shea, Widiger, & Klein, 1992). The reader is referred to Ilardi and Craighead (1994/1995) for the most cogently detailed examination of the relevant studies on treatment outcome; a much briefer overview of findings will be attempted here.

Studies on treatment outcome for personality disorder and depression, like the previously described investigations on comorbidity prevalence, fall into general categories based on empirical method. At least four studies have employed *naturalistic* designs, in which the treatment effects of Axis II disorder were observed outside the context of a controlled medication trial; these studies examined Axis II status as a moderator of treatment response across a wide range of somatic interventions (including various combinations of tricyclics, MAOIs, SSRIs, other psychotropic medications, and ECT). Charney et al. (1981) reported 76% rate of recovery for non-comorbid depressed patients receiving antidepressant medication therapy, compared with only 36% recovery for depressed patients suffering from comorbid personality disorder. In comparable studies, Pfohl et al., (1984) found 59% recovery for noncomorbid depressed patients, compared with 24% recovery for patients suffering from comorbid personality disorder; and Black, Bell, Hulbert, and Nasrallah (1988) reported 64% recovery for noncomorbid depressed patients, compared with only 26% for patients suffering from comorbid personality disorder. In a study that employed a somewhat different empirical design, M. D. Greenberg et al. (1995) found that Axis II dimensional ratings on Cluster A (odd-eccentric) pathology predicted diminished response to inpatient treatment for depression.

Although these studies are uniformly predictive of diminished somatic treatment response associated with Axis II disorder, the naturalistic designs present a number of problems for the interpretation of findings (see discussion in Ilardi & Craighead, 1994/1995). Most prominent is the possibility that comorbid patients were systematically less likely to receive "adequate" antidepressant trials compared with their non-comorbid counterparts—a finding that was reported in at least one of the preceding studies (Charney et al., 1981). By contrast, several other studies have undertaken empirical medication trials in which similar forms of treatment were prescribed for all depressed patients regardless of their Axis II status. Investigations of the tricyclic antidepressants have included Frank, Kupfer, Jacob, and Jarret (1987), Peselow, Fieve, and Di-Figlia (1992), Pilkonis and Frank (1988), and Shea et al. (1990). Similar investigations have focused on the monoamine oxidase inhibitors (MAOIs) (Davidson et al., 1985; Tyrer, Casey, & Gall, 1983) and the tetracyclics (Sato, Sakado, & Sato, 1993). With the sole exception of Davidson et al. (1985), all these studies have suggested that depressed patients with comorbid Axis II pathology experience diminished treatment effects by comparison with non-comorbid depressed patients.[8]

Any discussion of the specific results in these studies rapidly devolves into an examination of the minutiae of particular techniques for measuring outcome, distinctive criteria used for screening subjects, idiosyncratic statistical procedures used for data analysis, and the like. In reading such findings, the numbers and percentages from different studies are not, by in large, directly comparable. And although these studies bear generally on the subject of Axis II influence on somatic treatment response, several of the studies either involved joint treatments with imipramine and interpersonal psychotherapy (Frank et al., 1987; Pilkonis & Frank, 1988), or else examined results across several different forms of medication and psychotherapy treatment without finding any significant (treatment by comorbidity) interaction (e.g., Shea et al., 1990). Nevertheless, despite the conceptual difficulties in comparing individual studies, the consistency of the Axis II depression findings has been striking. As asserted by Ilardi & Craighead (1994/1995), "There is fairly strong evidence . . . that Axis II personality disorder comorbidity predicts negative outcomes, both acute and long-term, with pharmacological treatments for depression" (p. 214).

ANXIETY DISORDER AND PERSONALITY DISORDER

To date, the research literature on Axis II comorbidity and treatment outcome has mostly focused on unipolar major depression, a common variant of comorbidity that generally results in diminished treatment response

---

[8] Interestingly, with the notable exception of Shea et al. (1990), none of the cited medication treatment trials involved placebo-controlled, double-blind designs. This raises the possibility that experimenter-bias may have played a role in the results of some of these studies; cautious interpretation is indicated.

(Ilardi & Craighead, 1994/1995). Less attention has been focused on the prognostic significance of comorbidity between the Axis II personality disorders and the anxiety disorders, even though reviewers have reported substantial comorbidity rates in clinical samples (ranging from 27% to 65%; see review in Brown & Barlow, 1992). In recent years, there have been at least six studies examining somatic treatment outcome for anxiety disorders with comorbid Axis II disorder, and results from these studies will be reviewed.

Three studies have investigated the impact of Axis II comorbidity on outcome for somatic treatment of panic disorder. Reich (1988) examined the influence of Axis II comorbidity in a double-blind, placebo-controlled study of diazepam and alprazolam (Valium and Xanax). Positive diagnosis of several of the Axis II disorders (notably those in the *dramatic-erratic* cluster) predicted poorer response to treatment on several measures of outcome following an 8-week trial. In a similar study, Noyes et al. (1990) also investigated the impact of Axis II comorbidity in a double-blind, placebo-controlled study of diazepam and alprazolam. Although acute results were not reported following the initial 8-week treatment trial, the researchers did find that acute Axis II status strongly predicted several measures of outcome at a follow-up evaluation 2 to 4 years later. In a third related study, Green and Curtis (1988) investigated Axis II status as a concomitant to relapse of panic symptoms following the termination of medication in a controlled, double-blind trial of imipramine and alprazolam. These researchers found that subjects who relapsed following termination of treatment were significantly more likely to have met criteria for an initial comorbid Axis II personality disorder.

In addition to the results cited earlier, three other studies have investigated personality disorder as a predictor of poor somatic treatment response for anxiety disorders other than panic disorder. Tyrer et al. (1983) examined outcome in a trial of phenelzine for several groups of patients, including one group diagnosed with "anxiety neurosis" (an ICD-8 classification); the researchers found a significant relationship between poor outcome and comorbid personality disorder. Mavissakalian and Hamman (1987) explored the treatment effects of Axis II comorbidity for agoraphobia following a 16-week trial of imipramine, desipramine, or trazadone augmented by 8 weeks of self-directed exposure therapy. Here again, the researchers found that patients with higher dimensional ratings of Axis II pathology were far less likely to respond to treatment than were patients with lower Axis II ratings. Finally, Mavissakalian, Hamman, and Jones (1990) examined Axis II comorbidity treatment effects for obsessive-compulsive disorder in a

10-week trial of clomipramine. Mavissakalian et al. (1990) did not find a significant predictive effect for Axis II status, but did observe several suggestive but nonsignificant personality differences between responders and nonresponders to treatment.

Research on the prognostic significance of Axis II comorbidity and the anxiety disorders remains at an embryonic stage of development. Relatively few studies have been conducted, half of these have focused exclusively on panic disorder, and most of the studies involved some combination of methodological flaws, including the use of small empirical samples, absence of a placebo condition, or the employment of self-report measures for assessing Axis II status. Criticism notwithstanding, the available studies are reasonably consistent in suggesting poorer somatic treatment outcomes for anxiety patients who also exhibit comorbid Axis II pathology. A need for further investigation of these comorbidities is indicated.

ANXIETY DISORDER AND DEPRESSION

Because both depression and anxiety disorder appear strongly correlated with prevalence for Axis II disorders, it should come as little surprise that the two conditions are also strongly correlated with one another. Comorbidity data from clinical samples suggest 15% to 30% comorbidity rates for panic disorder in cases of acute major depression, and lifetime comorbidity rates approaching 50% for history of depressive episodes in patients presenting with an acute panic disorder or agoraphobia (see reviews in Brown & Barlow, 1992; Grunhaus, 1988; Noyes, 1990). On a more historical plane, it has long been noted that depression and anxiety are closely related emotional experiences (Grunhaus, 1988), and experiences that have sometimes proven difficult empirically to deconfound (e.g., see Feldman, 1993; Murray, 1989). Current interest in the comorbidity of depression and the anxiety disorders only represents the most recent manifestation of historical investigations into conditions such as *atypical* depression, *anxious* depression, or *secondary* depression (with associated anxiety). All these are putative subtypes of disorders associated with some mixture of anxious and depressive features; although diagnostic constructs and taxonomic systems have evolved over the years, research interest in the comorbidity of anxiety and depression has remained strong. Consequently, a substantial outcome literature has accumulated for somatic treatments for concurrent depression and anxiety.

Methodological problems, however, are even more striking here than in other areas of research on treatment outcome. Many of the studies in this literature, particularly those of pre-*DSM-III* vintage, employ obscure diagnostic categories, idiosyncratic assessment procedures, and arbitrary or inadequate measures of treatment response. Setting aside these problems, even the newer, post-*DSM-III* studies have frequently employed small sample sizes, or non-double-blind empirical designs, or empirical designs without placebo controls, or statistical analyses that do not permit comparison of treatment effects between patients with "pure" depression (or anxiety disorder) and patients suffering from comorbid disorders. Furthermore, many of these treatment studies neglected to describe their empirical methods in sufficient detail to permit post hoc reconstruction of exactly what was done. A particularly troubling example involves the design of several double-blind studies comparing the effects of phenelzine (an MAOI antidepressant) with imipramine (a tricyclic antidepressant). By contrast with the relatively benign tricyclics, the MAOIs are well known to produce a variety of adverse side effects, and they require significant dietary constraints to be consumed safely. None of the relevant treatment studies explains how these dietary issues were addressed in the context of an otherwise "double-blind" methodology. Recent findings about the fragility of double-blind designs even in standard antidepressant trials (Fisher & Greenberg, 1993) cause the current author to be less than sanguine about the blindness of the designs in the anxiety-depression studies.

Setting aside these concerns (for the moment), the pre-*DSM-III* literature contains a number of studies examining somatic treatment outcome for depressed patients with some degree of concurrent anxiety symptoms. The relevant studies include at least two naturalistic investigations (Davidson, Turnbull, & Miller, 1980; Paykel, 1972), and five medication trials, mostly double-blind (including investigations of imipramine, phenelzine, diazepam, and chlorpromazine; Paykel, Parker, Penrose, & Rassaby, 1979; Raskin, Schulterbrandt, Reatig, Crook, & Odle, 1974; Raskin, Schulterbrandt, Reatig, & McKeon, 1970; Ravaris et al., 1976; Robinson, Nies, Ravaris, & Lamborn, 1973). The most prominently reported finding in these studies was that "anxious" depressives tended to respond better to medication than to inert placebos. Of the five studies that attempted some comparison between anxious depressives (by any definition) and any other group of depressed patients, two studies found no difference in somatic response (Paykel, 1972; Raskin et al., 1970), two studies found that anxious depression exhibited a qualitatively different medication response pattern from other types of depression (Davidson et al., 1980; Raskin et al., 1974), and one study was ambiguous in its findings (Paykel et al., 1979). This treatment literature has been commonly interpreted to suggest that anxious depressions are less responsive to tricyclic medications, and more responsive to MAOIs (see Grunhaus, 1988). This thesis has been examined in a number of subsequent medication trials, several of which have supported claims of superiority for MAOIs (e.g., Davidson, Raft, & Pelton, 1987; Liebowitz et al., 1984; Liebowitz et al., 1985; Robinson et al., 1985), and others of which have contested the claims (e.g., Paykel, Rowan, Parker, & Bhat, 1982; Ravaris, Robinson, Ives, Nies, & Bartlett, 1980; Rowan, Paykel, & Parker, 1982; Sovner, 1981). Speaking purely from a methodological standpoint, most of these newer studies are no better in design than the ones that preceded them.

Apart from the investigations focusing on treatment response as a function of different medications, several other more recent studies have examined diagnostic comorbidity of anxiety disorder and major depression as a predictor for somatic treatment outcome. Of these, five (Noyes et al., 1990; Nutzinger & Zapotoczky, 1985; Pyke & Kraus, 1988; Van Valkenburg, Akiskal, Puzantian, & Rosenthal, 1984; Zitrin, Klein, & Woerner, 1980) suggested some degree of impaired treatment response associated with comorbid conditions and somatic treatments (in trials of medications such as alprazolam, diazepam, and various tricyclic antidepressants). By contrast, Buller, Maier, & Benkurt (1986) achieved more equivocal outcome findings; Liebowitz et al. (1984) found some evidence suggesting *improved* response to phenelzine treatment for depression with comorbid panic attacks; and Lesser et al. (1988) found that the presence of secondary major depressive disorder was not predictive of response to alprazolam treatment for panic disorder with agoraphobia.[9] Among the more recent comorbidity studies, Lesser et al. (1988) is by far the most methodologically rigorous, but its results are nevertheless marred by the exclusion of "primary depressives" (and several other diagnostic groups) from the research sample.

Research findings remain at a very early stage of development in regard to somatic treatment outcomes for comorbid anxiety disorder and major depression. Although many investigators have attempted to examine some combination of somatic treatments for some combination of anxious and depressive symptoms, findings have typically been confusing and ambiguous secondary to method inconsistencies in diagnosis, taxonomy, outcome measures, sample sizes, placebo controls, double-blind designs, and statistical techniques. Some studies since 1980 have suggested that comorbid diagnoses may often be associated with reduced treatment efficacy, but at

---

[9] Any interpretation of Lesser et al. (1988) must be tempered by their more general finding of *no* differences between outcome for alprazolam and placebo following 8 weeks of treatment. This general finding, though clearly displayed in a chart on p. 440 (Lesser et al., 1988), was otherwise omitted from discussion by the authors; seemingly, comorbidity predicted no treatment effects because there were no treatment effects to predict.

least one large-scale, recent trial has contested this (Lesser et al., 1988). Other studies have focused on the comparative efficacy of MAOIs as putatively superior to tricyclics for the treatment of "anxious depressions," again with somewhat ambiguous results. Perhaps the best conclusion is that comorbidity is fairly common between the anxiety disorders and major depression, and that caution is required in extending the findings of treatment trials on "pure" diagnostic cases to comorbid populations. Research methods have been especially problematic in studies that have focused on concurrent anxiety and depression: Consequently, a need is indicated for new, more rigorous outcome research on comorbidity between the two conditions.

ALCOHOL ABUSE AND MAJOR DEPRESSION

One of the most central areas of interest in recent comorbidity research involves the relationship between the *DSM* substance use disorders and the nonsubstance psychiatric disorders of Axis I. This interest has been reflected in several reviews touching on the topic (e.g., Liskow & Goodwin, 1986; O'Sullivan, 1984; Schulkit, 1986), as well as the recent NCS mandate (Kessler, 1994a) to study the epidemiological patterns of comorbidity between these two groups of conditions. Past research has shown that conditions such as alcohol abuse and major depression often occur with substantial comorbidity rates: Clinical samples have suggested that 30% to 40% or more of patients with alcohol disorders also meet criteria for history of major depression (see review in Schulkit, 1986). For current purposes, discussion will be limited to comorbidity between alcohol abuse and depression, a focus that has begun to generate controlled outcome trials for somatic treatments. It should be remembered, however, that this discussion takes place in the more general context of research on substance use and psychiatric comorbidity. Many of the same methodological issues will become relevant to the study of new forms of substance use comorbidity as treatment trials expand to focus on them.

As with the somatic outcome literature for other forms of comorbidity, research on alcoholism and depression has been hampered by numerous methodological problems. The ideal study would require a double-blind, placebo-controlled design, and would examine whether any difference in outcome (between medication and placebo) is itself dependent on the presence or absence of comorbid diagnosis.[10] None of the studies on alcoholism

---

[10] In a 2 × 2 ANOVA design in which main effects are examined for (drug vs. placebo) and (comorbid cases vs. "pure" cases), the crucial statistical analysis is the test of the *interaction:* Do comorbid patients, compared with "pure" patients, experience less of a response to treatment with medication?

and depression has yet met this standard. Once again, method problems include nonstandard assessment techniques, nonblind research designs, small empirical sample sizes, and obscure or inappropriate statistical procedures. Particularly noteworthy are studies that fail to adjust their statistics to compensate for running large numbers of significance tests (see discussion in Maxwell & Delaney, 1990), or else emphasize the results of secondary analyses apparently to obscure nonsignificant results on primary analyses. Although considerable interest has been expressed regarding somatic treatment response for combined alcoholism and depression, the empirical literature remains at an early stage of development.

Several investigators have undertaken "open-label" medication trials on patients suffering from some combination of depressive and alcohol related symptoms (e.g., Cornelius et al., 1993; Malka et al., 1992; Nunes et al., 1993). Not surprisingly, these studies (of fluoxetine, tianeptine, and imipramine) have obtained fairly positive treatment effects, with some amelioration both for depressive symptoms (Malka et al., 1992) as well as consumption of alcohol (Cornelius et al., 1993; Nunes et al., 1993). These results need to be viewed with caution, given the vulnerability of open trials to experimenter bias and expectancy effects. Although the authors of these studies acknowledged the inferential limits of their findings, they nevertheless suggested that medications could be useful for treating both depressive symptoms and alcohol consumption for patients suffering from both forms of pathology. This conclusion stands in contrast to a comparatively pessimistic review of earlier somatic treatment findings in studies on co-occurring alcoholism and depression (O'Sullivan, 1984).

In addition to these open trials, several researchers have also undertaken double-blind, placebo-controlled antidepressant medication trials to investigate outcome for patients with some combination of alcoholism and depressive symptoms (Cornelius et al., 1995; Kranzler et al., 1995; Mason, Kocsis, Ritvo, & Cutler, 1996; J. A. Shaw, Donley, Morgan, & Robinson, 1975; G. K. Shaw, Majumdar, Waller, MacGarvie, & Dunn, 1987). Results from these studies have been contradictory. Two studies found that medication served to ameliorate both depressive symptoms and alcohol consumption for patients with both forms of pathology (Cornelius et al., 1995; Shaw et al., 1987). One study found that medication ameliorated depressive symptoms but not alcohol consumption (Mason et al., 1996); and the two remaining studies found ambiguous or nonsignificant results (Shaw et al., 1975; Kranzler et al., 1995). Some of the inconsistency in these trials may have derived from methodological problems, including (in some cases) small sample sizes, high attrition rates, peculiar statistical tests, supplemental "counseling" interventions, or documented penetration of the double-blind. Although these studies are generally superior to their open-label counterparts, in no sense do they provide clear-cut findings about medication treatment effects for comorbidity.[11]

Studies on alcoholism and depression suffer from some of the same conceptual and methodological problems as do studies on anxiety disorders and depression. From the standpoint of investigating *DSM*-based diagnostic comorbidity, most of the reviewed studies are only indirectly relevant to the question of interest: Does comorbidity status predict poor somatic treatment response? Although current studies are potentially consistent with some somatic treatment effects both for depression and alcohol-related symptoms, the literature involves too many ambiguities and flaws for any conclusive interpretation. New studies will need to be undertaken in order directly to address the question.

SUMMARY

There are three major findings in the foregoing review. First, the sum of available empirical evidence suggests poorer somatic treatment outcome associated with several forms of comorbidity, including comorbidity between the personality disorders, the anxiety disorders, and major depression. Second (and notwithstanding the preceding), many of the available treatment outcome studies on co-occurring psychiatric conditions (particularly the studies on anxiety and depression, and on depression and alcoholism) have not run the appropriate statistical comparisons to determine whether comorbidity status is a negative prognostic factor. Consequently, many of these trials are, in actuality, only indirectly relevant to the study of comorbidity treatment effects. Third, the treatment outcome research literature is plagued with methodological flaws from which even the most rigorous double-blind trials have not been immune. Post hoc interpretation of empirical results becomes difficult when every study has to be microscrutinized to understand what was done and what was found. And even summary reviews can be misleading, when methodological details are downplayed and individual empirical trials are made to appear more comparable than they actually are. It is sincerely hoped that the current review has not erred in such a fashion.

For clinical purposes, it suffices to point out that available evidence on comorbidity suggests negative prognostic effects for many of the disorders and medications for which data are available. This conclusion is qualified by the small number of available empirical studies, together

---

[11] In particular, none of the available studies examined a direct contrast between the magnitude of antidepressant effects in a pure diagnostic sample, compared with a comorbid sample.

with the fact that many of these studies are "open-label" trials. Future research is likely to yield many more somatic treatment investigations targeting diagnostic comorbidity as moderator of outcome. However, empirical results are likely to remain obscure, barring the development of a much clearer set of standards in regard to assessment, measurement, and statistical techniques. By contrast with the optimism of other reviewers (e.g., Michels & Marzuk, 1993a, 1993b), the current author feels less than sanguine about recent progress in addressing these issues.

DISCUSSION

This chapter has presented some of the recent empirical findings on comorbidity, and briefly addressed their relevance to future research in psychiatry and the behavioral sciences. The major epidemiological and prognostic findings have been that psychiatric comorbidity is a common phenomenon, and that it likely predicts poor somatic treatment response for at least some forms of mental disorder. Overshadowing these findings, however, is this important point: Comorbidity outcome trials are so labyrinthine and (in general) so poorly conducted that it is often difficult to know what conclusions can legitimately be drawn from them. The prospect of deducing truth from the aggregation of such studies is rather like trying to find a single, silver needle in an entire field of haystacks. Only by burning the haystacks and sifting the ashes does any real hope emerge for locating the needle.

There is, among many researchers of somatic treatments, an enviable dedication to the employment of rigorous methods in studies of outcome (e.g., see Feinberg, 1992; Guze, 1989; Klein, 1996). Regrettably, as far as comorbidity medication trials are concerned, this commitment seems more to be honored in the breach than the observance. Empirical findings in this area are universally qualified by major methodological and taxonomic problems. Whereas high comorbidity prevalence has been reasonably well established despite conflicting "rates" and shifting taxonomy, comorbidity treatment effects remain far more ambiguous and difficult to study. And because findings on outcome can only be interpreted in light of the methods of individual studies, integration of these findings is a confusing and highly ambiguous task.

For comorbidity researchers, the obvious question becomes how to improve on previous empirical efforts. Following are some suggestions. Ideally, future studies should employ double-blind designs with active placebo controls, semistructured diagnostic interviews with independent (i.e., blind) ratings of treatment outcome, and statistical comparison of medication efficacy for pure versus comorbid diagnostic cases.

The contrast of particular interest involves the interaction between treatment type (medication vs. placebo) and comorbidity status (pure vs. comorbid) on some measure of treatment outcome: a contrast that corresponds to the interaction term in a 2×2 analysis of variance design. More complicated statistical analyses should be avoided when possible, *and clearly explained when necessary.*[12] Results of multiple significance tests should be adjusted to compensate for the increased likelihood of Type I error (see Maxwell & Delaney, 1990), and nonsignificant findings should be prominently reported, rather than downplayed in favor of supplementary statistical analysis. Details of procedures for sampling, measurement, and treatment should be clearly and concisely described, *so that the reader could duplicate the methods of the study based solely on its description.* As of today, there are no comorbidity studies that meet such standards.

For practicing clinicians, comorbidity raises important questions regarding how best to interpret research on treatment outcome. In context, it is important to realize that *all* treatment outcome studies involve comorbidity, regardless of whether the topic is explicitly mentioned. Some studies have focused on comorbidity directly, whereas other studies have tried to prevent it by diagnostic exclusion, and others have simply ignored it. Empirical findings may well depend on which of these procedures is followed, and interpretation of results must be tempered accordingly. In general, the extent to which empirical results can be extended to clinical populations depends first on the validity of the treatment trial, and second on the correspondence between empirical samples and clinical populations. Thus, if 50% (or more) of depressed patients suffer from concomitant personality disorder, panic attacks, alcohol abuse, PTSD, and so on, then treatment trials cannot exclude these conditions without limiting the generality of their findings. On the other hand, the application of general findings to specific comorbidity populations is also problematic until efficacy in these populations has been verified by specialized trials. Findings of generic efficacy for antidepressant medications do not necessarily ensure efficacy for the population of individuals suffering from major depression with concurrent obsessive-compulsive disorder, generalized anxiety disorder, and histrionic personality disorder. The practicing clinician should use caution in applying generic research findings to specific clinical cases.

To add further clinical confusion, it is also important to remember the effect that evolving taxonomy may exert on comorbidity findings: Shifting

---

[12] It would seem painfully obvious that any empirical study needs explicitly to state the *planned* statistical tests to be performed, as well as the rationale for using those particular statistical tests and comparisons. Evidently, however, the obvious has not been sufficiently painful.

diagnostic rules may potentially render earlier studies noncomparable to more recent studies. The strongest demonstration of this sort of effect may have been the revision of the schizophrenia categories in the *DSM-III*, a change that profoundly impacted the population of individuals who met criteria for the designation (e.g., Carson & Sanislow, 1993). More generally, it appears unlikely that there is strong diagnostic equivalence among such varied taxonomies as the Feighner criteria, the RDC, the ICD-8, and *DSM-I* through *DSM-IV*. In fact, assuming that these different criteria sets have any meaning at all, they presumably involve corresponding differences in populations of individuals who meet criteria for various forms of disorder. As alluded to earlier, several researchers have objected to the overrapid revision of *DSM* systems for precisely this reason (e.g., Carson, 1991; Kutchins & Kirk, 1993; Zimmerman, 1988, 1990; Zimmerman, Jampala et al., 1991). And for purposes of studying comorbidity and treatment outcome, these shifting diagnostic criteria have only served to lend additional ambiguity to an already chaotic subject matter.

Moving to a more theoretical plane, research on comorbidity raises questions regarding the putative independence of *DSM*-based disorder categories. It currently remains unclear at what point rising comorbidity rates would render valueless the fundamental distinctions of a diagnostic system. However, the most characteristic feature now associated with many forms of *DSM*-based disorder is high prevalence for other forms of disorder. This suggests that although diagnostic reliability may have improved with the introduction of the *DSM-III*, a new problem may have been introduced: diagnostic categories that are neither etiologically based nor parsimonious descriptors of real-world behavioral covariance.[13] It is not clear to what extent the *DSM-IV* field trials addressed this issue (i.e., with empirical research), but the historical development of the *DSM* taxonomy does not inspire strong confidence in its empirical, versus political, basis (see Frances, Mack, First, & Jones, 1995; Kirk & Kutchins, 1992, 1994; Klein, 1995; Kutchins & Kirk, 1993).

The study of comorbidity is a natural outgrowth of interest in psychiatric classification. The implicit assumption, that effective treatment

---

[13] An interesting perspective on this issue was offered by Hudson and Pope (1990), who cited nonspecificity of antidepressant response as suggesting a more meaningful, overarching diagnostic category that includes such conditions as major depression, bulimia, panic disorder, obsessive-compulsive disorder, ADHD, cataplexy, migraine, and irritable bowel syndrome. It is unclear how to reconcile this position with the seemingly contrary argument of other researchers that efficacy for somatic treatments can only be understood in terms of a web of increasingly complex comorbidity studies (e.g., Fyer, Liebowitz, & Klein, 1990), except that both sides seem to agree that the current diagnostic categories are, in some way, inadequate.

cannot occur in the absence of reliable and valid diagnosis, has led to repeated revisions of the *DSM* taxonomy to improve its reliability, or its validity, or some syntactic facet of its language. The same implicit assumption has led investigators to emphasize the heterogeneity of diagnostic classes such as "depression" or "schizophrenia," always with the implication that there is some ideal set of subtypes not yet defined, or some set of crucial taxonomic lines not yet drawn. And if only these elusive subtypes could once be identified, then diagnosis and somatic treatment would forever afterward assume unprecedented levels of clarity and effectiveness. Past progress in such diagnostic subtyping has not been impressive (e.g., Carson & Sanislow, 1993; R. P. Greenberg, Bornstein, Greenberg, & Fisher, 1992; Zimmerman & Spitzer, 1989), but investigators remain hopeful that the crucial set of subtypes or comorbidities may still lie just around the corner.

Meanwhile, research interest in comorbidity continues to increase, due in part to the prospect of endless new variations of comorbid disorder that might be isolated for detailed examination. As stated earlier, based on the roughly 300 diagnostic conditions of the *DSM-IV,* thousands of pairwise combinations of psychiatric disorders are potentially available for study. Left unmentioned were several *million* possible combinations of three comorbid disorders, several *hundred million* possible combinations of four comorbid disorders . . . and so on. *DSM*-based comorbidity reasoning, taken to its logical conclusion, might eventually lead some industrious young researcher to investigate somatic treatment outcome and neuropharmacology for patients with combined major depression, narcissistic personality disorder, transvestic fetishism, and trichotillomania—certainly a distinctive group of individuals, by any diagnostic standard! Again, there presumably comes a point beyond which the diagnostic system ceases to be very useful for classifying patients (reductio ad absurdum). Rampant comorbidity rates in large-scale epidemiological studies suggest that the point of absurdity may be more immediate and more pronounced than is generally recognized.

Future absurdities notwithstanding, the current literature on *DSM* comorbidity has already reached a critical stage of complexity. By "critical," it is meant that this literature cannot fully be understood except in terms of the extraordinarily convoluted methodological and taxonomic details of individual studies. Only with massive investment of time and energy can these details be integrated, and the resulting achievement is an unrewarding melange of results with few outstanding patterns (other than poor design and methods in many empirical studies). More ominous, however, is a foreseeable time when *no one* will truly understand the comorbidity literature, because "progress" will have resulted in complexity prohibitive to any meaningful integration of research results across minutiae of empirical designs, sampling techniques, taxonomic revisions, assessment procedures, exclusion criteria, outcome measures, statistical methods, and the like. In some ways, comorbidity is emblematic for the future of treatment outcome research more generally—a future that is uncertain at best. It remains to be seen whether interest in comorbidity will ultimately sweep researchers to unprecedented new insight, or instead break them on the epistemological rocks of an unyielding diagnostic system.

REFERENCES

Akiskal, H. S., Hirschfeld, M. D., & Yerevanian, B. I. (1983). The relationship of personality to affective disorders. *Archives of General Psychiatry, 40,* 801–810.

Akiskal, H. S., & Webb, W. L. (Eds.). (1978). *Psychiatric disorder: Exploration of biological predictors.* New York: S. P. Medical and Scientific Books.

Alnaes, R., & Torgersen, S. (1988). The relationship between *DSM-III* symptom disorders (axis I) and personality disorders (axis II) in an outpatient population. *Acta Psychiatrica Scandinavica, 78,* 485–492.

American Psychiatric Association. (1968). *Diagnostic and statistical manual of mental disorders* (2nd ed.). Washington, DC: Author.

American Psychiatric Association. (1980). *Diagnostic and statistical manual of mental disorders* (3rd ed.). Washington, DC: Author.

American Psychiatric Association. (1987). *Diagnostic and statistical manual of mental disorders* (3rd ed., rev.). Washington, DC: Author.

American Psychiatric Association. (1994). *Diagnostic and statistical manual of mental disorders* (4th ed.). Washington, DC: Author.

American Psychiatric Association, Committee on Nomenclature and Statistics. (1952). *Diagnostic and statistical manual of mental disorders.* Washington, DC: American Psychiatric Association Mental Hospital Service.

Black, D. W., Bell, S., Hulbert, J., & Nasrallah, A. (1988). The importance of axis II in patients with major depression: A controlled study. *Journal of Affective Disorders, 14,* 115–122.

Blashfield, R., Blum, N., & Pfohl, B. (1992). The effects of changing axis-II diagnostic criteria. *Comprehensive Psychiatry, 33,* 245–252.

Blazer, D. G., Kessler, R. C., McGonagle, K. A., & Swartz, M. S. (1994). The prevalence and distribution of major depression in a national community sample: The national comorbidity survey. *American Journal of Psychiatry, 151,* 979–986.

Brown, T. A., & Barlow, D. H. (1992). Comorbidity among anxiety disorders: Implications for treatment and *DSM-IV. Journal of Consulting and Clinical Psychology, 60,* 835–844.

Buller, R., Maier, W., & Benkurt, O. (1986). Clinical subtypes in panic disorder: Their descriptive and prospective validity. *Journal of Affective Disorders, 11,* 105–114.

Carson, R. C. (1991). Dilemmas in the pathway of the *DSM-IV:* Diagnoses, dimensions, and *DSM-IV:* The science of classification [Special issue]. *Journal of Abnormal Psychology, 100,* 302–307.

Carson, R. C., & Sanislow, C. A., III. (1993). The schizophrenias. In P. B. Sutker & H. E. Adams (Eds.), *Comprehensive handbook of psychopathology* (2nd ed., pp. 295–333). New York: Plenum Press.

Charney, D. S., Nelson, J. C., & Quinlan, D. M. (1981). Personality traits and disorder in depression. *American Journal of Psychiatry, 138,* 1601–1604.

Cornelius, J. R., Salloum, I. M., Cornelius, M. D., Perel, J. M., Ehler, J. G., Jarrett, P. J., Levin, R. L., Black, A., & Mann, J. J. (1995). Preliminary report: Double-blind, placebo-controlled study of fluoxetine in depressed alcoholics. *Psychopharmacology Bulletin, 31,* 297–303.

Cornelius, J. R., Salloum, I. M., Cornelius, M. D., Perel, J. M., Thase, M. E., Ehler, J. G., & Mann, J. (1993). Fluoxetine trial in depressed alcoholics. *Psychopharmacology Bulletin, 29,* 195–199.

Davidson, J., Miller, R., & Strickland, R. (1985). Neuroticism and personality disorder in depression. *Journal of Affective Disorders, 8,* 177–182.

Davidson, J., Raft, D., & Pelton, S. (1987). An outpatient evaluation of phenelzine and imipramine. *Journal of Clinical Psychiatry, 48,* 143–146.

Davidson, J., Turnbull, C. D., & Miller, R. D. (1980). A comparison of inpatients with primary unipolar depression and depression secondary to anxiety. *Acta Psychiatrica Scandinavica, 61,* 377–386.

Duggan, C. F., Lee, A. S., & Murray, R. M. (1990). Does personality predict long-term outcome for major depression? *British Journal of Psychiatry, 157,* 19–24.

Faravelli, C., Ambonetti, A., Pallanti, S., & Pazzagli, A. (1986). Depressive relapses and incomplete recovery from index episode. *American Journal of Psychiatry, 143,* 888–891.

Farmer, R., & Nelson-Grey, R. O. (1990). Personality disorders and depression: Hypothetical relations, empirical findings, and methodological considerations. *Clinical Psychology Review, 10,* 453–476.

Feighner, J. P., Robins, E., Guze, S. B., Woodruff, R. A., Winokur, G., & Munoz, R. (1972). Diagnostic criteria for use in psychiatric research. *Archives of General Psychiatry, 26,* 57–63.

Feinberg, M. (1992). Subtypes of depression and response to treatment. *Journal of Consulting and Clinical Psychology,60,* 670–674.

Feldman, L. A. (1993). Distinguishing depression and anxiety in self-report: Evidence from confirmatory factor analysis on nonclinical and clinical samples. *Journal of Consulting and Clinical Psychology, 61,* 631–638.

Fisher, S., & Greenberg, R. P. (1993). How sound is the double-blind design for evaluating psychotropic drugs? *Journal of Nervous and Mental Disease, 181,* 345–350.

Fogel, B. S., & Westlake, R. (1990). Personality disorder diagnoses and age in inpatients with major depression. *Journal of Clinical Psychiatry, 51,* 232–235.

Frances, A., Mack, A., First, M. B., & Jones, C. (1995). *DSM-IV:* Issues in development. *Psychiatric Annals, 25,* 15–19.

Frances, A., Widiger, T., & Fyer, M. R. (1990). The influence of classification methods on comorbidity. In J. D. Maser & C. R. Cloninger (Eds.), *Comorbidity of mood and anxiety disorders* (pp. 41–59). Washington, DC: American Psychiatric Press.

Frank, E., & Kupfer, D. J. (1990). Axis II personality disorders and personality features in treatment-resistant and recurrent depression. In S. P. Roose & A. H. Glassman (Eds.), *Treatment strategies for refractory depression* (pp. 207–221). Washington, DC: American Psychiatric Press.

Frank, E., Kupfer, D. J., Jacob, M., & Jarret, D. (1987). Personality features and response to acute treatment in recurrent depression. *Journal of Personality Disorders, 1,* 14–26.

Friedman, R. C., Aronoff, M. S., Clarkin, J. F., Corn, R., & Hurt, S. W. (1983). History of suicidal behavior in depressed borderline inpatients. *American Journal of Psychiatry, 140,* 1023–1026.

Fyer, A. J., Liebowitz, M. R., & Klein, D. F. (1990). Treatment trials, comorbidity, and syndromal complexity. In J. D. Maser & C. R. Cloninger (Eds.), *Comorbidity of mood and anxiety disorders* (pp. 669–679). Washington, DC: American Psychiatric Press.

Goethe, J. W., Szarek, B. L., & Cook, W. L. (1988). A comparison of adequately vs. inadequately treated depressed patients. *The Journal of Nervous and Mental Disease, 176,* 465–479.

Green, M. A., & Curtis, G. C. (1988). Personality disorders in panic patients: Response to termination of antipanic medication. *Journal of Personality Disorders, 2,* 303–314.

Greenberg, M. D., Craighead, W. E., Evans, D. D., & Craighead, L. W. (1995). An investigation of the effects of comorbid Axis-II pathology on outcome of inpatient treatment for unipolar depression. *Journal of Psychopathology and Behavioral Assessment, 17,* 305–321.

Greenberg, R. P., Bornstein, R. F., Greenberg, M. D., & Fisher, S. (1992). As for the kings: A reply with regard to depression subtypes and antidepressant response. *Journal of Consulting and Clinical Psychology, 60,* 675–677.

Greenberg, R. P., & Fisher, S. (1989). Examining antidepressant effectiveness: Findings, ambiguities, and some vexing puzzles. In S. Fisher & R. P. Greenberg (Eds.), *The limits of biological treatments for psychological distress* (pp. 1–37). Hillsdale, NJ: Erlbaum.

Grunhaus, L. (1988). Clinical and psychobiological characteristics of simultaneous panic disorder and major depression. *American Journal of Psychiatry, 145,* 1214–1221.

Guze, S. B. (1989). Biological psychiatry: Is there any other kind? *Psychological Medicine, 19,* 315–323.

Horowitz, L. M., & Malle, B. F. (1993). Fuzzy concepts in psychotherapy research. *Psychotherapy Research, 3,* 131–148.

Hudson, J. I., & Pope, H. G. (1990). Affective Spectrum Disorder: Does antidepressant response identify a family of disorders with a common pathophysiology? *American Journal of Psychiatry, 147,* 552–564.

Ilardi, S. S., & Craighead, W. E. (1994/1995). Personality pathology and response to somatic treatments for major depression: A critical review. *Depression, 2,* 200–217.

Joffe, R. T., & Regan, J. P. (1988). Personality and depression. *Journal of Psychiatric Research, 22,* 279–286.

Kessler, R. C. (1994a). Building on the ECA: The national comorbidity survey and the children's comorbidity survey. *International Journal of Methods in Psychiatric Research, 4,* 81–94.

Kessler, R. C. (1994b). The national comorbidity survey of the United States. *International Review of Psychiatry, 6,* 365–376.

Kessler, R. C., McGonagle, K. A., Zhao, S., Nelson, C. B., Hughes, M., Eshleman, S., Wittchen, H., & Kendler, K. S. (1994). Lifetime and 12-month prevalence of *DSM-III-R* psychiatric disorders in the United States. *Archives of General Psychiatry, 51,* 8–19.

Kessler, R. C., Sonnega, A., Bromet, E., Hughes, M., & Nelson, C. B. (1995). Posttraumatic stress disorder in the national comorbidity survey. *Archives of General Psychiatry, 52,* 1048–1060.

Kirk, S. A., & Kutchins, H. (1992). *The selling of DSM: The rhetoric of science in psychiatry.* Hawthorne, NH: Walter de Gruyter.

Kirk, S. A., & Kutchins, H. (1994). The myth of the reliability of *DSM. The Journal of Mind and Behavior, 15,* 71–86.

Klein, D. F. (1995). What's new in *DSM-IV? Psychiatric Annals, 25,* 461–474.

Klein, D. F. (1996). Preventing hung juries about therapy studies. *Journal of Consulting and Clinical Psychology, 64,* 81–87.

Klerman, G. L. (1990). Approaches to the phenomena of comorbidity. In J. D. Maser & C. R. Cloninger (Eds.), *Comorbidity of mood and anxiety disorders* (pp. 13–37). Washington, DC: American Psychiatric Press.

Koenigsberg, H. W., Kaplan, R. D., Gilmore, M. M., & Cooper, A. M. (1985). The relationship between syndrome and personality disorder in *DSM-III:* Experience with 2,462 patients. *American Journal of Psychiatry, 142,* 207–212.

Kranzler, H. R., Burleson, J. A., Korner, P., Del Boca, F. K., Bohn, M. J., Brown, J., & Liebowitz, N. (1995). Placebo-controlled trial of fluoxetine as an adjunct to relapse prevention in alcoholics. *American Journal of Psychiatry, 152,* 391–397.

Kutchins, H., & Kirk, S. A. (1993). *DSM-IV* and the hunt for gold: A review of the treasure map. *Research on Social Work Practice, 3,* 219–235.

Leaf, P. J., Myers, J. K., & McEvoy, L. T. (1991). Procedures used in the epidemiologic catchment area study. In L. N. Robins & D. A. Regier (Eds.), *Psychiatric disorders in America: The epidemiologic catchment area study* (pp. 11–32). New York: Free Press.

Lesser, I. M., Rubint, R. T., Pecknold, J. C., Rifkin, A., Swinson, R. P., Lydiard, R. B., Burrows, G. D., Noyes, R., Jr., & DuPont, R. L., Jr. (1988). Secondary depression in panic and agoraphobia: 1. Frequency and response to treatment. *Archives of General Psychiatry, 45,* 437–443.

Libb, J. W., Stankovic, S., Freeman, A., Sokol, R., Switzer, P., & Houck, C. (1990). Personality disorders among depressed outpatients as identified by the MCMI. *Journal of Clinical Psychology, 46,* 277–284.

Liebowitz, M. R., Quitkin, F. M., Stewart, J. W., McGrath, P. J., Harrison, W., Rabkin, J., Tricamo, E., Markowitz, J. S., & Klein, D. F. (1984). Phenelzine v. imipramine in atypical depression. *Archives of General Psychiatry, 41,* 669–677.

Liebowitz, M. R., Quitkin, F. M., Stewart, J. W., McGrath, P. J., Harrison, W., Rabkin, J., Tricamo, E., Markowitz, J. S., & Klein, D. F. (1985). Effect of panic attacks on the treatment of atypical depressives. *Psychopharmacology Bulletin, 21,* 558–561.

Lilienfeld, S. O., Waldeman, I. D., & Israel, A. C. (1994). A critical examination of the use of the term and concept of *comorbidity* in psychopathology research. *Clinical Psychology: Science and Practice, 1,* 71–83.

Liskow, B. I., & Goodwin, D. W. (1986). Pharmacological treatment of alcohol intoxication, withdrawal, and dependence: A critical review. *Journal of Studies on Alcohol, 48,* 356–370.

MacEwan, G. W., & Remick, R. A. (1988). Treatment resistant depression: A clinical perspective. *Canadian Journal of Psychiatry, 33,* 788–792.

Magee, W. J., Eaton, W. W., Wittchen, H., McGonagle, K. A., & Kessler, R. C. (1996). Agoraphobia, simple phobia, and social phobia in the national comorbidity survey. *Archives of General Psychiatry, 53,* 159–168.

Malka, R., Lôo, H., Ganry, H., Souche, A., Marey, C., & Kamoun, A. (1992). Long-term administration of tianeptine in depressed patients after alcohol withdrawal. *British Journal of Psychiatry, 160*(Suppl. 15), 66–71.

Marton, P., Korenblum, M., Kutcher, S., Stein, B., Kennedy, B., & Pakes, J. (1989). Personality dysfunction in depressed adolescents. *Canadian Journal of Psychiatry, 34,* 810–813.

Mason, B. J., Kocsis, J. H., Ritvo, E. C., & Cutler, R. B. (1996). A double-blind, placebo-controlled trial of desipramine for primary alcohol dependence stratified on the presence or absence of major depression. *Journal of the American Medical Association, 275,* 761–767.

Mavissakalian, M., & Hamann, M. S. (1987). *DSM-III* personality disorder in agoraphobia II: Changes with treatment. *Comprehensive Psychiatry, 28,* 356–361.

Mavissakalian, M., Hamman, M. S., & Jones, B. (1990). *DSM-III* personality disorders in obsessive-compulsive disorder: Changes with treatment. *Comprehensive Psychiatry, 31,* 432–437.

Maxwell, S. E., & Delaney, H. D. (1990). *Designing experiments and analyzing data: A model comparison perspective.* Belmont, CA: Wadsworth.

Mezzich, J. E., Fabrega, H., & Coffman, G. A. (1987). Multiaxial characterization of depressive patients. *Journal of Nervous and Mental Disease, 175,* 339–346.

Michels, R., & Marzuk, P. M. (1993a). Progress in psychiatry (Part 1). *New England Journal of Medicine, 329,* 552–560.

Michels, R., & Marzuk, P. M. (1993b). Progress in psychiatry (Part 2). *New England Journal of Medicine, 329,* 628–638.

Murray, E. J. (1989). Measurement issues in the evaluation of psychopharmacological therapy. In S. Fisher & R. P. Greenberg (Eds.), *The limits of biological treatments for psychological distress* (pp. 39–67). Hillsdale, NJ: Erlbaum.

Noyes, R., Jr. (1990). The comorbidity and mortality of panic disorder. *Psychiatric Medicine, 8,* 41–66.

Noyes, R., Jr., Reich, J., Christiansen, J., Suelzer, M., Pfohl, B., & Coryell, W. A. (1990). Outcome of panic disorder: Relationship to diagnostic subtypes and co-morbidity. *Archives of General Psychiatry, 47*, 809–818.

Nunes, E. V., McGrath, P. J., Quitkin, F. M., Stewart, J. P., Harrison, W., Tricamo, E., & Ocepek-Welikson, K. (1993). Imipramine treatment of alcoholism with comorbid depression. *American Journal of Psychiatry, 150*, 963–965.

Nutzinger, D. O., & Zapotoczky, H. G. (1985). The influence of depression on the outcome of cardiac phobia (panic disorder). *Psychopathology, 18*, 155–162.

O'Sullivan, K. (1984). Depression and its treatment in alcoholics: A review. *Canadian Journal of Psychiatry, 29*, 379–384.

Parker, G. (1987). Are the lifetime prevalence rates in the ECA study accurate? *Psychological Medicine, 17*, 275–282.

Paykel, E. S. (1972). Correlates of a depressive typology. *Archives of General Psychiatry, 27*, 203–210.

Paykel, E. S., Parker, R. R., Penrose, R. J. J., & Rassaby, E. R. (1979). Depressive classification and prediction of response to phenelzine. *British Journal of Psychiatry, 134*, 572–581.

Paykel, E. S., Rowan, P. R., Parker, R. R., & Bhat, A. V. (1982). Response to phenelzine and amitriptyline in subtypes of outpatient depression. *Archives of General Psychiatry, 39*, 1041–1049.

Peselow, E. D., Fieve, R. R., & DiFiglia, C. (1992). Personality traits and response to desipramine. *Journal of Affective Disorders, 24*, 209–216.

Pfohl, B., Stangl, D., & Zimmerman, M. (1984). The implications of *DSM-III* personality disorders for patients with major depression. *Journal of Affective Disorders, 7*, 309–318.

Pilkonis, P. A., & Frank, E. (1988). Personality pathology in recurrent depression: Nature, prevalence, and relationship to treatment response. *American Journal of Psychiatry, 145*, 435–451.

Pyke, R. E., & Kraus, M. (1988). Alprazolam in the treatment of panic attack patients with and without major depression. *Journal of Clinical Psychiatry, 49*, 66–68.

Raskin, A., Schulterbrandt, J. G., Reatig, N., Crook, T. N., & Odle, D. (1974). Depression subtypes and response to phenelzine, diazepam, and a placebo: Results of a nine-hospital collaborative study. *Archives of General Psychiatry, 30*, 66–74.

Raskin, A., Schulterbrandt, J. G., Reatig, N., & McKeon, J. J. (1970). Differential response to chlorpromazine, imipramine, and placebo. *Archives of General Psychiatry, 23*, 164–173.

Ravaris, L., Nies, A., Robinson, D. S., Ives, A., Lamborn, K. R., & Korson, L. (1976). A multiple-dose, controlled study of phenelzine in depression-anxiety states. *Archives of General Psychiatry, 33*, 347–350.

Ravaris, L., Robinson, D. S., Ives, J. O., Nies, A., & Barlett, D. (1980). Phenelzine and amitriptyline in the treatment of depression: A comparison of present and past studies. *Archives of General Psychiatry, 37*, 1075–1080.

Regier, D. A., Farmer, M. E., Rae, D. S., Locke, B. Z., Keith, S. J., Judd, L. L., & Goodwin, R. K. (1990). Comorbidity of mental disorders with alcohol and other drug abuse: Results from the epidemiologic catchment area (ECA) study. *Journal of the American Medical Association, 264,* 2511–2518.

Regier, D. A., & Robins, L. N. (1991). Introduction. In L. N. Robins & D. A. Regier (Eds.), *Psychiatric disorders in America: The epidemiologic catchment area study* (pp. 1–10). New York: Free Press.

Reich, J. H. (1988). *DSM-III* personality disorders and the outcome of treated panic disorder. *American Journal of Psychiatry, 145,* 1149–1152.

Reich, J. H., & Green, A. I. (1991). Effect of personality disorders on outcome of treatment. *Journal of Nervous and Mental Disease, 179,* 74–82.

Reich, J. H., & Noyes, R., Jr. (1987). A comparison of *DSM-III* personality disorders in acutely ill panic and depressed patients. *Journal of Anxiety Disorders, 1,* 123–131.

Robins, L. N., Helzer, J. E., Croughan, J. L., & Ratcliff, K. S. (1981). National Institute of Mental Health diagnostic interview schedule: Its history, characteristics, and valididty. *Archives of General Psychiatry, 38,* 381–389.

Robins, L. N., Locke, B. Z., & Regier, D. A. (1991). An overview of psychiatric disorders in America. In L. N. Robins & D. A. Regier (Eds.), *Psychiatric disorders in America: The epidemiologic catchment area study* (pp. 328–366). New York: Free Press.

Robins, L. N., & Regier, D. A. (Eds.). (1991). *Psychiatric disorders in America: The epidemiologic catchment area study.* New York: Free Press.

Robinson, D. S., Kayser, A., Corcella, J., Laux, D., Yingling, K., & Howard, D. (1985). Panic attacks in outpatients with depression: Response to antidepressant treatment. *Psychopharmacology Bulletin, 21,* 562–567.

Robinson, D. S., Nies, A., Ravaris, L., & Lamborn, K. R. (1973). The monoamine oxidase inhibitor, phenelzine, in the treatment of depressive-anxiety states: A controlled clinical trial. *Archives of General Psychiatry, 29,* 407–412.

Rounsaville, B. J., Dolinsky, Z. S., Babor, T. F., & Meyer, R. E. (1987). Psychopathology as a predictor of treatment outcome in alcoholics. *Archives of General Psychiatry, 44,* 505–513.

Rowan, P. R., Paykel, E. S., & Parker, R. R. (1982). Phenelzine and amitriptyline: Effects on symptoms of neurotic depression. *British Journal of Psychiatry, 140,* 475–483.

Sanderson, W. C., Wetzler, S., Beck, A. T., & Betz, F. (1992). Prevalence of personality disorders in patients with major depression and dysthymia. *Psychiatry Research, 42,* 93–99.

Sato, T., Sakado, K., & Sato, S. (1993). Is there any specific personality disorder or personality disorder cluster that worsens the short-term treatment outcome of major depression? *Acta Psychiatrica Scandinavica, 88,* 342–349.

Schulkit, M. (1986). Genetic and clinical implications of alcoholism and affective disorder. *American Journal of Psychiatry, 143,* 140–147.

Shaw, G. K., Majumdar, S. K., Waller, S., MacGarvie, J., & Dunn, G. (1987). Tiapride in the long-term management of alcoholics of anxious or depressive temperament. *British Journal of Psychiatry, 150,* 164–168.

Shaw, J. A., Donley, P., Morgan, D. W., & Robinson, J. A. (1975). Treatment of depression in alcoholics. *American Journal of Psychiatry, 132,* 641–644.

Shea, M. T., Glass, D. R., Pilkonis, P. A., Watkins, J., & Docherty, J. P. (1987). Frequency and implications of personality disorders in a sample of depressed outpatients. *Journal of Personality Disorders, 1*, 27–42.

Shea, M. T., Pilkonis, P. A., Beckham, E., Collins, J. F., Elkin, I., Sotsky, S. M., & Docherty, J. P. (1990). Personality disorders and treatment outcome in the NIMH treatment of depression collaborative research program. *American Journal of Psychiatry, 147*, 711–718.

Shea, M. T., Widiger, T. A., & Klein, M. H. (1992). Comorbidity of personality disorders and depression: Implications for treatment. *Journal of Consulting and Clinical Psychology, 60*, 857–868.

Shrout, P. E. (1994). The NIMH epidemiologic catchment area program: Broken promises and dashed hopes? *International Journal of Methods in Psychiatric Research, 4*, 113–122.

Slater, E., & Roth, M. (1969). *Clinical psychiatry* (3rd ed.). Baltimore: Williams & Wilkins.

Sovner, R. D. (1981). The clinical characteristics and treatment of atypical depression. *Journal of Clinical Psychiatry, 42*, 285–289.

Spitzer, R. L., Endicott, J., & Robins, E. (1978). Research diagnostic criteria: Rationale and reliability. *Archives of General Psychiatry, 35*, 773–782.

Spitzer, R. L., & Williams, J. B. (1994). American psychiatry's transformation following the publication of the *DSM-III*. *American Journal of Psychiatry, 151*, 459–460.

Tyrer, P., Casey, P., & Gall, J. (1983). Relationship between neurosis and personality disorder. *British Journal of Psychiatry, 132*, 404–408.

VanValkenburg, C., Akiskal, H. S., Puzantian, V., & Rosenthal, T. (1984). Anxious depressions: Clinical, family history and naturalistic outcome—Comparisons with panic disorder and major depressive disorder. *Journal of Affective Disorders, 6*, 67–82.

Wakefield, J. C. (1992). Disorder as harmful dysfunction: A conceptual critique of *DSM-III-R's* definition of mental disorder. *Psychological Review, 99*, 232–247.

Weissman, M. M. (1993). The epidemiology of personality disorders: A 1990 update. *Journal of Personality Disorders, 7*, 44–62.

Weissman, M. M., Prusoff, B. A., & Klerman, G. L. (1978). Personality and the prediction of long-term outcome for depression. *American Journal of Psychiatry, 135*, 797–800.

Wencel, H. E. (1995). *The use of pharmacologic probes for testing physiological and psychiatric disease hypotheses: A methodological critique.* Unpublished master's thesis, Duke University, Durham, NC.

Widiger, T. A., & Shea, T. (1991). Differentiation of axis I and axis II disorders. *Journal of Abnormal Psychology, 100*, 399–406.

Wilson, H. S., & Skodol, A. E. (1988). Special report: *DSM III-R:* Introduction and overview of changes. *Archives of Psychiatric Nursing, 2*, 87–94.

Wilson, M. (1993). *DSM-III* and the transformation of American psychiatry: A history. *American Journal of Psychiatry, 141*, 542–545.

Wolman, E. B. (Ed.). (1978). *Clinical diagnosis of mental disorders: A handbook.* New York: Plenum Press.

World Health Organization. (1990). *Composite international diagnostic interview* (CIDI) (Version 1.0). Geneva, Switzerland: Author.

Zimmerman, M. (1988). Why are we rushing to publish *DSM-IV? Archives of General Psychiatry, 45,* 1135–1138.

Zimmerman, M. (1990). Is *DSM-IV* needed at all? *Archives of General Psychiatry, 47,* 974–976.

Zimmerman, M. (1994). Diagnosing personality disorders: A review of issues and research models. *Archives of General Psychiatry, 51,* 225–245.

Zimmerman, M., Jampala, V. C., Sierles, F. S., & Taylor, M. A. (1991). *DSM-IV:* A nosology sold before its time? *American Journal of Psychiatry, 148,* 463–467.

Zimmerman, M., Pfohl, B., Coryell, W. H., Corenthal, C., & Stangl, D. (1991). Major depression and personality disorder. *Journal of Affective Disorders, 22,* 199–210.

Zimmerman, M., & Spitzer, R. L. (1989). Melancholia: From *DSM-III* to *DSM-III-R. American Journal of Psychiatry, 146,* 20–28.

Zitrin, C. M., Klein, D. F., & Woerner, M. G. (1980). Treatment of agoraphobia with group exposure in vivo and imipramine. *Archives of General Psychiatry, 37,* 63–72.

Zuckerman, D. M., Prusoff, B. A., Weissman, M. M., & Padian, N. S. (1980). Personality as a predictor of psychotherapy and pharmacotherapy outcome for depressed outpatients. *Journal of Consulting and Clinical Psychology, 48,* 730–735.

CHAPTER 3

Costly Compromises: A Critique of the Diagnostic and Statistical Manual of Mental Disorders

ROBERT C. CARSON

IN THE CONTEMPORARY era, virtually all American-based research on the efficacy of various treatment interventions in psychopathology, including those involving psychoactive drugs, is carried out on groups of patients defined according to criteria specified in the current version of the *Diagnostic and Statistical Manual of Mental Disorders* (*DSM-IV*; American Psychiatric Association [APA], 1994). The scientific adequacy of that research is therefore dependent to a remarkable extent on the scientific adequacy of the *DSM* effort. The reliability, validity, and generalizability of conclusions deriving from such research is ensured only to the extent of the established reliability and validity of the taxonomic system according to which particular patient groups are identified. This chapter undertakes a critical examination of the *DSM* in light of the crucial role it must play in advancing successful interventions in mental disorder.

CLASSIFICATION OF MENTAL DISORDERS

Human progress in overcoming ignorance with respect to natural phenomena has very often begun, it would seem, with the development of conceptual systems that classified objects of observation into groups whose members shared certain identical or highly similar properties. By isolating that same or similar property among otherwise diverse phenomena, the astute observer performs, as it were, one of the elemental methods of empirical science: a controlled observation markedly enhancing the likelihood of discovering identical or highly similar processes, even perhaps causal ones, associated with the shared characteristic(s) in an otherwise heterogeneous array of observed phenomena.

On logical grounds alone, it is a powerful investigational strategy. It is not, however, in itself incorruptible, nor does it guarantee that the *essential* underlying mechanisms responsible for the similarities observed will be accurately identified. The history of science and of its "natural philosophy" predecessors is replete with poorly formulated classifications of observed phenomena, and with associated notions of underlying mechanisms now known to be manifestly erroneous. As Kurt Lewin (1935) years ago pointed out in a seminal paper, no less a figure than Aristotle—a relentless taxonomist—managed to so misuse the method that it required centuries of work by more precise and quantitatively oriented observers, such as Galileo, to correct Aristotle's misconceptions about nature.

The invention of taxonomies in the various domains of science is thus an evolving process, often intimately associated with advances in understanding, and in the prediction and control of events. Not uncommonly in the history of science, scientific revolutions of the sort described by Kuhn (1970) have involved dramatic transformations of the manner in which the phenomena of a field are conceived to be organized; that is, in the taxonomy employed for allocating observed phenomena into newly apparent, or discovered, niches. Nevertheless, as Kuhn (1970) demonstrated, established frameworks for ordering the data of a field can be, and often are, highly resistant to alteration in the face of observations highlighting their inadequacies. The "revolution" comes only after the appearance of a more integrative and generative organizational schema, as with the absorption of classical Newtonian physics by quantum mechanics.

It is a main thesis of this chapter that the *Diagnostic and Statistical Manual of Mental Disorders* (APA, 1994) represents a prescientific stage of development with respect to an attempt to bring taxonomic order to aberrant behavioral phenomena, deemed *psychopathological* and hence the imputed manifestation of one or another form of mental disorder. I will argue that the *DSM* approach to organizing the phenomena of disordered behavior is fundamentally flawed to the degree that research advance in the field is seriously hampered by its pervasive influence. It persists, I suggest, not because it is a productive, generative instrument for ordering the pertinent observations, but because it and its Kraepelinian and psychodynamic forebears have had no serious competition over roughly the past century, doubtless due in part to the deliberate—and sociopolitically potent—employment of a medical disease metaphor in constructing the system. Millon (1991), in fact, explicitly notes that "the current state of psychopathologic nosology and diagnosis resembles that of medicine a century ago" in being "overwhelmingly descriptive" (p. 245). The chapter ends with some suggestions of directions in which we might move to overcome this impasse.

"MENTAL DISORDER" AS DEFINED BY *DSM-IV*

As will be seen, and has been abundantly addressed by a host of commentators, the present *DSM* is beset with many technical, essentially psychometric, problems. To begin at the beginning, however, I must question the very definition of mental disorder as promulgated by the *DSM*. That definition reads as follows:

> In the *DSM-IV*, each of the mental disorders is conceptualized as a clinically significant behavioral or psychological syndrome or pattern that occurs in an individual and that is associated with present distress (e.g., a painful symptom) or disability (i.e., impairment in one or more important areas of functioning) or with a significantly increased risk of suffering death, pain, disability, or an important loss of freedom. In addition, this syndrome or pattern must not be merely an expectable and culturally sanctioned response to a particular event, for example, the death of a loved one. Whatever its original cause, it must currently be considered a manifestation of a behavioral, psychological, or biological dysfunction in the individual. Neither deviant behavior (e.g., political, religious, or sexual) nor conflicts that are primarily between the individual and society are mental disorders unless the deviance or conflict is a symptom of a dysfunction in the individual, as described above. (APA, 1994, pp. xxi–xxii)

Here, the basic medical metaphor is incorporated into the definition of the field of inquiry. According to the scenario envisioned, mental disorder can exist only "in" an individual, presumably ruling out the myriad behavioral aberrations that appear to be the product of social and interpersonal influences operative within relationships among persons who do not individually qualify as mentally disordered. Moreover—and this distinction is emphasized—the "syndrome or pattern" of problematic behavior displayed by the subject individual can be considered a manifestation of "mental disorder" *only* if it is due to an underlying "behavioral, psychological, or biological dysfunction." An important implication here is that behavioral deviance deriving from, say, an entirely normal (in terms of intact learning mechanisms, etc.) acquisition of behavior patterns consistent with an individual's developmental experience could not be a mental disorder.

Given the centrality of the notion of "dysfunction" (obviously suggestive of the symptom/underlying disease metaphor), it is somewhat disconcerting to discover that this term is in fact never defined in the *DSM-IV*. The imputed dysfunction cannot in fact be the problematic behavior itself, as that would be an entirely circular proposition, in fact a tautology. In addition, many defenders of the *DSM* point pridefully to its "descriptive," "atheoretical," and "operational," character, which would seem inconsistent with the positing of a (presumably) unique but still for the most part entirely obscure underlying "dysfunction" for each of the disorders recognized.

What, then, can be the nature of these critical dysfunctions that produce corresponding mentally disordered behavior? Astutely recognizing the "missing link" defect of the *DSM* definition of mental disorder, Wakefield (1992a, 1992b) has attempted to fill this yawning conceptual gap—in the process suggesting a more concise rendering of that definition, as follows:

> A mental disorder is a mental condition that (a) causes significant distress or disability, (b) is not merely an expectable response to a particular event, and (c) is a manifestation of a mental dysfunction. (Wakefield, 1992b, p. 235)

Even more simply, Wakefield (1992a, 1992b) suggests that the essence of the definition is the notion of "harmful dysfunction," noting that the term "harmful" of necessity will often involve value considerations—concerning which more will be said. The term dysfunction in this analysis is intended to specify a more objective or at least objectifiable concept that embodies the idea of an internal mechanism failing to perform according to "design." But in fact this idea (as Wakefield acknowledges) obviously has its own scientific and philosophical perplexities, not excluding teleologic ones, both sacred and profane. The upshot is that we continue to lack a clear, rational, and reliable means of deciding, for the majority of instances of unexpectable reactions involving attributed harm to the individual, which are and which are not manifestations of mental disorder "in" the abnormally behaving person.

The force of the latter conclusion is enhanced when investigators consider the knotty problem of values, which by their nature are not subject to empirical verification or disconfirmation. In medicine generally, there are almost always objective indicators of what is "harmful" or an "illness" in terms of the functional integrity of the biological system. In "mental disorders," on the other hand, what is declared to be harmful has far less clear-cut empirical anchors and is apt to vary from culture to culture and even from individual to individual. Romme and Escher (1989) report on a "congress" of hallucinators in the Netherlands whose members consider themselves free of mental disorder (see also Bentall, 1990, for a discussion of hallucinations in purportedly "normal" individuals).

As Gorenstein (1992) has demonstrated in his excellent analysis of the concept of mental illness, scientific and valuational issues in the field have in fact become "hopelessly intertwined," such that the medical model of deviant behavior no longer functions merely as an instrument of science "but as a pretext for promulgating certain values and policies concerning the handling of deviant individuals." He goes on to note that these values and policies were then "erroneously presumed to be validated by science" (p. 11). Gorenstein argues (correctly in my judgment) that the scientific and the at least equally difficult "policy" issues of the field can and must be separated if scientific advance is to be assured. That will not be easy to achieve, and the conceptualization of mental disorder underlying the *DSM* would appear to be less than facilitative in this regard. It is not very convincing "science," and it does not offer a value-free pathway for identifying mentally disordered individuals. The latter point is somewhat menacingly made by reflecting that the criterial phrase "an important loss of freedom" in the *DSM* definition reproduced earlier may be interpreted as referring to mental hospital commitment consequent to establishment of a "diagnosis" interpreted as warranting it.

THE "NEW LOOK" IN PSYCHIATRIC DIAGNOSIS

Prior to the *DSM-III* (1980), psychiatric diagnosis in the United States was largely based on vague narrative descriptions of what were regarded as the central features of the then-recognized mental disorders, which were relatively few in number. The second edition of the *Diagnostic Statistical Manual of Mental Disorders* (*DSM-II*; APA, 1968) contained 26 diagnoses having major numerical codes, whose quality may be illustrated by the diagnostic criteria for schizophrenia:

> This large category includes a group of disorders manifested by characteristic disturbances of thinking, mood, and behavior. Disturbances of thinking are marked by alterations of concept formation which may lead to misinterpretation of reality and sometimes to delusions and hallucinations, which frequently appear psychologically self-protective. Corollary mood changes include ambivalent, constricted and inappropriate emotional responsiveness and loss of empathy with others. Behavior may be withdrawn, regressive and bizarre. The schizophrenias, in which the mental status is attributable to a *thought* disorder, are to be distinguished from the Major affective illnesses . . . which are dominated by a *mood* disorder. The *Paranoid states* . . . are distinguished from schizophrenia by the narrowness of their distortions of reality and by the absence of other psychotic symptoms. (p. 33)

Such a criterion statement, replete with imprecise professional jargon and lacking in quantitative distinctions as to intensity or duration of the "symptoms" displayed, leaves much room for idiosyncratic diagnostician judgment and interpretation. The result, in the case of schizophrenia as well as other imputed disorders, was widespread inconsistency in application of the various diagnoses, not uncommonly accompanied by the development of locale-specific norms for rendering diagnoses in different clinics and hospitals, sometimes within the same community. It also encouraged a sort of guru-like approach to diagnosis. I recall from my own clinical training in the mid-1950s a senior mentor who assured me that he could "smell" schizophrenia if it were present "in" a patient, an olfactory sensitivity my cohorts and I seemed unable to acquire.

Rampant unreliability (i.e., interdiagnostician disagreement) of psychiatric diagnosis, to the point of professional embarrassment, was, however, only the most critical of a number of serious problems the *DSM-III* and subsequent editions of the manual attempted to address, not always very successfully. A persistent difficulty, to be discussed, has been that of achieving a true separation of the various disorders recognized within this very categorically organized classification system. The 1968 *DSM-II* was the first attempt to deal with this issue by explicitly encouraging multiple concurrent psychiatric diagnoses, where the relevant criteria are met, for the same patient. As will be seen, the solving of the "overlap" problem in this manner has had some seriously misleading consequences, which persist in the *DSM-IV.*

To return to the reliability problem, the 1980 *DSM-III* constituted a radical departure from earlier diagnostic practice by attempting, insofar as possible, to purge the diagnostic process of subjective and judgmental elements. It did so by requiring that a list of relatively explicit observational criteria be met for the clinician legitimately to render any particular *DSM*-recognized diagnosis. Borrowing from the logical positivist tradition in epistemology, this approach was termed one of diagnostic "operationism." It has persisted through *DSM-III-R* (1987) and *DSM-IV* (1994), as has the multiaxial system introduced with the other changes in *DSM-III.* Meanwhile, the number of recognized diagnoses has exploded, owing both to the addition of new diagnoses and elaborate subdivision of older ones. The *DSM-IV* contains nearly 300 separately coded diagnoses.

As suggested, a major function of the 1980 *DSM-III*, with its new "operational" trappings, was to have been that of substantially improving psychiatric diagnostic reliability. How well was that goal approximated? It turns out that there is no simple answer to this seemingly straightforward question, in part because Kappa, the statistic normally employed to assess interdiagnostician agreement and one that corrects for chance agreements, is subject to procedural variations that may substantially affect its magnitude. In a masterful analysis of the field trial data for *DSM-III,* Kirk and Kutchins (1992) have demonstrated that, with modest exceptions, the reliability of *DSM-III* diagnoses failed to meet the apparently fair quality benchmark of acceptability (Kappa = .70) adopted by its own framers. These authors also note, however, that the problem of diagnostic reliability was nevertheless declared "solved" by major figures in the field with the publication of *DSM-III.* And indeed a reasonably thorough literature search of the topic (by the present author) confirmed that this once-compelling issue now largely (and surprisingly) seems to be ignored. Diagnostic unreliability probably remains a significant problem, although there is good evidence that such reliability may be enhanced by the employment of structured diagnostic interviews and other methods that reduce the multisource variance determining diagnostic conclusions (Wiens, 1991). It is doubtful that such methods are widely employed in routine clinical work, nor are they always used in the selection of research subjects.

As suggested elsewhere (Carson, 1991), the pre-1980 preoccupation with diagnostic reliability, in any event, may have been excessive relative to more central concerns. A "reliable" diagnosis that conveys little or no useful information beyond behavioral concordance with its own criteria is, at best, an exceedingly modest achievement. The truly critical issue is that of validity—the degree to which the reliable diagnosis provides explanatory and predictive power, including (preferably) actuarial information about differential outcomes where various intervention options are employed (Garfield, 1993). A quarter-century ago, the "neo-Kraepelinians" Robins and Guze (1970) published a proposed set of criteria for evaluating the validity of a psychiatric diagnosis. These included clinical description, laboratory studies, delimitation from other disorders, follow-up study, and family study. Very few if any of the diagnoses appearing in the latest incarnation of the *DSM (IV)* could reasonably be said in fact to meet those criteria. Probably the important diagnosis *schizophrenia,* again, would most closely approximate such a standard. However, careful analyses of this diagnosis (Carson, 1991, 1996a; Carson & Sanislow, 1993) provide little reason to be complacent about the essential psychopathological meaning of the term. Andreasen and Carpenter (1993), scholars far more sympathetic to the disease model than this author, refer to schizophrenia as a "provisional construct." There remains doubt, therefore, that the validity of even this crucially important and well-studied diagnostic entity has in fact been adequately demonstrated. Guze (1995) has described the creation of *DSM* diagnoses as more "sociopolitical" than scientific in character, and so it would appear to be.

TECHNICAL FEATURES OF *DSM-IV*

Like all its predecessors, the *DSM-IV* taxonomic system shares certain technical inconsistencies and weaknesses that limit its ability to function in a scientifically productive manner. Chief among these is its thoroughly Aristotelian format, to be discussed, which is in turn dictated by (a) excessive concern with clinical pragmatism (Carson, 1991), and (b) the empirically indefensible sociopolitical aim of claiming mental disorder to be entirely within the purview of the profession of medicine, conceived exclusively as an applied biological science (Carson, 1996a).

Related to the latter persuasion has been the maintenance of the medical-disease-like categorical format through all the *DSMs*, including the latest edition, despite mounting evidence that aberrant behaviors purported to be the product of underlying mental disorders are stubbornly resistant to arraying themselves into neat, tightly bounded syndromes (see, e.g., Adams & Cassidy, 1993; Carson, 1996b; Clark, Watson, & Reynolds, 1995; Frances et al., 1991). The notion of "category" in science is subject to a number of rather technical considerations that are often poorly understood and hence are another source of confusion concerning the logical status of *DSM* diagnoses. The interested reader is referred to Adams and Cassidy (1993), Millon (1991), and Poland, Von Eckardt, and Spaulding (1994), who provide detailed discussion of these issues. Here I shall merely highlight the pertinent features of the *DSM-IV* effort.

A *conjunctive* category is one in which each item of a criterion set is unique to that category. Where the same or very similar attributes are shared among several categories, the latter are said to be *disjunctive* in character. Maximal precision of classification is obtained with conjunctive categories, but as pointed out by Wittgenstein many years ago (1953), nature seems to be very ungenerous in providing true conjunctive categories for its constituent phenomena. Perhaps nowhere is this more true than in the case of human personality and behavior. Among phenomena known to be multiply determined, as here, discontinuous boundaries, i.e., conjunctive categories, are a highly unlikely outcome; or, as I have put it in a previous context, "all of the [potential] spaces are very likely to be filled" (Carson, 1996b, p. 241), thus tending to make for a relatively "seamless" observational domain.

A concrete example of the implausibility of the conjunctive category ideal in this field is provided in the widespread occurrence of high levels of anxiety and depression as central features across the entire domain of psychopathology, as well as their frequent co-occurrence in individual cases of disorder (see, e.g., Watson et al., 1995). These manifestations appear to share a status not unlike that of fever in general medicine, rather than being, in themselves, categories of disorder, as the *DSM* would have it.

Related to the conjunctive/disjunctive distinction is the issue of whether the rules governing category identification are to be *monothetic* or *polythetic* in their formulation. In a monothetic system, all the defining features of the category *must* be present for a given instance to be included in the category; that is, the individual criterial items are individually necessary and jointly sufficient. By contrast, polythetic systems permit category inclusion where only a subset of possible or ideal features of the category are present.

Monothetic inclusion criteria produce high homogeneity among members of the category. Polythetic criteria produce an essentially prototypal category whose members may differ considerably in the manner in which their "sameness" is manifested. An attempt was made in the 1980 *DSM-III* to employ, where deemed possible, monothetic decision rules to enhance within-category homogeneity among disorders. The result was a serious curtailment of patients qualifying for *any* specific diagnosis, an unacceptable proportion (where the rules were rigorously applied) falling between the cracks or receiving Not Otherwise Specified (NOS) diagnoses. The monothetic thrust was therefore abandoned in 1987 with the adoption of *DSM-III-R*—and so, necessarily, was the goal of within-category psychopathological homogeneity (Clark et al., 1995).

By and large, therefore, the *DSM-IV*, based on a puzzling, inconsistent, and probably inappropriately medically oriented definition of mental disorder, is a disjunctive, polythetic category-based taxonomic system of doubtful reliability and unproven validity. Its categories, which do not provide clear lines of demarcation—quite possibly an unattainable ideal (Carson, 1996b)—in fact must be considered to contain highly heterogeneous samples of patients (see, e.g., Clark et al., 1995; Poland et al., 1994). That being the case, the notion of a common or shared underlying disorder, or "dysfunction," of unitary epigenesis that will account for membership in the class would appear to be at best an injudicious hope and at worst a seriously misleading encouragement to the waste of precious research resources in pursuit of what appear to be largely chimerical objectives.

There are growing complaints as well that *DSM* diagnoses employed in the selection of patients for field trials, and in the organization of manuals attempting to specify recommended forms of treatment, regularly fail to capture aspects of the individual patient's problem that are critical to effective treatment planning. In an era of managed care and demands for "empirically validated therapies," the constraints imposed by the *DSM*'s failings in this regard could well prove to have serious economic repercussions for the mental health professions (see, e.g., Goldfried & Wolfe, 1996).

THE REIFICATION OF ILLUSION

These serious, fundamental deficiencies notwithstanding, it is routine in clinical practice as well as in the professional literature—particularly that emanating from psychiatry—to accord *DSM* diagnoses a respect and an influence in decision making that can in no sense be considered merited by the scientific quality of the taxonomic system from which they derive. That system is explicitly oriented, in the main, to clinical practicality, a goal that is not necessarily consistent with scientific rigor. To a large extent, this misplaced confidence appears due to a pronounced conceptual drift, apparently widely shared among mental health professionals, toward reification of the diagnostic entities so inadequately—perhaps even casually—constructed in the process of producing successive versions of the diagnostic manual. As suggested elsewhere (Carson, 1991, 1994, 1996b), the erroneous assumption that a *DSM* diagnosis represents a coherent "nomological unity" (Poland et al., 1994) in the same sense as does a medical diagnosis of, say, appendicitis is perhaps nowhere better illustrated than in the current fascination with "comorbidity" among psychiatric diagnoses.

Before proceeding, however, fairness dictates noting that the dangers of such reification have been repeatedly emphasized by the major coordinators of the *DSM-IV* effort, both in the manual itself (APA, 1994) and in collateral publications (e.g., Frances et al., 1991; Frances, Widiger, & Fyer, 1990). Frances et al. (1991) state the problem succinctly:

> The limitations of the categorical model result in a high prevalence of boundary patients, the need for boundary categories (schizoaffective, mixed anxiety-depression), and an artifactually elevated rate of essentially definitional comorbidity. (p. 408)

In a taxonomic system characterized by indistinct and unstable boundaries, with marked interpenetration among its supposedly (but questionably) valid and discriminable categories, high levels of comorbidity would be an expected and unavoidable outcome.

Nevertheless, with "meteoric speed," according to one observer, the pursuit of new comorbidities among psychiatric diagnoses has in the past decade reached unprecedented proportions. In the typical instance, in my experience, the purveyors of these "new discoveries" provide not the slightest hint of recognition that what they have discovered is almost always a triviality necessitated by the failure of the *DSM* format to identify unique and discriminable forms of mental disorder. It seems increasingly likely that no such coherent, mutually distinguishable entities exist in the domain of psychopathology.

The medical metaphor in psychopathology, with its trappings of separable disorders and allegedly specifically targeted prescription drugs and the like appears to this observer to be in tatters. On the latter point, consider Prozac, once touted as a new-generation antidepressant and now routinely used in the treatment of at least a half-dozen "other" disorders, and apparently for some psychological conditions that are not officially disorders at all (Kramer, 1993). And yet, I acknowledge that I see no hope in the immediate future of discarding this manifestly inadequate approach to ordering the phenomena of aberrant and self-defeating behavior. Kirk and Kutchins (1992), in their title, refer to the "selling" of the *DSM*. If such a characterization has any merit, one has to admire the skill and perseverance of the marketing personnel. They have succeeded in foisting on their professional colleagues, and on an unsuspecting public, a pernicious product having few if any truly redeeming features apart from maintenance of a poorly defended analogy with medical disease. Unfortunately, there is no accompanying warranty for compensating those injured by its use, which in a curious twist may include a large proportion of an entire generation of psychiatric residents.

ARISTOTELIANISM: ITS COSTS IN KNOWLEDGE ADVANCEMENT

As developed by Lewin (1935) in his classic paper, the essence of Aristotelianism is that of conflating the "behavior" of objects with their internal, intrinsic, and presumably permanent properties, which are potentially discoverable by discerning similarities in the manner in which different objects behave under the same or roughly comparable conditions. Thus, the class of "light" objects are discriminable from the class of "heavy" objects by virtue of the observations that the former tend to rise and the latter to fall. Such events as rising or falling were thus attributed entirely to the objects' inherent characteristics, rather than to any presumed relationship between the nature of the object (such as its mass) and any external influences (such as gravity or air currents) that might be impinging on it. (I deliberately ignore here, by the way, the relativistic complexities of seeming to treat mass as separable from gravity.)

I have developed the argument elsewhere (Carson, 1996a) that typological systems in psychology relating to the personalities and characteristic behavior of persons routinely flirt with the limitations of the Aristotelian mode of thought, insofar as they divert attention from an appreciation of person-situation dynamics. They tend to obfuscate the context-dependent nature of virtually all significant human behavior. The *DSM* taxonomic system, in my judgment, suffers the same fate—

except that here the relationship proceeds beyond mere flirtation to embrace, if not illicit union. The effects of this explicit and exclusive centering of the problematic behavior "in" the person include the undynamic and intellectually stultifying quality of the resultant diagnoses (schizophrenic persons hallucinate because it is in the nature of schizophrenia for them to do so), but much else that is troublesome as well.

Noteworthy among these more extended effects is that the *category*, rather than its diverse members, becomes the focus of research effort. The typical outcome is so routine as to be disheartening: A *publishable* result is one in which the criterion and control groups show a statistically significant mean difference on some (often theoretically opaque) measure or other, where the two distributions of scores are in fact markedly overlapping. A common consequence is that over time the accumulation of such small differences, should they prove replicable, permits investigators to formulate "risk factors" for the disorder in question. Such risk factors typically account for minuscule portions of psychopathological outcome variance, and they are almost never specific to particular outcome diagnoses (see, e.g., Coie et al., 1993). One suspects, in light of this too familiar scenario, that etiologically oriented research in psychopathology has somehow become derailed. I subscribe to that somewhat dire assessment and, in addition, attribute much of the blame to the fundamental misdirections of the *DSM* effort.

HOW TO RECOUP

Assuming that science is eventually self-correcting, and that investigators may therefore look forward one day to casting off the medical yoke I believe to be the premiere constraint on progress in psychopathological research, it is possible to predict with a reasonable degree of assurance the directions in which solutions to the heretofore described conundrums are to be found. I offer my own version of these in the form of two somewhat related principles, as follows:

1. It is extremely likely, to the point of virtual certainty, that significant aspects of human behavior, normal or abnormal, will never be reducible to any strong (i.e., conjunctive, monothetic) version of a category-based taxonomy. As we have had ample occasion to learn in our experience over the years with the *DSM*, anything less than a strong version (which appears unattainable without a drastic increase in uncodable or nonspecific cases) tends to create more problems than it solves in terms of category interpenetration (rampant "comorbidity") and within-category heterogeneity. Accordingly, the categorical format for organizing the phenomena of mental disorder will sooner or later have to be abandoned as unworkable. This

point has already been conceded for at least the Axis II Personality Disorders by the Chair of the *DSM-IV* Task Force (Frances, 1993). There exists a more promising approach, as follows.

2. In describing the triumph of Galileian over Aristotelian mechanics, Lewin (1935) cogently noted that this advance, like most others in the history of science, was dependent on the substitution of dimensional for categorical models of representation, thus opening the way for powerful mathematical analyses. I think it will not be otherwise for the field of psychopathology, although I do not minimize the difficulties of (a) determining what critical dimensions are involved, and (b) how they shall best be measured. As to the first of these, a reasonable place to begin would be an attempt to identify what dimensions underlie "normal" behavior or successful coping, about which, at present, incredibly little is known in a systematic way. With reasonably successful progress in achieving the goal of dimensionalization, treatment planning would be transformed from a type of empirical guessing game (let's see if *this* works) in which "diagnosis," per se, often seems minimally relevant, into a rational procedure of strengthening deficits and modulating excesses.

The Millennium is practically upon us; I suggest it is time to seize the day and move determinedly toward a resolution of this significant roadblock to satisfactory progress in the management of disordered behavior.

REFERENCES

Adams, H. E., & Cassidy, J. F. (1993). The classification of abnormal behavior: An overview. In P. B. Sutker & H. E. Adams (Eds.), *Comprehensive handbook of psychopathology* (2nd ed., pp. 3–26). New York: Plenum Press.

American Psychiatric Association. (1968). *Diagnostic and statistical manual of mental disorders* (2nd ed.). Washington, DC: Author.

American Psychiatric Association. (1980). *Diagnostic and statistical manual of mental disorders* (3rd ed.). Washington, DC: Author.

American Psychiatric Association. (1987). *Diagnostic and statistical manual of mental disorders* (3rd ed., Rev.). Washington, DC: Author.

American Psychiatric Association. (1994). *Diagnostic and statistical manual of mental disorders* (4th ed.). Washington, DC: Author.

Andreasen, N. C., & Carpenter, W. T., Jr. (1993). Diagnosis and classification of schizophrenia. *Schizophrenia Bulletin, 19*(2), 199–214.

Bentall, R. P. (1990). The illusion of reality: A review and integration of psychological research on hallucinations. *Psychological Bulletin, 107*(1), 82–95.

Carson, R. C. (1991). Dilemmas in the pathway of the *DSM-IV*. *Journal of Abnormal Psychology, 100*(3), 302–307.

Carson, R. C. (1994). Reflections on SASB and the assessment enterprise. *Psychological Inquiry, 5*(4), 317–319.

Carson, R. C. (1996a). Aristotle, Galileo, and the *DSM* taxonomy: The case of schizophrenia. *Journal of Consulting and Clinical Psychology, 64,* 1133–1139.

Carson, R. C. (1996b). Seamlessness in personality and its derangements. *Journal of Personality Assessment, 66*(2), 240–247.

Carson, R. C., & Sanislow, C. A., III. (1993). The schizophrenias. In P. B. Sutker & H. E. Adams (Eds.), *Comprehensive handbook of psychopathology* (2nd ed., pp. 295–333). New York: Plenum Press.

Clark, L. A., Watson, D., & Reynolds, S. (1995). Diagnosis and classification of psychopathology: Challenges to the current system and future directions. *Annual Review of Psychology, 46,* 121–153.

Coie, J. D., Watt, N. F., West, S. G., Hawkins, J. D., Asarnow, J. R., Markman, H. J., Ramey, S. L., Shure, M. B., & Long, B. (1993). The science of prevention: A conceptual framework and some directions for a national research program. *American Psychologist, 48*(10), 1013–1022.

Frances, A. (1993). Dimensional diagnosis of personality—Not whether, but when and which. *Psychological Inquiry, 4*(2), 110–111.

Frances, A., First, M. B., Widiger, T. A., Miele, G. M., Tilly, S. M., Davis, W. W., & Pincus, H. A. (1991). An A to Z guide to *DSM-IV* conundrums. *Journal of Abnormal Psychology, 100*(3), 407–412.

Frances, A., Widiger, T., & Fyer, M. R. (1990). The influence of classification methods on comorbidity. In J. D. Maser & C. R. Cloninger (Eds.), *Comorbidity of mood and anxiety disorders* (pp. 42–59). Washington, DC: American Psychiatric Press.

Garfield, S. L. (1993). Methodological problems in clinical diagnosis. In P. B. Sutker & H. E. Adams (Eds.), *Comprehensive handbook of psychopathology* (2nd ed., pp. 27–46). New York: Plenum Press.

Goldfreid, M. R., & Wolfe, B. E. (1996). Psychotherapy practice and research: Repairing a strained alliance. *American Psychologist, 51*(10), 1007–1016.

Gorenstein, E. E. (1992). *The science of mental illness.* San Diego, CA: Academic Press.

Guze, S. B. (1995). (Review of *DSM-IV*, no title). *American Journal of Psychiatry, 152*(8), 1228.

Kirk, S. A., & Kutchins, H. (1992). *The selling of DSM: The rhetoric of science in psychiatry.* New York: Aldine de Gruyter.

Kramer, P. D. (1993). *Listening to Prozac: A psychiatrist explores antidepressant drugs and the remaking of the self.* New York: Viking Penguin.

Kuhn, T. S. (1970). *The structure of scientific revolution* (2nd ed.). Chicago: University of Chicago Press.

Lewin, K. (1935). The conflict between Aristotelian and Galileian modes of thought in contemporary psychology. In *A dynamic theory of personality: Selected papers* (D. K. Adams & K. E. Zener, Trans., pp. 1–42). New York: McGraw-Hill.

Millon, T. (1991). Classification in psychopathology: Rationale, alternatives, and standards. *Journal of Abnormal Psychology, 100*(3), 245–261.

Poland, J., Von Eckardt, B., & Spaulding, W. (1994). Problems with the *DSM* approach to classifying psychopathology. In G. Graham & G. L. Stephens (Eds.), *Philosophical psychopathology* (pp. 235–260). Cambridge, MA: MIT Press.

Robins, E., & Guze, S. B. (1970). Establishment of diagnostic validity in psychiatric illness: Its application to schizophrenia. *American Journal of Psychiatry, 126*(7), 983–987.

Romme, M. A. J., & Escher, A. D. (1989). Hearing voices. *Schizophrenia Bulletin, 15*(2), 209–216.

Wakefield, J. C. (1992a). The concept of mental disorder: On the boundary between biological facts and social values. *American Psychologist, 47*(3), 373–388.

Wakefield, J. C. (1992b). Disorder as harmful dysfunction: A conceptual critique of *DSM-III-R*'s definition of mental disorder. *Psychological Review, 99*(2), 232–247.

Watson, D., Clark, L. A., Weber, K., Assenheimer, J. S., Strauss, M. E., & McCormick, R. A. (1995). Testing a tripartite model: 2. Exploring the symptom structure of anxiety and depression in student, adult, and patient samples. *Journal of Abnormal Psychology, 104*(1), 15–25.

Wiens, A. N. (1991). Diagnostic interviewing. In M. Hersen, A. E. Kazdin, & A. S. Bellack (Eds.), *The clinical psychology handbook* (2nd ed., pp. 345–361). New York: Pergamon Press.

Wittgenstein, L. (1953). *Philosophical investigations*. New York: Macmillan.

Part Two

EFFICACIES OF PSYCHOACTIVE DRUGS FOR ADULTS

CHAPTER 4

Mood-Mending Medicines: Probing Drug, Psychotherapy, and Placebo Solutions

ROGER P. GREENBERG and SEYMOUR FISHER

NTIDEPRESSANT MEDICATIONS are widely accepted by practitioners, the public, and the media as effective tools for combating depression. The apparent simplicity of the treatment for both patient and clinician is a significant factor in its appeal. Furthermore, by suggesting that the causation and control of emotional states can be largely independent of environmental circumstances, individuals are freed from the burdens of assigning responsibility for their feelings to themselves or others and are insulated from the need to expend much effort to undo their negative emotions. Practitioners, too, have ample reasons for hailing biochemical solutions for depressive conditions. The treatments are easy to implement, are a ready response to patient demands to do something concrete, cloak clinicians in a mantle of medical respectability, and are nicely supported by well-financed pharmaceutical and insurance industries. In short, there is strong motivation to believe in the power of the pill for treating affective disorders and substantial social desirability in declaring that despondency can be quickly derailed by medicinal remedies.

In a previous review (Greenberg & Fisher, 1989), we attempted to find out how well antidepressants live up to the common perceptions of proven effectiveness. Our analysis of the research evidence raised many questions about the true magnitude of antidepressant effects and the mechanisms that create the results. Overall, a reading of the literature left us less certain about antidepressant potency and more doubtful about the unique merits of psychopharmacological solutions for despair compared with some of the verbal psychotherapy approaches.

The aim of this chapter is to summarize what we learned in our past inspection of the scientific studies, update the material with more recent research, broaden the discussion to the research on "newer" antidepressants such as fluoxetine (i.e., Prozac), assess the comparative efficacy of drugs and psychotherapeutic approaches for depression, examine the empirical literature on the treatment of bipolar disorders, and touch on potentially significant biasing factors in the ways in which antidepressants are tested.

SOME BASIC INFORMATION ABOUT DEPRESSION

There is little doubt that unipolar depression is a significant and widespread problem. Prevalence estimates range between 3% and 13%, with some depressive symptoms experienced by up to 20% of the adult population at any moment in time (Amenson & Lewinsohn, 1981; Kessler et al., 1994; Oliver & Simmons, 1985). Estimates of lifetime incidences of depression range between 20% and 55% with women evidencing rates double those of men. Only a minor percentage of depressions (i.e., 9% to 18%) can be linked to a recognizable physical disorder (Hall, Popkin, Devaul, Fallaice, & Stickney, 1978; Koranyi, 1979). Similarly, only a small amount of the variance in scores on depression scales (i.e., 16%) can be attributed to genetic factors (Gatz, Pederson, Plomin, Nesselroade, & McClearn, 1992) and increases since World War II in rates of dysthymia, depressive adjustment disorder, and major depression cannot be explained on the basis of hereditary variables (Blehar, Weissman, Gershon, & Hirschfeld, 1988).

Demonstrating that affective disordered patients show quantifiable defects in brain structure or function has also proven to be problematic (DePue & Iacono, 1989). Thus, despite a lot of conjecture about a biological basis for mood disorders, there is as yet no convincing consistent evidence for any biochemical theory of causation. Although this fact is often camouflaged amidst weighty scientific discussion in most textbooks, ultimately there is usually an acknowledgment of the uncertainty that is characteristic of current biological explanations (Breggin, 1991). For example, the *Comprehensive Textbook of Psychiatry* emphasizes that research is "still preliminary" and findings cannot be "nicely fitted into any one theoretical framework" (Schildkraut, Green, & Mooney, 1989, pp. 877–878). Likewise, the *Textbook of Psychiatry* published by the American Psychiatric Press concludes, "As it is true for most other major disorders in psychiatry, the etiology of affective illness is still unknown" (Hirschfeld & Goodwin, 1988, p. 417).

We, as well as others (e.g., Antonuccio, Danton, & DeNelsky, 1995; Fisher & Greenberg, 1989; Muñoz, Hollon, McGrath, Rehm, & VandenBos, 1994), have looked at the ephemeral explanations and inconsistent data and raised concerns about the biomedical biases that typically frame depression as a "medical illness" requiring biological interventions as first-line treatments. Nonetheless, almost half of the people treated for depression in the United States are attended to by primary care physicians with drugs being the most common treatment administered (Narrow, Regier, Rae, Manderscheid, & Locke, 1993).

HOW EFFECTIVE ARE "STANDARD" ANTIDEPRESSANT DRUGS?

On the surface, questions about the helpfulness of established antidepressants appear straightforward and uncomplicated. However, reading through the existing literature makes it clear that answers can shift depending on how the questions are posed, how the evidence is interpreted, and whether several methodological factors are taken into account. To some degree, answers are contingent on how the problem is set up. For instance, if the question asked is: Do antidepressants appear beneficial to the majority of individuals who receive them in studies? The answer is likely to be yes. After sifting through many reviews of antidepressant efficacy, we concluded that within any given study more than half of the patients given drug treatment are often deemed to have improved (Greenberg & Fisher, 1989). This observation has been a cornerstone argument for advocates of antidepressant drug treatments. However, given the intrinsic risks involved when taking pharmacologically active substances, it is important to raise questions about the *relative* worth of antidepressants when compared with placebo and psychotherapy treatments. If drug treatments do not afford substantial benefits over less physically chancy alternatives, perhaps more caution would need to be exercised in their application. Findings about comparative worth may muddy the enthusiasm for unbridled drug use. We must also ask about how valid tests of antidepressant outcome have been. As will be demonstrated, there is now reason to be suspect about the objectivity of antidepressant results because investigations are more open to bias than the scientific community and the public have believed.

The double-blind treatment trial has come to be viewed as essential for establishing the relative efficacy of antidepressants and determining that the effects rest more on the pharmacological ingredients of the compounds than on the psychological and social components involved in the treatment relationship. The research design is supposed to be a buffer against the possibility of subjective biases tilting the outcome of results. The double-blind requires that neither the treating clinician nor the patient know whether an active medication or a pill with biochemically inert ingredients is being delivered.

The importance of study design for determining antidepressant treatment outcome is well documented. Wechsler, Grosser, and Greenblatt (1965) in a review of 103 publications found that drug effects were related to the type of research design. Treatments were more effective when there were no placebo controls employed. The work on imipramine, the treatment most frequently studied, accentuated this point. Only 1 of the 9 studies comparing imipramine to placebo found the drug to be effective for at least 65% of the patients. In contrast, imipramine was at least 65% effective in 7 out of 9 studies without a control group and 11 out of 17 reports in which it was compared with another active agent. Like Wechsler and his colleagues, A. Smith, Traganza, and Harrison (1969) also discovered that the type of research design was a principal factor governing the rate of reported improvement. The more strictly controlled the study, the smaller the drug improvement rate became. After screening more than 2,000 articles and 490 antidepressant drug trials (a "comprehensive overview" of the literature) they concluded that the methodology of an antidepressant clinical trial is more important than the drug being studied for determining outcome. They decided that "the differences between the effectiveness of antidepressant drugs and placebo are not impressive" (p. 19).

In general, authors have scanned the research literature and come away with varying degrees of enthusiasm for the idea that antidepressants produce results that are unequivocally superior to outcomes attained with placebo. In examining past reviews (Greenberg & Fisher, 1989), we concluded that several reached positive conclusions about the results of antidepressants in placebo-controlled trials (Cole, 1964; Davis, 1965; Davis, Klerman, & Schildkraut, 1968; Klein & Davis, 1969; Klerman & Cole, 1965; Morris & Beck, 1974), whereas others were more cautious, equivocal, or modest in their judgments (Atkinson & Ditman, 1965; Brady, 1963, as cited in Beck, 1967; Friedman, Granick, Cohen, & Cowitz, 1966; McNair, 1974; Rogers & Clay, 1975; A. Smith et al., 1969; Wechsler et al., 1965).

The range of opinion about the relative effectiveness of antidepressants may be largely attributed to diversity of study results and the relatively modest level of drug superiority in those reports that are supportive of medication. Even reviews that are most positive show that 30% to 40% of the studies reveal no difference between response to drugs and placebo (M. L. Smith, Glass, & Miller, 1980). When assessing percentage of improvement, proponents of medication usually conclude that about one-third of patients do not show improvement with drug treatment, one-third display improvement with placebos, while the remaining third are believed to show improvement with medications that would not have been achieved with placebo. Thus, even with a positive spin on the data, about two-thirds of the patients—those who do not respond to anything and those responding to placebo—would do as well or better with placebo as with treatment by active medication.[1] Statistical meta-analyses, which have compressed the results of large numbers of studies, have also indicated modest advantages for standard antidepressants over placebo. M. L. Smith et al. (1980) calculated that the average antidepressant-treated individual falls at the 66th percentile of the placebo control group. Put another way, the typical placebo treated patient does better than 34% of those treated with antidepressants. Taking drugs rather than placebos improved the average depressed person's outcome by about 16 percentile points. The modesty of the effect is highlighted by the finding that antidepressants produced smaller effects than other major types of psychotropic medications (i.e., antipsychotics and antianxiety agents).

Another meta-analysis, produced by a group of researchers in Australia and New Zealand, also evaluated the results of controlled antidepressant trials (Quality Assurance Project, 1983). Using different criteria for study inclusion, data handling, and outcome measures, slightly higher effect sizes were obtained than those reported by M. L. Smith et al. (1980). However, both "neurotic" and "endogenous" depressions were reported to be most responsive to nondrug treatments. Psychotherapy achieved higher effectiveness levels with neurotic depressions, and electroconvulsive therapy achieved better results with depressions labeled endogenous.

Several reviews we examined in the past found that the percentage of depressed patients improving on drugs was only moderately higher than the percentage of patients improving on placebo (Greenberg & Fisher, 1989). In a review of 16 especially well-controlled studies displaying differences between standard antidepressant drugs (imipramine or amitriptyline) and placebo, we found that the majority (62%) revealed no difference in the percentage of patients benefiting from the active drug. The median drug-placebo difference in the studies was 21% (Greenberg & Fisher, 1989). Other reviews conducted more recently confirm our conclusions about the smallness of the difference. For example, the Depression Guideline Panel

---

[1] The percentage of patients showing improvement, which most studies report, is not equivalent to rates of recovery or substantial improvement. The latter rates would be lower. For example, in a past review the median rate of substantial improvement on antidepressants in 7 controlled study samples was calculated to be only 25% (Greenberg & Fisher, 1989, p. 15).

(DGP) set up by the Agency for Health Care Policy and Research indicated the level of drug-placebo differences was on the order of 18% to 25% (DPG, 1993) and a meta-analysis performed by Trivedi and colleagues (reported in Frank, Karp, & Rush, 1993) showed drug-placebo differences of about 18%. Our reaction to these findings is mirrored by the comment of psychiatrist Walter Brown (1994b) who, after studying the relevant reports, stated tongue-in-cheek, "That's not an astonishing effect" (p. 288).

Incidentally, Dr. Brown, like us, was also struck by the high rate of responsivity to placebo by depressed patients. He demonstrated across three separate trials that, on average, patients on placebos were improving at a rate that exceeded the conventional criterion of a greater than 50% drop in Hamilton Depression Scale scores (Brown, Johnson, & Chen, 1992). It is now known that depressed patients often respond to placebo. Several reviews demonstrate improvement rates of 30% to 40% depending on study conditions (Bialik, Ravindran, Bakish, & Lapierre, 1995; Greenberg & Fisher, 1989; Klerman, 1986; Morris & Beck, 1974; Rogers & Clay, 1975; A. Smith et al., 1969). When we surveyed the 16 especially well-controlled studies mentioned earlier, we found a good deal of variability in response to either antidepressants or placebo with placebo response rates ranging as high as 91% (Greenberg & Fisher, 1989). The well-known National Institute of Mental Health Collaborative Study of Depression Treatment (Elkin et al., 1989) similarly showed that most depressed patients treated with placebo and routine clinical management improved significantly and did as well as those treated with active medication or psychotherapy.

The consistency of a substantial rate of placebo response among the depressed leaves little doubt that psychosocial factors are important for achieving a therapeutic response, even when active medications are being used (an observation documented in detail in Chapter 1). Furthermore, the evidence for placebo potency is so apparent that it even raises the possibility of placebos being sanctioned as a recognized effective treatment. In fact, after reviewing the pertinent literature, this provocative proposal was actually made by Walter Brown (1994a, 1994b)[2] and seriously debated by several respected scientist clinicians (Dunner, 1994; Klein, 1994; A. J. Rush, 1994; Shea, 1994). As suggested in a later section of this chapter, the power of the placebo might be amplified even further by augmenting biochemically inert pills with substances producing body sensations.

---

[2] Brown (1994a, 1994b) excluded from his placebo treatment proposal patients who were actively suicidal or evidenced high levels of severity, melancholic features, long episode durations or certain "biological" features such as pituitary-adrenocortical overactivity and short REM latency.

Under such conditions, drug-placebo outcome differences diminish even more, possibly to the point of being nondetectable (Greenberg & Fisher, 1989; Thomson, 1982).

ARE NEW GENERATION ANTIDEPRESSANTS MORE BENEFICIAL THAN THE OLD STANDARDS?

The introduction of new types of antidepressants in the 1980s raised the possibility of significant improvements in outcome over the previously established drugs. Therefore, the class of medications known as serotonin reuptake inhibitors (SSRIs) has attracted much hopeful attention. Through a combination of skillful marketing and expansive media coverage, one of the drugs in this class, fluoxetine (Prozac), became the most widely prescribed antidepressant in the United States within a few years of reaching the market in 1987. Labeled a "wonder drug" by the media (Schumer, 1989), fluoxetine sales generated more money by 1989 than had been generated by *all* other antidepressants combined just 2 years earlier (Cowley, Springer, Leonard, Robins, & Gordon, 1990).

Is there reason to believe that these new drugs do a better job of subduing depression than the older ones had? In a word, the answer is no. In a meta-analysis of all the double-blind, placebo-controlled efficacy trials of fluoxetine, we discovered a relatively modest effect size that was quite comparable to the effect sizes obtained in previous meta-analyses of tricyclic antidepressant outcome (Greenberg, Bornstein, Zborowski, Fisher, & Greenberg, 1994). An array of other meta-analyses and reviews have examined the comparability of new generation antidepressants to tricyclics (e.g., Anderson & Tomenson, 1994; Anstay & Brodaty, 1995; Baldessarini, 1989; Bech, 1993; J. G. Edwards, 1992, 1995; Kasper, Fuger, & Moller, 1992; Nierenberg, 1994; Paykel & Priest, 1992; Song et al., 1993; Workman & Short, 1993). The invariable conclusion reached by these investigations is that all antidepressants—new and old—produce equivalent outcomes. A summary comment by J. G. Edwards (1995) is representative of the many reviews that have been done. He stated:

> It is hoped that an antidepressant superior in effectiveness to, or more rapid in onset of action than, the older TCAs imipramine and amitriptyline, will one day be synthesised. However, to date none of the newer antidepressants—including the SSRIs—has been shown consistently to have such advantages over TCAs. (p. 143)

With the establishment of relatively comparable efficacy rates between old and new drugs, it became necessary to demonstrate other types of advantages to motivate a switch. Attention has focused on differences in the magnitude of side effects and the possibility of the old drugs being more frequently used to commit suicide because of their higher toxicity in overdose. It is somewhat amusing that the introduction of a new class of antidepressants and the desire to market them brought to the fore so many concerns about the drawbacks of the older medications.

SIDE EFFECTS AND TREATMENT DISCONTINUATION

Side effects are a significant part of the antidepressant experience. Yet, despite a voluminous amount of scientific data, side effects are typically considered only peripherally in most studies (Dewan & Koss, 1989). Generally, side effects are considered a nuisance factor by investigators. Concerns are attenuated because many side effects are transitory, occur with low mortality, and might be dealt with by lowering dosage or adding another drug. From the perspective of the patient, side effects may be more troublesome and cause for concern than they are to the drug administrators (Fisher & Greenberg, 1989). Surprisingly, side effects might also play a positive role in the treatment of depression in some instances because they can serve as distractions. Research has shown that highlighting somatic distress can frequently diminish psychological discomfort (Fisher & Greenberg, 1989).

Although there are debates about whether the new generation of antidepressants should be given in preference to the old standards because of differences in problems with side effects (e.g., J. G. Edwards, 1992, 1995; Harrison, 1994; Nelson, 1994; Ostrow, 1985; Owens, 1994; Pies, 1995), there is no doubt that they differ in the *types* of side effects they are most likely to produce. Reviews indicate that the most common side effects produced by standard tricyclic antidepressants are sedation, anticholinergic actions (e.g., dry mouth, constipation, blurred vision, sweating, urinary retention), cardiac arrhythmias, and orthostatic hypotension (which can lead to dizziness, falls, and physical injuries). Sexual dysfunction and delirium have also been associated with standard antidepressants (see reviews by Dewan & Koss, 1989; J. G. Edwards, 1995).

The newer SSRI antidepressants cause less sedation, anticholinergic effects, and cardiac complications than the standard tricyclics (J. G. Edwards, 1995; Gram, 1994; Owens, 1994). However, nausea, diarrhea, loss of weight, tremors, agitation, anxiety, and insomnia are commonly associated with SSRI treatment (J. G. Edwards, 1995; Gram, 1994; Nelson, 1994). There have also been some reports linking SSRIs with extrapyramidal symptoms including akathesia, dystonia, dyskinesia, and other parkinsonian symptoms (Arya, 1994). Although sexual dysfunction side effects have been frequently unrecognized and underreported, research indicates significant rates of 30% to 40% while using traditional antidepressants with even higher rates being documented for the SSRIs (e.g., Balon, Yeragani, Pohl, & Ramesh, 1993; Gitlin, 1994; Hsu & Shen, 1995; Jacobsen, 1994; Jani & Wise, 1988; Pollack, Reiter, & Hammerness, 1992).

Should the new drugs be preferred to the old on the basis of side effect differences? The question has not been answered consistently by different reviewers (Edwards, 1992; Harrison, 1994; Nelson, 1994; Ostrow, 1985; Owens, 1994). Despite the frequent suggestion that SSRIs improve treatment compliance and comfort because of being less troublesome to patients, *all* antidepressants have been found to produce recurring side effects. Many patients find SSRIs disagreeable to take, just like they do the tricyclic antidepressants.

Treatment discontinuation rates have been used as an index for gauging the relative tolerability of older versus newer antidepressants. At least four meta-analyses and two reviews have examined the issue of dropout comparisons between SSRI and tricyclic drug trials (Anderson & Tomenson, 1995; Gram, 1994; Montgomery et al., 1994; Montgomery & Kasper, 1995; Nelson, 1994; Song et al., 1993). One analysis concluded that the dropout rates were comparable in 58 studies. About one third of the patients dropped out in the SSRI trials and one third dropped out in studies of tricyclics and related antidepressants. Slightly more dropouts in the tricyclic group were attributed to side effects (18.8% vs. 15.4%: Song et al., 1993). Montgomery and colleagues presented two additional meta-analyses (one of 42 studies and another with an augmented sample of 67 studies). Unlike Song et al., they excluded all trials using non-tricyclic comparators. Treatment dropout due to lack of effectiveness was similar for both groups. However, these investigators attributed a somewhat smaller percentage of dropouts to side effects in the SSRI group (15% vs. 19%: Montgomery et al., 1994; Montgomery & Kasper, 1995). Anderson and Tomenson (1995), noting that the Montgomery group did not analyze total dropout rates, conducted an additional meta-analysis of 62 studies comparing treatment discontinuation with SSRIs and tricyclics. They found that more patients taking tricyclic antidepressants dropped out than patients taking SSRIs, both overall and due to side effects.

In a review of four large multicenter studies, Nelson (1994) found no overall differences in discontinuation rates between SSRIs and tricyclics. For each class of drugs, more than 40% of the patients dropped out of treatment. Dropouts due specifically to side effects appeared to be somewhat higher for the tricyclic group in three of the studies. Nelson cautioned about the dangers of comparing discontinuation rates between studies because of the influence of idiosyncratic study factors such as possible differences in the efforts made to retain patients. He also noted that results can be biased because, although the studies were all double-blind, treating clinicians determined the reasons for dropout. Clinicians may be unblinded by their awareness of the types of side effects produced. Side effects are, he stated, "the best clues to the drug administered" (p. 629). More will be said about the lack of blindness issue later in this chapter.

To complicate interpretation of the dropout data further, Gram (1994), in reviewing the evidence on fluoxetine, notes that dropout rates were high (30% to 60%) in several studies. Tolerability (measured by dropout rates due to adverse effects) was higher among patients treated with tricyclics than fluoxetine, but only in North American samples, not in European studies. Gram speculates that possible dissimilarities in tricyclic dosage levels and differences in patient populations (inpatients vs. outpatients) might account for the discrepant findings.

The bottom line, after considering all relevant analyses, is that substantial numbers of patients drop out of treatment no matter which type of antidepressant they are taking, but SSRIs may offer a slight advantage for some people in terms of side effect tolerability. Is the overall difference meaningful? Nelson (1994) concludes: "The literature does support the clinical impression that the SSRIs are better tolerated than the TCAs, but the findings are not as dramatic as some clinicians might expect . . . the overall number of patients completing treatment with these two drug classes was relatively similar" (p. 631). Anderson and Tomenson (1995) sum up the results by pointing out that the differences were "comparatively small" and "of uncertain importance clinically and when cost effectiveness is considered" (p. 1436).[3]

Suicide

What about suicide potential? Do antidepressants lower the probability of suicide? Are newer drugs less likely to be used to commit suicide as a result of being less toxic in overdose? Because depression is implicated as a risk factor for suicide (Black & Winokur, 1990; Buda & Tsuang, 1990; Hirschfeld & Davidson, 1988), researchers have been interested in the possible impact of antidepressants on suicidal acts and suicidal ideation. Some might

---

[3] Treatments with SSRIs are several times the cost of equivalent treatments with tricyclic antidepressants. Some argue that the benefits of the newer drugs are not worth the added cost (e.g., Owens, 1994), while others either feel that they are worth it or that, in theory, cost differences may be narrowed by taking other factors, such as drug-monitoring expense, into account (e.g., Jonsson & Bebbington, 1994; Harrison, 1994). Still others assert that cost should not be a consideration at all in weighing relative effectiveness, because calculations can differ depending on individual patient circumstances (e.g., Pies, 1995). Finally, Hotopf, Lewis, and Normand (1996), after an extensive review of all relevant studies and their limitations, conclude SSRIs are not a cost-effective alternative to tricyclics.

expect that the reported progress in psychopharmacological treatments would have diminished the likelihood of suicide. Unfortunately, research findings do not support this expectation. Suicide rates have increased in the general population during recent decades (Diekstra, 1989), although it is not certain that the trend applies specifically to those with affective disorders. Researchers do know that during the past 30 to 40 years, with drug therapies available, there has been no decrease in the suicide rate for those with affective disorders (Buchholtz-Hansen, Wang, Kragh-Sorenson, and the Danish University Antidepressant Group, 1993). Paradoxically, as a result of a series of case reports published in the late 1980s and early 1990s, concerns were raised that SSRIs might actually worsen suicide risk for some patients (e.g., Damluji & Ferguson, 1988; Dasgupta, 1990; King et al., 1991; Masand, Gupta, & Dewan, 1991; Teicher, Glod, & Cole, 1990).

In trying to reach some judgments about the relationship between antidepressants and suicide, we examined a recent sample of meta-analytic and narrative overviews (e.g., American College of Neuropsychopharmacology Task Force, 1993; Beasley et al., 1992; Buchholtz-Hansen et al., 1993; J. G. Edwards, 1995; Kapur, Mieczkowski, & Mann, 1992; Montgomery, 1993). Our synthesis of this material led to the following conclusions.[4]

First, relatively few people (perhaps less than 1%) commit suicide during a period when they are taking antidepressants (J. G. Edwards, 1995). Moreover, when suicides do occur, antidepressant overdose is unlikely to be the method of choice (J. G. Edwards, 1995). However, in the small percentage of patients who do use antidepressants to kill themselves, it is more likely that tricyclic drugs rather than SSRIs will be involved because of their higher toxicity and lethality in overdose (J. G. Edwards, 1995; Jick, Dean, & Jick, 1995; Kapur et al., 1992; Kathol & Henn, 1983).

It should be emphasized, as J. G. Edwards (1995) carefully documents, that patients treated with tricyclics do not have a higher suicide rate than those treated with SSRIs. Similarly, Beasley and his colleagues (1992), in a meta-analysis of 17 double-blind clinical trials, found that the number of suicidal acts did not differ in groups of patients treated with tricyclics, SSRIs, or even placebos. Buchholtz-Hansen et al. (1993) also reported no differences in suicide rates between groups of patients

---

[4] Much of the existing data on suicide and depression come from Europe where there are existing network databases. There are no comparable databases in the United States, rendering it difficult to determine risk for suicidal behavior associated with specific drugs. Estimates, based on extrapolations from some known figures for numbers of prescriptions in the United States, suggest that suicide attempts in the United States with fluoxetine may be fewer than would be expected in the depressed population (American College of Neuropsychopharmacology Task Force, 1993). However, because of the nature of the data, the conclusion is an educated speculation.

on and off antidepressant medications. Two additional sources of data are consistent with the conclusion of no difference in suicide rates between antidepressant and placebo-treated patients (no matter which class of antidepressants is looked at). The American College of Neuropsychopharmacology Task Force (1993) reviewed data supplied by two pharmaceutical manufacturers comparing a variety of antidepressants with placebos. Within each data source (Ns respectively 4,668 patients and 3,902 patients), there were no differences in rates of suicide between patients randomized to treatment with any one of a number of antidepressants or placebo during double-blind controlled trials and follow-up periods of continuation pharmacotherapy.

Indications are that individuals intent on committing suicide will find the means to do so (see J. G. Edwards, 1995). Utilizing several European studies, J. G. Edwards (1995), makes the case that the most prevalent methods of suicide may change from time to time, with availability of a method being a significant factor in its use. Limiting a method's availability may reduce deaths from that particular usage, but there then appears to be a counterbalancing increase in other (frequently more violent) methods. The result is a suicide rate that remains relatively constant. The presence of an antidepressant drug is not likely to determine that suicide will or will not occur, but it might influence how the suicide will be carried out for those intent on killing themselves (particularly if the older standard antidepressants are available).

Although there is yet no hard consistent evidence that drug treatments decrease the probability of suicide, there are some indications that antidepressants may help to decrease thoughts about suicide. A few studies report greater reduction in suicidal ideation when SSRI or tricyclic treated patients are compared with those receiving placebos (American College of Neuropsychopharmacology Task Force, 1993; Beasley et al., 1992; Montgomery & Pinder, 1987; Muijen, Roy, Silverstone, Mehmet, & Christie, 1988; Wakelin, 1988). J. G. Edwards (1992) suggests that results from studies of this type be viewed with caution because they rely on "suicide items" from depression rating scales to assess suicidal ideation. He notes that such scales are not accurate in measuring severity of suicidal intent and they do not predict subsequent suicidal behavior.

WHAT IS THE "TRUE" ANTIDEPRESSANT-PLACEBO RESPONSE DIFFERENCE?

As indicated, antidepressant drugs have been shown to be more effective than placebo in many studies. However, on average, the level of effectiveness beyond placebo has been modest. Some have viewed the indications of limited success and suggested that "true" drug-placebo differences may actually be larger than many studies show. The larger differences are thought to be obscured by problems common to the majority of studies. A lack of clear consistent inclusion criteria for creating homogeneous groups of depression subtypes and the failure to ensure adequate dosage levels are two factors prominently mentioned as reasons for the lack of success in demonstrating larger differences between antidepressant and placebo treated groups (e.g., Feinberg, 1992; Klein, Gittleman, Quitkin, & Rifkin, 1980). On the other hand, we and others have raised the possibility that antidepressant-placebo improvement rate differences might actually be even smaller than the modest findings suggest because of researcher ineffectiveness in adequately controlling for bias in treatment trials (e.g., Fisher & Greenberg, 1993; Greenberg & Fisher, 1989, 1994; Thomson, 1982).

THE ENDOGENOUS-NEUROTIC DISTINCTION

Would depression subtyping increase drug-placebo outcome differences? Assertions about subtyping depression usually stress that depression is a heterogeneous illness, and therefore, subtyping is necessary to create homogeneous groups that would be differentially responsive to drug treatments. The common distinction made is between depressions labeled endogenous or melancholic and those designated as neurotic or reactive. Broadly speaking, the former are believed to be based on biological abnormalities that may be inherited while the latter are felt to be more likely triggered by environmental events (Feinberg, 1992). The separation of the depressed into discrete homogeneous groupings in order to highlight those for whom medications work best has appeal. However, efforts to substantiate the usefulness of the distinction have proven to be frustrating and disappointing (Greenberg, Bornstein, Greenberg, & Fisher, 1992b). Lack of agreement and arbitrariness mark the efforts to establish a reliable and meaningful distinction. Katschnig, Nutzinger, and Schanda (1986) classified 176 depressed inpatients using nine different systems for assessing endogenous depression. They reported considerable disparities among the definitions for subtyping depression. Depending on which definition was used, the percentage of patients identified as endogenous ranged from 25% to 75%. Philipp and Maier's (1985) analysis of eight different systems produced similar results (with endogenous depressions ranging from 27% to 62% of their inpatient sample). In both studies, the criteria of the *Diagnostic and Statistical Manual of Mental Disorders* (*DSM-III*; American Psychiatric Association [APA], 1980) produced the lowest frequency of endogenous depression.

Problems in finding evidence for reliability also arose for a committee appointed by the American Psychiatric Association to review research on the validity of the *DSM-III* criteria for melancholia (Zimmerman &

Spitzer, 1989). They were unable to uncover a single study of *DSM-III* melancholia that addressed the issue of interrater reliability or used a test-retest design. Eventually political considerations predominated and the committee strayed from the idea of finding useful criteria by means of an empirical approach. Unable to arrive at unanimity, the committee vote split on whether to eliminate depression subtyping altogether.

The creation of a homogeneous depression classification is made more difficult by the association of the category with symptom severity. In at least nine studies, patients given the endogenous label have been found to display more severe symptoms than those not so labeled (Zimmerman & Spitzer, 1989). This observation has led some to conclude that the endogenous classification represents merely a different intensity level of depression rather than a different subcategory of the disorder (Lewis, 1934; Zimmerman, Coryell, & Pfohl, 1986).

Even if the evidence of unreliability in identifying endogenous depressions is ignored, the diagnosis, however it is made, does not appear to predict biological treatment outcome. The American Psychiatric Association committee reviewed 12 studies in trying to find out whether patients classified as endogenous are more prone than the nonendogenous to be antidepressant responders. None of the studies showed an association between the classification and treatment outcome (Zimmerman & Spitzer, 1989). This conclusion parallels that of Katschnig et al. (1986) who reported no differences over a 2- to 3-year period on a large variety of outcome measures applied to a sample of patients with disorders labeled neurotic or endogenous depression. No differences in outcome emerged no matter which of nine different classification systems was used. Brugha, Bebbington, MacCarthy, Sturt, and Wykes (1992), in a naturalistic study of outpatient treatment for depression, also found equivalent levels of improvement with antidepressant treatment no matter whether depressions were labeled endogenous or neurotic. Unexpectedly, over a 4-month period, the two types of depression showed similar levels of improvement with or without antidepressant treatment.

To add to the evidence regarding subtyping and outcome, we reviewed a meta-analysis we had done on 22 placebo controlled studies of tricyclic and newer antidepressants (Greenberg, Bornstein, Greenberg, & Fisher, 1992a, 1992b). Severity of depression (as indexed by comparisons of studies of inpatients with studies of outpatients) had no association with outcome. Furthermore, comparing the five studies that called their samples endogenous with the five defining their samples as neurotic also showed no differences in outcome. Both samples displayed modest to minimal effects depending on the outcome measure used. Another study embedded in the original meta-analysis used a sample of mixed subtyping (Rickels

& Case, 1982). An analysis of that study again revealed that subtyping was unrelated to outcome.

Most studies of various forms of psychotherapy have also not produced differences in outcome based on making a distinction between endogenous and nonendogenous subtyping (Beck, Hollon, Young, Bedrosian, & Budenz, 1985; Blackburn, Bishop, Glen, Whalley, & Christie, 1981; Hollon et al., 1992; Kovacs, Rush, Beck, & Hollon, 1981; Simons & Thase, 1992; Sotsky et al., 1991; Thase, 1983), although a few have (Gallagher & Thompson, 1983; McKnight, Nelson-Gray, & Barnhill, 1992).

In summary, our review of the literature does not support the idea that depression subtyping in terms of an endogenous-neurotic distinction is predictive of outcome. It is possible, though, as some have suggested (Bielski & Friedel, 1976; Friedel, 1983), that individual symptoms, rather than diagnostic subtypes, may turn out to be better predictors of treatment response.[5] For now, discriminating among the common depression subtypes does not appear to be as promising a strategy for enhancing antidepressant effectiveness rates as many hoped it would be.

DOSAGE AND BLOOD LEVELS

What about drug dosage level? It is surmised that some studies do not achieve maximum drug-placebo differences because the medication dosages used are not high enough (Klein et al., 1980). Support for this idea has come from a few researchers (Quitkin, Rabkin, Ross, & McGrath, 1984). Yet, the work of others challenges this speculation. For example, Wechsler and his colleagues (1965) uncovered no relationships between dosage level (or length of treatment) and percentage of improvement in a sizable number of studies. Also, a large-scale meta-analysis of antidepressant efficacy studies conducted by Australian and New Zealand researchers (Quality Assurance Project, 1983) revealed no relationship between dosage level and effect size (a measure of outcome magnitude).

Although it seems both logical and reasonable to suggest that drugs be administered in dosages that are sufficient for achieving therapeutic effects (see overview by Quitkin, 1985), surprisingly little controlled

---

[5] There is some indication that severe depressions accompanied by delusions or hallucinations (i.e., psychotic depressions) respond much more poorly to antidepressants or to placebos than nonpsychotic major depressions do and that these differences are not attributable to severity of depression (Schatzberg & Rothschild, 1992). Initial findings suggest that such symptom presentations respond better to electroconvulsive therapy (ECT) or to a combination of antidepressant and antipsychotic medications. However, the bulk of the evidence on treating psychotic depressions somatically results from open trials and retrospective reports. Therefore, to dispel doubt about effectiveness, further substantiation from additional better controlled trials is required.

experimental work comparing antidepressant dosages has been done. For an earlier review, we were able to locate only two studies (of the older standard antidepressants) specifically pertinent to this issue (Greenberg & Fisher, 1989). One of the studies (Watt, Crammer, & Elkes, 1972) produced evidence that a higher dose was more therapeutic than a lower dose (150 vs. 300 mg of desmethylimipramine). However, raters of outcome in the study were not blind to dosage level and the higher dose produced recovery in only 50% of the patients. A second study (G. M. Simpson, Lee, Cuculic, & Kellner, 1976) compared the use of a 300 mg dose of imipramine with a 150 mg dose and demonstrated only a borderline edge for the higher dose.

A more recent European publication examined the issue of dosage for 130 outpatients treated for depression either by general practitioners or by psychiatrists in hospital practice (Brugha et al., 1992). This was a naturalistic study in which clinicians were free to treat patients by whatever means they believed would be most helpful. Outcome was evaluated over a 4-month period. Most patients improved whether they received antidepressants or not. Looking only at those receiving antidepressants, there was no significant difference in outcome between those placed on higher or lower antidepressant doses. The lack of statistical significance for dosage differences remained even when other variables such as depression severity, duration, compliance, patient age, and gender were taken into account.

Results of studies with the newer SSRI antidepressant fluoxetine reveal no effect linked to dose. Gram (1994), in his review of the research on fluoxetine, identified three such studies (Dunlop, Dornseif, Wernicke, & Potvin, 1990; Wernicke, Dunlop, Dornseif, Bosomworth, & Humbert, 1988; Wernicke, Dunlop, Dornseif, & Zerbe, 1987). Consistent across the studies, there was no relationship between dose and effect. A 5 mg dose per day was as effective as any of the higher doses. Gram (1994) also pointed out work done on 1,100 depressed outpatients who were tried on increased doses of fluoxetine (60 mg) when they did not respond to 3 weeks of treatment with a lower dose (20 mg). The higher dose proved to be no more effective than the lower dose had been.

The limited evidence for added benefits with larger antidepressant doses has not deterred recommendations for their use. A respected researcher-clinician made the following recommendation: "Aggressive increases in doses of antidepressants may be appropriate when moderate doses seem to be inadequate. . . . This impression is offered even without the availability of well-designed, systematic, and conclusive dose-response studies of most antidepressants" (Baldessarini, 1989, p. 123).

Would examining the evidence on blood plasma levels rather than dosage size show better relationships with outcome? The question is a natural outgrowth of the fact that dosage and blood plasma levels do not seem to be highly related. Yet, attempts to link outcome with blood plasma levels have not fully clarified the picture. While a number of studies have revealed an association between outcome and plasma levels for some drugs, the inconsistency of results and the magnitude of the relationships discovered raise some uneasiness. The evidence is complicated by wide biochemical and pharmacokinetic variations in each individual's response to medications (e.g., Moller et al., 1985). After reviewing this area of study, G. H. Simpson, Edmond, and White (1983) conclude: "Efforts to relate plasma levels to therapeutic outcome have, in general, been disappointing" (p. 27), and these relationships, although "extensively studied since 1962, remain controversial" (p. 29).

Treatment outcome and the blood level concentrations of drugs have been moderately related in studies of some clinical groups while showing no consistent relationship in others (American Psychiatric Association [APA] Task Force, 1985; Glassman, Perel, Shostak, Kantor, & Fleiss, 1977; Reisby et al., 1977). Blackwell (1982) reported that treatment response correlated with plasma level in only one third of the patients he studied. Different conclusions have also been reached for different drugs. Based on the limited available studies, clinical response and blood level measurement have shown a level of consistency for some drugs (e.g., imipramine) and none with others (e.g., amitriptyline) (APA Task Force, 1985). Even when significant correlations are found, they account for only a small part of the "drug effect" (Glassman et al., 1977; Reisby et al., 1977). Regarding the newer SSRI antidepressants, there is consensus among several researchers that no relationship has been demonstrated between plasma concentrations of the drugs and therapeutic response (Glassman, 1994; Gram, 1994; Kelly, Perry, Holstead, & Garvey, 1989; Preskorn, Silkey, Beber, & Dorey, 1991).

There is also some debate about whether only certain types of depression will show a relationship between plasma level and therapeutic response. Freidel (1982), for example, after acknowledging that only the antidepressants nortriptyline and imipramine have shown some relationship between outcome and plasma level, goes on to suggest that the relationship holds only for those patients with endogenous types of diagnoses. He would expect no relationship in those who fall into other subcategories of depression such as psychotic, atypical, neurotic, or reactive. Even this idea, however, does not receive consistent support. A carefully done study of 90 inpatients—85% diagnosed as endogenous—revealed virtually no significant relationships of any kind between measures of plasma concentration and several measures of clinical response to amitriptyline or imipramine (Kocsis, Hanin, Bowden, & Brunswick, 1986).

Glassman (1994) in a candid revealing paper assesses the studies that have looked at antidepressant plasma levels and contrasts their results with the work of his research group in the 1970s. He points to the technical difficulties involved in securing accurate measurements and emphasizes how hard it is to carry out a study in which there is assurance that the many other variables that can affect depression, aside from blood levels of the medication, have been eliminated. He notes that the research would require the selection of relatively pure samples of acute (not chronic), noncomorbid, severe, previously not treated depressed patients, who are not refractory to antidepressant treatment. Such patients would then need to be hospitalized for weeks with placebo responders eliminated and all potentially therapeutic factors, other than drug ingestion, controlled. In fact, he doubts that such a study could be done under modern conditions. Glassman acknowledges that the results of antidepressant plasma level studies of outpatients have been "very disappointing" and raises questions about how generalizable the results his group obtained in the 1970s are to other types of patients today. He writes nostalgically:

> Where it was possible to demonstrate a relationship [between blood levels and outcome, the patients of the 1970s studies were] remarkably similar. . . . They were almost entirely inpatients, they were almost entirely severely depressed unipolar patients, and they were almost entirely patients in their 50s and 60s. . . . As soon as you go away from that sample, we are extrapolating those results to a population that has not actually been studied . . . what you cannot expect is that you are going to see, in your clinical populations, the same powerful relationships that you see in studies specifically designed to examine blood level relationships. The reason for that is, in well-designed blood level studies an enormous effort has gone into selecting a population where all variables that might influence outcome, except for blood levels, have been removed. That simply is not true or possible in clinical populations. (p. 27)

Although unintended, Glassman's article is a tribute to the strength of psychosocial variables effects on depression and an affirmation of the idea that blood level measurement in clinical practice is unlikely to lead to improved medication effectiveness rates.

Study Designs and Generalizability

In contrast to speculation that antidepressant treatment superiority might be larger than the modest figures reported in most drug trials is the suggestion that research trials actually inflate the apparent benefits beyond what most patients are likely to experience. Support for this idea comes from a close look at the way most antidepressant trials are carried out. Scrutiny of the research evidence raises the possibility of bias in the results of many studies and promotes questions about how well findings are apt to match the realities of everyday clinical practice.

The acknowledged standard for evaluating the effectiveness of antidepressant drugs (as well as other psychotropic agents) is to administer either the medications or inert pills called placebos to patients randomly assigned to the treatment and control groups. It is critical that both patients and research personnel remain blind to the nature of assignments to the active and control conditions. The double-blind design was created to ensure that researchers' biases are held in check. It had become apparent that sound, objective assessments of outcome are unlikely if the desires of the research participants are allowed to influence the results (e.g., Lasagna, 1955). Without scrupulous restraint, drug trials become susceptible to detrimental effects of participant expectation and bias. As controls designed to safeguard objectivity in research trials become more meticulous, the apparent efficacy of psychotropic drugs decreases. The possibility of undue influence appears especially important in studies of psychotropic drugs because outcome is usually measured by judgments about feelings and behaviors rather than by measures of physiological change. Multiple studies have established the reasonableness of the double-blind design strategy (e.g., Fisher & Greenberg, 1989; Ross & Olson, 1981) and research design has proved to have a paramount influence on how antidepressant drug trials turn out (A. Smith et al., 1969; Wechsler et al., 1965).

Can investigators feel secure that research on psychotropic drugs is shielded from bias? Is the double-blind design truly double-blind? In an extensive search of the literature to shed light on this issue, we uncovered reports attesting to the fragility of the double-blind schema. Almost all studies of psychiatric drug effectiveness make no effort to certify that subjects and clinicians are actually unaware of whether active drugs or placebos are being administered. It is simply assumed that the use of a double-blind design guarantees that blindness is occurring. As we burrowed deeper into the literature, however, we began to uncover a scattering of projects where efforts were made to find out if the double-blind had been breached. Most often this was done by asking patients and clinicians to guess whether the treatment that had been delivered was a drug or a placebo. Our initial finding of a few studies of this type grew to 26, then 29 and now more than 30 (Fisher & Greenberg, 1993; Greenberg & Fisher, 1989, 1994). These reports confirmed the vulnerability of the double-blind and documented that it is almost always breached. For every supposedly double-blind study showing that participants could not accurately guess whether drugs or placebos were being dispensed, there were 9 to 10 reports revealing that the double-blind had been penetrated. The undeniable conclusions drawn from this finding were that data on the efficacy of psychotropic drugs are tainted and that judgments previously drawn about the magnitude of antidepressant effects are now untrustworthy. We were left with a sense of uncomfortable uncertainty.

How is the double-blind penetrated? One positive answer to this question is to attribute the unblinding to the active drug's ability to produce more beneficial changes than the placebo (e.g., Henker, Whalen, & Collins, 1979; Rickels, Raab, & Carranza, 1965). Thus, contrasting patterns of responsivity might make apparent what is supposed to remain hidden. However, several studies have indicated that the "side effects" of active drugs, which occur with greater frequency, duration, and specificity than do those for placebo, may be a major reason for the unblinding process (e.g., Engelhardt & Margolis, 1967; Marini, Sheard, Bridges, & Wagner, 1976; Rabkin et al., 1986; Rickels et al., 1966). Investigators have noted the important role played by side effects in this regard (e.g., Letemendia & Harris, 1959; Oxtoby, Jones, & Robinson, 1989).

The possible confounding of results by side effects is well illustrated by a meta-analysis of fluoxetine outcome that we and our colleagues conducted (Greenberg et al., 1994). All double-blind, placebo-controlled trials of fluoxetine were entered into the analysis. Results showed a relatively modest effect size for fluoxetine outcome that was no greater than effect sizes obtained by previous meta-analyses of tricyclic antidepressants. To see whether side effects might have influenced ratings of outcome by transforming the double-blind into a transparent design, we compared study effect sizes with the percentage of patients reporting side effects in each study. Correlations between the percentage of patients reporting side effects and the effect size outcome measures were significant whether outcome ratings were made by clinicians or by patients. The greater the number of drug treated patients who experienced side effects, the better the outcome was judged to be. The findings reinforced concerns about the possibility of biased outcome ratings as a result of penetration of the double-blind through information leaked by side effects.

As detailed elsewhere (Greenberg & Fisher, 1989), the double-blind design, as currently conducted, has a major flaw. The placebo, an inert substance, simply does not create the array or magnitude of body sensations that match those elicited by active drugs. Differential cues, therefore, allow those involved in the study to discriminate active from inactive substance and may permit the understandable prodrug zeal to mold outcome ratings in the direction of researcher and patient hopes and expectations.

Two strategies for making study designs blinder should be mentioned. The employment of each strategy has demonstrated a shrinkage in the apparent superiority of antidepressant treatment outcome. One strategy involves using active placebos (which create body sensations) rather than inert placebos as comparison treatments in studies. Reviews of the modest number of studies employing this strategy reveal that even a small increase in body sensations produced by an active placebo is enough to create outcome ratings that are substantially equivalent to those produced for active drugs (see Greenberg & Fisher, 1989; Thomson, 1982).[6] For example, Thomson appraised all the double-blind, placebo-controlled studies completed between 1958 and 1972 that he could find. He noted that 68 used an inert placebo as a control while 7 employed an active one (atropine), which produced an array of body sensations. Comparing study outcomes, he discovered that tricyclic antidepressants had a superior therapeutic effect in 59% of the studies in which an inert placebo comparison occurred, but only one study (14% of the designs) showed the antidepressant to be superior when an active placebo was employed. The difference was significant. A few additional studies have shown results consistent with those reported by Thomson (Greenberg & Fisher, 1989).

Another strategy attempts to reduce potential bias by increasing design complexity (Greenberg et al., 1992a). We analyzed study results in which designs involved comparing newer antidepressants (under double-blind conditions) to *both* older standard antidepressants and a placebo. Presumably, in this context researchers would be more interested in the impact of the new drug than the old standard drug. Under these conditions, we assumed there would be lowered motivation for biasing or magnifying results for the older accepted drug. Also anticipated was that the complexity of testing two drugs simultaneously (each with its own distribution of side effects) and a placebo in the same trials would make it more difficult to prejudge outcome or focus bias. We speculated that the more complex design would be "blinder" than designs that simply compared one drug and a placebo. It was presumed that in such a design there would be less researcher interest in establishing the magnitude of the standard, already established, antidepressant. This analysis was derived from 22 trials in which a newer antidepressant, a standard antidepressant, and a placebo were compared. As predicted, a meta-analysis of efficacy measures showed that effect sizes for the older antidepressants were only one-half to one-quarter the size of those found in earlier, less complex investigations focusing only on the older antidepressants. The findings strengthen the impression of possible bias affecting outcome, even in trials where the double-blind is supposed to protect the results from contamination.

Aside from the possibly inflated estimates of outcome produced by studies in which blindness has been compromised, there are several

---

[6] Although this conclusion is generally true, there are complexities regarding the use of active placebos (see Chapter 1).

other reasons for believing that antidepressant research results may not accurately predict the real-world outcomes most patients are likely to experience. One prominent reason for concern is that the practitioners, patients, and settings most often studied are not representative of the conditions under which most patients receive antidepressant treatment. Most frequently, treatment outcome research is carried on in highly specialized health care settings in which both patients and providers are highly select and homogenized in terms of their characteristics. A sizable percentage of patients often treated for depression are eliminated from studies because they do not meet strict research criteria for inclusion or because they exhibit disorders in addition to depression (see Chapter 2). Also, ethnic or cultural variables are rarely taken into account or even reported by most studies, despite the evidence that these factors influence drug metabolism, treatment compliance, and treatment-seeking behavior (see reviews by Lin, Poland, & Nakasaki, 1993; Muñoz et al., 1994). Similarly, Antonuccio et al. (1995), in their review comparing psychotherapy and medication outcomes, note the inattention given to gender in analyses of comparative outcomes. They suggest that the results of comparative treatment studies (which use mainly female subjects) may not readily generalize to men. Finally, two reviews document the paucity of double-blind placebo controlled trials evaluating the impact of antidepressants on older patients. Gerson, Plotkin, and Jarvik (1988) discovered that between 1964 and 1986 such reports appeared on only 60 elderly patients. Updating this finding for studies published from 1987 to 1992, Anstay and Brodaty (1995) were able to locate only three placebo-controlled, double-blind trials conducted on the elderly.

Viewing the restricted and constricted sampling, Muñoz et al. (1994) conclude that generalization of study results to typical primary care settings, providers, and patients requires a "sizeable leap" (p. 46). A similar conclusion is reached by the Depression Guideline Panel (DPG) of the Agency for Health Care Policy and Research. They state: "Although randomized trials provide the best evidence for the efficacy of a treatment in a specific type of patient, their applicability to the community at large may be limited by the trials' stringent enrollment criteria, unique treatment settings, and unrepresentative clinical procedures" (DPG, 1993, p. 17).

Conclusions about the effects of antidepressant drugs tend to be based on groups of patients who not only match rigorous diagnostic criteria to "purify" the sample, but also survive a series of filtering processes that increasingly deplete the size and representativeness of the group. After selection, many patients are eliminated from the research along the way because they show some response to an initial washout trial or placebo (perhaps 20%)[7] or drop out because of adverse effects or concerns about lack of efficacy (perhaps 35% or more) (Fisher & Greenberg, 1989). Thus, final treatment samples are made up of a series of "leftover" patients who have outlasted several debarring processes. The degree to which these samples are affected by differences in prevailing local conditions is unknown. However, multicenter studies not infrequently show a difference in outcome when the same drug is applied to similarly selected patients in different settings (Greenberg & Fisher, 1989). Under apparently parallel conditions, some centers may produce positive results while others do not (e.g., Feighner, Aden, Fabre, Rickels, & Smith, 1983; Greenblatt, Grosser, & Wechsler, 1964). The upshot of these observations is that antidepressant results can be significantly impacted by psychosocial factors having nothing to do with the biochemical ingredients of the drug being studied. The unique conditions prevailing during any set of antidepressant trials may cloud the likelihood of generalizing from research results to predict outcome for a specific patient sitting in a practitioner's office. This conclusion is consistent with the observation of Thase and Kupfer (1996) that 80% to 90% of the outcome variance in treating depressions of mild to moderate severity can be accounted for by "nonspecific factors" such as clinical support. It is also in accord with findings from the National Institute of Mental Health Treatment of Depression Collaborative Research Program (Krupnick et al., 1996), which demonstrated that the level of the therapeutic alliance (broadly defined as the collaborative bond between clinician and patient) exerted a significant and "very large effect" on outcome. In fact, to the surprise of the researchers, ratings of the relationship proved to be as important for antidepressant outcome as they were for psychotherapy or placebo outcome.

The source of outcome ratings is another possible distorting factor in determining the size of an antidepressant effect. In a meta-analysis of antidepressant studies that were presumably blinder because of greater design complexity, we found small but significant antidepressant effects when outcome was determined by clinician ratings but no advantage for antidepressants beyond the placebo effect when patients rated their own outcomes (Greenberg et al., 1992a). These results were consistent with past studies and reviews indicating that clinician ratings of antidepressant outcome tend to be more liberal than patient ratings and are more likely

---

[7] Research has not supported the value of the washout procedure. Three studies indicate that an initial phase to eliminate (or washout) placebo responders does not lower the placebo response rate in a trial (Greenberg, Fisher, & Riter, 1995; Reimherr, Ward, & Byerley, 1989; Trivedi & Rush, 1994).

subject to bias (B. C. Edwards et al., 1984; Lambert, Hatch, Kingston, & Edwards, 1986; Murray, 1989). At times, advocates of antidepressant treatment, in attempting to give greater weight to the somewhat more positive outcomes hinted at by clinician rating scales, theorize that clinician-rated measures may have better psychometric properties than patient-rated measures. There is no evidence to support this contention. In actuality, Murray (1989), in reviewing the evidence contrasting the two most widely used measures of each type (i.e., the Hamilton Rating Scale for Depression, Hamilton, 1960, and the Beck Depression Inventory, Beck, Ward, Mendelson, Mock, & Erbaugh, 1961), concluded that the patient-rated measure has better psychometric properties and is most likely a more objective outcome measure.

The material reviewed in this section corroborates the contention that antidepressant drug trials create a false sense of security about their objectivity. The double-blind design is a semifiction that can be rendered transparent by the side effect profiles associated with antidepressants. Without the use of active placebos and/or other efforts to ensure study objectivity, one cannot be sure about the level of unique benefits that antidepressants may afford over placebos. Moreover, study design features, such as the purification of patient samples, the elimination of large numbers of subjects, and the reliance on outcome measures that are reactive to the raters' desires (e.g., global rating scales) may deceptively enhance success rates for medication trials while reducing the ability to generalize the results to the patient population at large. The "true" magnitude of the antidepressant advantage is uncertain.

ANTIDEPRESSANT COMPARISONS WITH PSYCHOTHERAPY TREATMENTS

In a previous inspection of the literature, we did an extensive analysis of the comparative efficacy of antidepressant and psychotherapeutic treatments for depression (Greenberg & Fisher, 1989). The psychotherapy treatments of interest were those specifically designed to deal with depression. Such models included cognitive therapy, interpersonal psychotherapy, and social skills training. The review uncovered a good deal of empirical support for the success of psychosocial approaches in dealing with depression. Moreover, the psychotherapy treatments fared quite well in direct outcome comparisons with medication. Most of the time, psychotherapy treatment results proved to be equal or superior to the outcomes obtained with drug treatments. For example, eight trials were discovered that pitted antidepressant drugs against depression-specific psychotherapies in the same studies. Five of the eight reports indicated that psychotherapy was superior to the drug in promoting substantial change (Bellack, Hersen, & Himmelhoch, 1981; Beutler et al., 1987; Blackburn et al., 1981, General Practice Sample; McLean & Hakstian, 1979; A. J. Rush, Beck, Kovacs, & Hollon, 1977). The remaining three trials found psychotherapy to be equivalent to medication in fostering improvement (Blackburn et al., 1981, Hospital Outpatient Sample; Murphy, Simons, Wetzel, & Lustman, 1984; Weissman et al., 1979). None of the trials showed the drug treatments to be superior.

Looking at these findings, we wondered if adding drugs to psychotherapy would produce better results. Eleven trials addressing this issue were located. In nine of the trials, adding drugs to psychotherapy produced no additional benefits for treatment outcome (Beck et al., 1985; Bellack et al., 1981; Beutler et al., 1987; Blackburn et al., 1981, General Practice Sample; DeRubeis, 1983; Murphy et al., 1984; Roth, Bielski, Jones, Parker, & Osborn, 1982; A. J. Rush & Watkins, 1981; Wilson, 1982). The other two trials suggested that combining psychotherapy with drugs produced advantages over either treatment alone (Blackburn et al., 1981, Hospital Outpatient Sample; DiMascio et al., 1979; Weissman et al., 1979). In finding the combination treatment preferable, Weissman and her collaborators suggested that psychotherapy and drugs had their impacts on different aspects of the clinical presentation. Whereas drugs appeared to influence mainly sleep and appetite, psychotherapy's effects were more wide-ranging affecting mood, apathy, suicidal ideation, work, and interest. Some evidence was later presented for differential treatment response between those classified as having situational depressions and those diagnosed with endogenous depressions (Prusoff, Weissman, Klerman, & Rounsaville, 1980). Those with situational depressions appeared to respond best to interpersonal therapy, with drugs providing no added benefits. A combination of interpersonal psychotherapy and medication was deemed best for those with the endogenous classification.

Another analysis available to us at the time of our previous review also focused on studies (published between 1974 and 1984) that contrasted combined treatments with either psychotherapy or medication delivered alone (Conte, Plutchik, Wild, & Karasu, 1986). Seventeen reports on 11 patient samples were analyzed with a statistical procedure that weighted studies based on their design adequacy. It was concluded that combined treatment was "slightly" more effective than the application of either drugs or psychotherapy alone. However, it was acknowledged that the results could also be interpreted to mean that most often combined treatments offer no advantage over the individual treatments delivered singly. The likelihood was four times greater that psychotherapy would be equal to the combined treatment than be inferior to it, and it was twice as likely that drug treatment would equal the combined treatment than fall short of its results.

Also available to us for our past review (Greenberg & Fisher, 1989) was a meta-analysis conducted by Steinbrueck, Maxwell, and Howard (1983). This work statistically compressed the results of 56 outcome studies examining the relative effectiveness of psychotherapy and drug therapy in the treatment of unipolar depression in adults. Although each treatment had to be compared with a control group, the psychotherapy and the drug therapy did not have to occur in the same studies to be included. Effect sizes completed for each study were the measures of treatment effectiveness used for comparison purposes. Psychotherapy outcome was judged to be superior to drug therapy outcome with an average effect size that was twice as large. However, because data on the two types of treatment were drawn from studies conducted under different conditions, caution is required in interpreting the results. Outcome differences might be accounted for on the basis of differences in study characteristics rather than differences in treatment modes. Some of the differences may have favored psychotherapy outcome (e.g., lack of double-blind procedures in psychotherapy studies), whereas others may have biased results toward more favorable drug outcomes (e.g., studied drug treatments lasted almost twice as long on average as psychotherapy treatments, 7 weeks vs. 4 weeks). Therefore, although the results pointed to psychotherapy superiority, there was no way to be sure that the demonstrated advantage was due only to treatment differences.

Advocates of biological treatment have sometimes tried to downplay the modest showing of antidepressants relative to psychotherapy and placebo treatments in many studies, by suggesting that medications are likely to be more effective in "real life" because of the greater freedom physicians would have to change dosages or drugs. Two studies address this speculation and each produced evidence that antidepressants may be even less uniquely efficacious in everyday practice than they are in drug trials. Teasdale, Fennell, Hibbert, and Amies (1984) looked at the treatment outcomes for 34 general practice patients with a major depressive disorder (91% were classified as definite or probably endogenous major depressive disorder based on the Research Diagnostic Criteria). Patients were assigned randomly to either the treatment they would normally receive (which relied on antidepressant medication) or a course of the usual treatment plus cognitive psychotherapy. The patients receiving the combined treatment did significantly better than those receiving the typical medical treatment, as measured by blind and independent assessments of symptom severity (i.e., the Hamilton Rating Scale for Depression and the Montgomery Asberg Depression Scale). Patients receiving the cognitive treatment also rated themselves as less depressed than those receiving routine treatment. At termination, only 23% in the usual treatment condition rated themselves as not depressed (on the Beck Depression Inventory) as compared to 82% of the psychotherapy patients. If improvement criteria were relaxed to include those who were mildly depressed post-treatment, 58% of the usual treatment sample were judged to have benefited. Follow-up results 3 months later showed the usual treatment group eventually reached the recovery level of the combined treatment group.

Another study (unavailable for the Greenberg & Fisher, 1989, review) presented data on outpatients with major depression treated as their physicians saw fit, unconstrained by having to follow a research protocol (Brugha et al., 1992). The 119 patients were almost evenly divided between those classified as endogenous depression and those classified as neurotic depression. Outcome over a 4-month period proved to be unrelated to whether or not tricyclic drugs had been prescribed. Furthermore, neither the type nor severity of depression played a role in the results. Dosage level was not a significant factor either. The authors concluded that significant improvement took place for the majority of patients; but, "this improvement was not related to drug treatment" (p. 10).

An additional pertinent point should be reiterated regarding trials in which psychotherapy is compared with drug treatment. Hollon and DeRubeis (1981) suggest that the psychotherapy-plus-placebo combination used to represent psychotherapy in many comparative trials may actually create misleading results. Using data from several comparative studies, they found that psychotherapy alone appeared to be a more potent treatment than psychotherapy-plus-placebo. One explanation for this, consistent with our experience, is that perhaps patients taking placebos (or medications for that matter) are less inclined to invest themselves in psychosocial treatment while they await the "magical" biochemical solution to their discomforts. In any event, if the observation of Hollon and DeRubeis proves to be correct, reviews of the literature may underestimate psychotherapy effects when compared with medication.

Overall, our previous overview of the research literature (Greenberg & Fisher, 1989) left us cautiously optimistic about the relative merits of psychosocial treatments for depression and inclined to support their use as the initial treatments of choice for most cases of depression. We concluded:

> A growing number of carefully done trials comparing active, focused psychotherapies (such as cognitive or interpersonal therapy) to antidepressant drug treatment suggests that depressed outpatients receiving psychotherapy do at least as well, and sometimes better, then those receiving drugs. Although drugs may help patients with their sleep disturbances, research

shows they are often less efficient than psychotherapy in helping patients with depression and apathy . . . and frequently ineffective in aiding patients in their social adjustment, interpersonal relationships, or work performance. . . . In contrast, psychotherapy with similar depressed outpatients has led to improvements in overall adjustment, interpersonal communication, and work performance while reducing interpersonal friction and anxious rumination. (p. 16)

Several additional independent reviews of the comparative efficacy of antidepressant and psychotherapy treatments have appeared since the publication of our analysis of the literature (Greenberg & Fisher, 1989). The later reviews have presented the evidence in both narrative (Antonuccio, 1995; Antonuccio et al., 1995; Clarkin, Pilkonis, & Magruder, 1996; Muñoz et al., 1994; Persons, Thase, & Crits-Christoph, 1996; Thase & Kupfer, 1996) and meta-analytic form (Dobson, 1989; Hollon, Shelton, & Loosen, 1991; Robinson, Berman, & Neimeyer, 1990; Wexler & Cicchetti, 1992). The reviews overlap to some degree in the studies covered. Yet, their appraisals of the effects of contrasting treatments for depression delivered to thousands of patients are arrived at independently. Despite diverse approaches for the reviews, the main conclusion reached by virtually all reexaminations of the evidence is strikingly reminiscent of our 1989 judgment: To the degree it has been scientifically tested, depression-specific psychotherapies have turned out to be either equally effective or more effective than drugs for most cases of depression.

Several meta-analyses have appeared since Steinbrueck et al., (1983, described earlier) concluded that psychotherapy was significantly more potent than medications in treating depression with an effect size that was twice as large. Dobson (1989) confined his meta-analytic review to only comparisons between cognitive therapy and other therapeutic modalities. Comparisons were made on the basis of a single common outcome measure, the Beck Depression Inventory, which is a patient-rated measure. Eight studies involving 721 patients contrasted cognitive therapy with tricyclic antidepressants. Cognitive therapy was found to be superior with the average treated patient doing better than 70% of drug-treated patients.

Robinson et al. (1990), in a meta-analytic survey of controlled studies, did not confine themselves only to cognitive therapy studies or to one measure of outcome. They were able to find 15 studies that provided the pertinent comparisons between psychotherapy, medication, or the two in combination. In the initial analyses, psychotherapy was more effective than pharmacotherapy in treating depression. Combination treatment did not differ from the outcomes of either treatment alone. The review then went on to suggest that the discovered differences in outcome might be an artifact of researcher allegiance to one or another treatment method. Introductory comments for each study were used to rate researcher allegiance. When the allegiance factor was controlled statistically, all approaches (including variants of psychotherapy) produced equivalent benefits. Commenting on investigator allegiance, Antonuccio et al. (1995) caution that if allegiance correlates with a third variable like scientific rigor or efficacy, statistically controlling for allegiance may inappropriately handicap studies that are well designed or show large effects of a particular treatment. Allegiance effects have also been addressed by Gaffan, Tsaousis, and Kemp-Wheeler (1995). They focused on this factor in reanalyzing the studies in Dobson's (1989) meta-analytic review and contrasting the results with a sample of more recently published research. They concluded that Dobson's results were indeed inflated by researcher allegiance. However, unlike Robinson et al., even after taking allegiance into account, the superiority of cognitive treatment to medication remained, albeit at a lower level. Gaffan and colleagues also noted that the more recently published set of studies showed no effect of researcher allegiance.

A meta-analytic review by Hollon et al. (1991) also compared the impact of cognitive therapy and tricyclic medication over nine randomized controlled studies involving 542 patients. They concluded that cognitive therapy is comparable to medication treatments for acute depressive episodes and that combined therapy offers no advantages over either approach delivered singly (although additional larger scale studies are needed to solidify this conclusion). Finally, they suggested that cognitive therapy, with or without drugs, may be more beneficial for reducing the risk of relapse after termination. Conclusions of this analysis were presented tentatively because of study and design limitations, low power, and the possibility of differential rates of retention for the various treatments.

Wexler and Cicchetti (1992) were particularly interested in the practical implications for outpatient treatment that might be drawn from well-designed outcome studies. With this aim, seven studies (comprising 513 patients) were reviewed and comparisons were made between psychotherapy, pharmacotherapy, and combined treatment on success rates, failure rates, and dropout rates. Overall, combined treatment showed no advantage over psychotherapy alone and only a small advantage over drug treatment alone. However, when dropout rates were considered along with success rates, both psychotherapy alone and combined treatments proved to be substantially better than the drug alone treatment. They concluded that in the absence of special considerations, psychotherapy should be the recommended treatment of first choice for depression because it is less costly than combined treatments and exposes patients to fewer side effects. Putting the treatments in a larger context, they reasoned that of every 100 patients presenting with major depression, only 29 will be treated success-fully by medications alone. Of 100 similar patients, 47 would be expected to recover successfully if treated by either psychotherapy alone or by com-bined treatment. Negative outcomes (defined by dropouts or no response) would be expected in 52 out of any 100 patients treated by medication alone. Negative outcomes would be expected in only 30 patients treated by psychotherapy alone or 34 patients receiving combined treatment.

After scanning the available scientific evidence, the authors of three major narrative reviews agree, in concert with us, that the benefits of psy-chotherapy for the treatment of depression are frequently underrated. Muñoz et al. (1994) offer a reasoned, well-documented, balanced, and diplomatically worded challenge to the biologically skewed recommen-dations contained in the Depression in Primary Care Guidelines pub-lished by the Agency for Health Care Policy and Research. They conclude, "With the exception of psychotic depressions, psychotherapy is at least as effective as pharmacotherapy and is free from complications for most pa-tients. Moreover, psychotherapy may provide a greater breadth of bene-fits than pharmacotherapy" (p. 57).

Persons et al. (1996), following a consummate review of the research lit-erature, also voice concerns about the treatment guidelines issued by the Depression Guideline Panel (1993) as well as those published by the American Psychiatric Association (APA; 1993). They reach the judgment that the American Psychiatric Association Guideline "understates the value of cognitive, behavioral, brief psychodynamic, and group therapies" and "overvalues the role of combined psychotherapy-pharmacotherapy regimens" (p. 283). Both treatment guidelines are appraised as deficient because they "understate the value of psychotherapy alone in the treat-ment of more severely depressed outpatients" (p. 283).

Similar sentiments are expressed by Antonuccio et al. (1995) following a thorough review of the research literature. They state:

> In our view, there is a tendency to underestimate the power and cost-effectiveness of a caring, confidential psychotherapeutic relationship in the treatment of depression. If we as therapists can learn to be patient in deal-ing with the emotional suffering of depressed individuals and help guide them through it with specific psychotherapeutic strategies, as many as 50% to 80% will respond within 8 to 16 weeks of treatment, without drugs and without the associated medical risks. For those who do not respond to psy-chotherapy, the costs and benefits of drug treatment or combined treatment can then be carefully weighed. . . . Despite the conventional wisdom, the data suggest that there is no stronger medicine than psychotherapy in the treatment of depression, even if severe. (p. 582)

THE NATIONAL INSTITUTE OF MENTAL HEALTH TREATMENT OF DEPRESSION PROGRAM AND THE ISSUE OF SEVERITY

Even though several of the research analyses mentioned previously included findings from the National Institute of Mental Health (NIMH) Treatment of Depression Collaborative Research Program (TDCRP) (Elkin et al., 1989), no discussion of comparative effects of psychotherapy and antidepressants would be complete without explicit acknowledgment of this work. It is the 800-pound gorilla of comparative projects. Undoubtedly one of the largest, most ambitious and most publicized investigations of outcome within the mental health field, it has been the basis for more than 35 publications appearing in professional journals. The complexity of the research design—involving multiple treatment centers, multiple outcome measures, multiple ways of construing the subject sample, and multiple comparisons of four treatments—has fueled debates about the nature and interpretation of the data. The debates culminate in a five-paper interchange in the *Journal of Consulting and Clinical Psychology* (Elkin, Gibbons, Shea, & Shaw, 1996; Jacobson & Hollon, 1996a, 1996b; Klein, 1996; McNally, 1996).

The design of the TDCRP involved the random assignment at three different sites of 250 unipolar depressed patients (45% of those initially screened) to four treatment conditions: cognitive-behavior therapy; interpersonal psychotherapy; imipramine plus clinical management; and a pill-placebo plus clinical management control condition. A total of 239 patients actually entered the treatments, which were planned to last 16 weeks, with a range of 16 to 20 sessions. Four scales were used to measure outcome at several points during treatment. These included clinician-rated measures (an abbreviated version of the Hamilton Depression Scale and the Global Assessment Scale) and patient-rated measures (Beck Depression Inventory and the Hopkins Symptom Checklist-90 total score). Outcome analyses were conducted on three overlapping samples of patients ranging from those who completed at least 15 weeks of treatment ($n = 155$) to those who received at least 3.5 weeks of treatment ($n = 204$) to all patients who entered treatment ($n = 239$).

It is not surprising that questions of interpretation would arise with so many ways to frame the data. Some of the findings have a "now you see it, now you don't" quality because they appear for some outcome measures with some sample configurations, but not for others. Nonetheless, the researchers involved in this project sought conclusions through attempts to derive meaning from the pattern of results. There is something for everyone in this data. The good news is that all the study treatment conditions including placebo plus clinical management, appeared to produce significant and equivalent benefits for patients during the time they were in treatment (Elkin et al., 1989; Ogles, Lambert, & Sawyer, 1995). Puzzled by the strong placebo showing, the researchers attributed some of the positive effect to its being embedded in a context of clinical management, which was equated with supportive psychotherapy. Yet, the researchers were still uncomfortable with the failure to differentiate the outcomes for each treatment. They decided to perform some "secondary" or "exploratory" analyses on subject samples that were divided on the basis of depression severity. The use of the terms *secondary* and *exploratory* and the failure to state a priori hypotheses raised concerns for some critics about the possibility of the severity results being due only to chance because of the many previously unplanned comparisons being made.

Analyzing the results according to the severity level of depression revealed some differences favoring the drug treated and interpersonal psychotherapy groups over the placebo group, but only in the more severely depressed patients. Those with mild to moderate depressions (the majority of the subjects) did equally well with all treatments. Furthermore, even in the more severely depressed group, there remained little indication of differences in outcome among the three active treatment conditions. In a later analysis, with the use of a newer, more powerful statistical technique, additional significant differences emerged suggesting possible unique benefits for the severely depressed treated by the medications, particularly in comparison with either placebo or cognitively treated patients (Elkin et al., 1995).

Cognitive therapy advocates viewed with suspicion the relatively poor showing of cognitive therapy with the severely depressed because of conflicting findings from other research (Jacobson & Hollon, 1996a). They questioned whether cognitive treatment had been delivered in an optimal fashion and pointed to indications that one of the three treatment centers had achieved much better results with cognitive therapy, equivalent to those with drug therapy (Jacobson & Hollon, 1996b). It was noted that the study had no validated measures to ensure that the treatments were delivered in an equally skilled, competent fashion. The merits of the arguments were debated with dueling statistics, which did not resolve the differing viewpoints (Elkin et al., 1996; Jacobson & Hollon, 1996a, 1996b).

In any event, despite some unanswered questions, spottiness in the results, and lack of consistency with some other research, psychiatric groups writing guidelines for the treatment of depression (APA, 1993; DGP, 1993) made this project the centerpiece for the assertion that antidepressant medications should be the first-line treatment for severe depression. In reacting to this assertion, Jacobson and Hollon (1996a) caution that this is only one study and that treatment guidelines should reflect results of the entire empirical literature, rather than being overly tied to one investigation. This opinion is also voiced by other reviewers (Antonuccio et al., 1995; Muñoz et al., 1994; Persons et al., 1996) and is even endorsed by Elkin and her colleagues (1996).

Lost in the disputes, to some degree, is the TDCRP finding that, regardless of severity level, all treatment outcome differences vanished by the time of an 18-month follow-up (Shea et al., 1992). The results at that point were disappointing. The percentage of patients who completed treatment, recovered from major depression, and did not relapse for an 18-month period were as follows: cognitive behavior therapy 30%, interpersonal psychotherapy 26%, placebo 20%, and imipramine 19%. If all patients (including those who dropped out) are considered, the results look even worse. In each group, only a minority of the patients benefited from the treatment in the long run. In addition, patients receiving the antidepressant were most likely to seek treatment following termination, produced the highest probability of relapse, and exhibited the fewest weeks of reduced or minimal symptoms during the follow-up period. This project demonstrated a poor prognosis over time for patients who were treated with antidepressants (or any of the other approaches for that matter). The follow-up data led the authors to conclude that 16 weeks of treatment is not sufficient for most patients to achieve recovery and lasting improvement with the types of treatment administered.

What about the issue of severity in the context of the rest of the research literature? Are severely depressed patients likely to do better with antidepressants than with psychotherapy? Most studies reporting data relevant to this issue were conducted with outpatient subjects. The usual finding in these investigations has been that there is no indication that psychotherapy produces results that are inferior to antidepressants in patients whose depressions are labeled either more severe or endogenous (Blackburn et al., 1981; Hollon et al., 1992; Kovacs, Rush, Beck, & Hollon, 1981; McLean & Taylor, 1992; Murphy et al., 1984).

The investigation by Hollon et al. (1992) is representative of the findings concerning severity of depression and outcome that have emerged from most trials directly comparing psychotherapy and antidepressants. A cohort of 107 unipolar depressed outpatients were randomly assigned to 12 weeks of treatment with cognitive therapy alone, an antidepressant (imipramine) alone, or combined treatment. Severity in this study was strictly defined in a manner consistent with the NIMH TDCRP Project and care was taken to make sure that the antidepressant therapy was adequately delivered. The two types of treatment produced equivalent outcomes on both clinician and patient-rated measures, even for the most severely depressed patients. Poorer response was predicted by the level of initial severity for those treated by drugs, but not for those treated with cognitive psychotherapy. Combined treatments were not better than either of the therapies delivered alone.

Only a few studies suggest, in contrast to those previously listed, that antidepressants may add something positive to psychotherapy in the treatment of the severely depressed. Thase et al. (1994) contrasted the outcome results for outpatients treated with cognitive therapy alone, interpersonal therapy alone, or a combination treatment of medication and interpersonal therapy. In this study, level of severity did affect outcome for the different treatments. Among the less severe depressives, both psychotherapy alone and the combination treatment produced equivalent benefits. However, for the more severely depressed, the combined treatment outperformed either of the psychotherapies. A similar result appeared in a paper by Prusoff et al. (1980), which we mentioned earlier. In this work, depressions labeled endogenous showed indications of a better response when treated with a combination of interpersonal therapy and drugs, whereas depressions labeled situational responded just as well to the psychotherapy alone as they did to the combination treatment.

After assessing the evidence on severity in comparative trials of antidepressants and psychotherapy (as well as surveying the material presented in the "Endogenous-Neurotic Distinction" section of this chapter), we are inclined to agree with the conclusions drawn by other investigators who have appraised similar empirical work (Antonuccio et al., 1995; Persons et al., 1996; Muñoz et al., 1994). At least for depressed outpatients,[8] no matter what the level of severity, there is reason to believe that a trial of psychotherapy alone should be considered as a first treatment option for a period of months, with the possibility of adding medications if the patient remains unresponsive. An additional reason to consider psychotherapy is that some types of psychosocial treatment may help stave off relapse, a topic to be discussed in the next section.

RELAPSE

There is little doubt that a diagnosis of major depression is frequently accompanied by uncertain prospects for the future. As noted in a past review, depressed people are often subject to a return of their discomforting symptoms after a period of recovery (Greenberg & Fisher, 1989). In fact, a

---

[8] There is minimal research literature on the comparative effects of drugs and psychotherapy on inpatients and those classified as either psychotic depression or melancholic depression.

survey of the research literature indicates that about 50% of depressed patients relapse within 2 years of recovery (Belsher & Costello, 1988). Relapse becomes less likely, however, the longer an individual remains well. Since the introduction of antidepressants, the high rates of relapse observed when medications are terminated have resulted in recommendations for increasing lengths of treatment. From initial standards for medication treatments that lasted only until symptoms remitted, periods of treatment have lengthened, even to the point of experts advocating indefinite periods of medication for patients who have experienced repeated bouts of depression (e.g., Fava & Kaji, 1994; Frank et al., 1990; Kupfer et al., 1992; Prien & Kupfer, 1986; Reynolds et al., 1992; Thase & Sullivan, 1995). Previous treatment with drugs does not appear to reduce later risk (Hollon, Evans, & DeRubeis, 1990).

Research is beginning to suggest that there may be ways to remain free of depression without the cost and side-effect risk associated with prolonged antidepressant use. Initial results from several studies have encouraged reviewers in the optimistic belief that treatment with cognitive-behavioral therapy may be more effective than antidepressants in lowering the probability of relapse (e.g., Antonuccio et al., 1995; Greenberg & Fisher, 1989; Hollon et al., 1991; Muñoz et al., 1994).[9] Although the relevant studies vary in their degree of experimental control, measures, and sample sizes, they provide consistent evidence for the potential long-term benefits of cognitive therapy treatments.

Five studies have been reported showing, to one degree or another, that after treatment is terminated, outpatients who had responded to cognitive therapy are less likely to relapse than those who had responded to antidepressant treatment (Blackburn, Eunson, & Bishop, 1986; Evans et al., 1992; Kovacs et al., 1981; Shea et al., 1992; Simons, Murphy, Levine, & Wetzel, 1986). Overall, previous cognitive therapy reduced the relapse rate by half in these investigations. An additional study, examining the long-term course for depressed inpatients, also found that adding cognitive therapy to medication treatment reduced the relapse rate by half in the year following treatment cessation (Miller, Norman, Keitner, Bishop, & Dow, 1989). In the one study comparing patients who terminated cognitive therapy to those continuing treatment on medications, cognitive therapy proved to be at least as beneficial for preventing relapse (Evans et al., 1992). In the 2 years following 3 months of treatment, patients receiving

---

[9] Only a couple of reports have examined the potential prophylactic effects of interpersonal psychotherapy, and they have not shown the benefits revealed by the studies of cognitive therapy (Shea et al., 1992; Weissman, Klerman, Prusoff, Sholomskas, & Padian, 1981).

cognitive therapy showed less than half the relapse rate of those receiving 3 months of medication alone. Moreover, patients who had 3 months of cognitive therapy proved to be as resistant to relapse as patients who continued on 15 months of medication.

The initial evidence on the prophylactic potential of cognitive therapy is promising, although further controlled research is needed to solidify the positive conclusions that have been drawn (Hollon et al., 1992). It should also be pointed out that many patients in the brief psychotherapy trials studied did not both respond to treatment and remain well for extended periods. Therefore, numerous patients may require more extended periods of psychotherapy. The development of "continuation" psychotherapy, like "continued" medication, may be required for difficult, resistant cases following short-term therapy (Thase & Simons, 1992; Thase & Sullivan, 1995).

BIPOLAR DISORDER

The manic-depressive syndrome occupies a central position in psychiatric nosology. In contrast to unipolar depressives, the manic-depressive (bipolar) displays cycles of alternating affects. Detailed criteria for diagnosing manic depressive states are provided by various versions of the DSM; but, in essence, they depict cyclic shifts between feeling significantly depressed and feeling irrationally elated or excited. Lithium has for some time been considered one of the most effective therapeutic agents for controlling manic-depressive symptomatology. It was first tried by Cade (1949). Early evidence for its effectiveness was almost entirely anecdotal.

In the 1970s, however, a series of controlled studies appeared that apparently demonstrated a high level of success for lithium in treating manic-depressive symptoms, particularly with reference to preventing their recurrence after clinical recovery. This series comprised roughly 10 studies that have been enumerated and described by F. K. Goodwin and Jamison (1990) and others (Moncrieff, 1995; Vestergaard, 1992). Typically, the studies were double-blind and often involved comparing pairs of groups of bipolar patients who had been clinically stabilized on lithium: One patient was continued on lithium and the other taken off lithium and placed on placebo. In some instances, the patients were not initially on lithium and were randomly assigned to lithium or placebo. About a third of the studies could be dismissed because they were based on small inadequate samples. However, the remainder were impressive because not only did they involve reasonably large numbers of patients but they also came up with striking therapeutic differences between lithium and placebo. F. K. Goodwin and Jamison (1990) indicated that the average relapse rate in these studies for patients on placebo was 81% whereas the average for those remaining on lithium was 34%. Thus, there was a hefty 47% difference reported. Indeed, the results were so impressive that lithium became the standard therapeutic agent for bipolars. It was hailed as the equivalent of a magic bullet. More contemporary studies have not lived up to such early glowing reports. Increasing disappointments with lithium in the course of everyday clinical practices have led to the supplementary use of a range of other drugs (e.g., antipsychotics, carbamazepine). Further discussion of this matter will be offered shortly.

Looking back at the dazzling data reported by the studies of lithium in the 1970s, one can see that they were not appraised with sufficient critical caution. At that time, there was limited awareness of the exaggerated placebo effects that inflate the apparent effectiveness of active drugs when they are newly introduced by loyal enthusiasts. Roberts (1995) has documented this point well. It is also true that there was only slight awareness at that time of the vulnerability of the double-blind to penetration by bias (e.g., Fisher & Greenberg, 1993). Actually, there is documentation of lithium's specific vulnerability in this respect because of clues provided by its characteristic side-effects (e.g., polyuria, weight gain, tremor) (Marini et al., 1976; Stallone, Mendlewicz, & Fieve, 1975). One could reasonably ask whether a significant amount of enhancing bias might have been present in the early enthusiastic findings concerning lithium. The combination of that unique "new treatment" enthusiasm with the probable opportunity to circumvent the double-blind guarantee of blindness would not bode well for objectivity.[10] There was reason to wonder whether the glowing findings of the early lithium studies might be exaggerated.

With this perspective, we examined several of the early major investigations in some detail to ascertain how their designs might or might not have rendered them specifically susceptible to distorting influences. We chose to appraise those five studies that were based on fairly substantial numbers of patients and also that seriously applied controls, such as random assignment and versions of the double-blind (viz., Baastrup, Poulsen, Schou, Thomsen, & Amdisen, 1970; Coppen et al., 1971; Dunner, Stallone, & Fieve, 1976; Prien, Caffey, & Klett, 1973; Stallone, Shelley, Mendlewicz, & Fieve, 1973).

One of the first points to impress us was that in all five instances the major criterion for defining therapeutic success of lithium versus placebo

---

[10] There is another matter to consider with respect to the double-blind issue. Numerous studies concerned with the effects of discontinuing lithium have been based on a design in which bipolar patients who have been taking lithium for an extended period are either continued on lithium or taken off and put on placebo instead. Because the placebo is disguised to look like the active medication, it is assumed that the patients do not know they have been switched. However, it would be amazing if patients who have had many months to observe the impact of lithium on their bodies did not quickly detect the alterations in body experiences initiated by discontinuing the active agent and starting on a placebo.

was how frequently patients were considered to have relapsed as indicated by the severity of manic-depressive symptoms they developed during a period of observation. The basic design in these studies revolved about identifying bipolar patients who had recovered (as the result of lithium treatment) from previous manic-depressive symptoms; then randomly assigning them to taking either lithium or placebo; finally monitoring their clinical states to ascertain when sufficiently disabling exacerbations occurred requiring hospitalization. Actually, in four studies relapse was considered to have occurred if the supervising psychiatrist simply felt that the patient's condition required "supplementary treatment." In one of the studies, however, (Coppen et al., 1971), particular care was taken to supplement the clinical relapse criterion with ratings of adjustment on standardized scales.

In any case, evaluating the success of lithium versus placebo primarily in terms of whether each patient's supervising clinician considered hospitalization to be necessary appears to be a risky and unreliable procedure. Even more problematic is equating clinical success or failure with the vaguely defined judgment whether the patient required "supplementary treatment." The decision whether to hospitalize a psychiatric patient is highly subjective and variable as a function of local standards. Consider the drastic changes in standards of hospitalization that evolved as managed care programs have gained power. The decision whether to hospitalize a patient is the end result of such multiple factors as the tolerance of the treating psychiatrist for potential complications (e.g., suicide), the need or lack of need to fill hospital beds, the tolerance of the patient's family for deviant behaviors, contemporary treatment standards, and so forth. It seems likely that if, in the course of a research protocol dealing with bipolars, the psychiatrist rendering decisions whether to hospitalize specific individuals was able to see through the double-blind and was also motivated to find results favorable to lithium, it would not be difficult to rationalize delaying the hospitalization of the treatment group (on lithium) and speeding up the hospitalizations of the placebo patients. A basic bias of this sort could have pervaded the 1970s studies and consistently given lithium an advantage over placebo.

Apropos of this point, it is telling that in one of the largest and most influentially decisive of the 1970 studies (viz., Prien et al., 1973) the psychiatrists who decided whether to hospitalize the lithium versus placebo patients were actually not blind concerning each patient's treatment status. Prien et al. were aware of the potential problem this raised concerning the integrity of the study. They commented:

Major treatment decisions such as hospitalization were made by the treatment physician who knew the identity of the patient's medications. This raises the question of physician bias and its effect on treatment outcome. A major concern is the possibility that the physician may have been quicker to hospitalize placebo patients than lithium carbonate patients, resulting in placebo patients being less severely ill at the time of hospitalization. Such a finding would make it difficult to interpret (the) data. (p. 340)

Prien et al., however, proceeded to dismiss this really serious defect in the research design by noting that blind evaluations obtained from other raters (e.g., psychologists) did not indicate any gross differences in the degree of disturbance between the lithium and placebo patients at the time of hospitalization. Aside from the real question whether these so-called blind raters were truly blind, detailed data are not provided concerning the degree of disturbance in the nonrelapsed lithium patients. It is not known whether they were significantly more disturbed than the nonrelapsed placebo patients. But even more importantly, the investigators state that the dosage levels of placebo patients were "rarely manipulated," whereas "about half of the severely relapsed patients on lithium carbonate had their dosage increased prior to hospitalization" (Prien et al., 1973, p. 341); and, further, "About one-sixth of the nonrelapsed patients on lithium carbonate had their dosage increased for poor clinical response. *This probably prevented relapse in some cases* [italics added]" (p. 341). Such comments are revealing because they indicate that the supervising psychiatrists were actively doing more to prevent relapses in the lithium than the placebo samples. Prien et al. try to minimize this defect in the design by noting that even if all the lithium patients whose dosages were manipulated were dropped from the data analysis there would still be a significant difference (although reduced) in relapse outcome between the lithium and placebo groups. However, this is simply post hoc damage control. Once targeted differences are identified in treatment strategies by the psychiatrists vis-à-vis the two classes of patients, it is certain that significant bias was exercised and we cannot rule out other serious ways in which it may have influenced the entire experiment. A study so obviously infiltrated by bias is simply not scientifically trustworthy.[11]

Moncrieff (1995) has leveled analogous criticisms at the Prien et al. findings. Thus, he noted:

---

[11] Other criticisms could be raised concerning the early bipolar studies. Lithium often could not be shown to reduce depressive (compared with manic) episodes; and limited attention was given to the effects of high dropout rates on the overall results (Himmelhoch, 1994; Moncrieff, 1995). G. M. Goodwin (1995), on the other hand, feels that the defects in the early studies have been exaggerated and do not vitiate the basic lithium versus placebo differences that were reported.

The trouble with . . . the Prien et al. (study) is that it was not double-blind. The treating psychiatrists, responsible for diagnosing and managing relapse, were aware of the identity of subjects' medication. They were also instructed to increase the dose of lithium when a patient on lithium started to show symptoms. The importance of this issue is that it means the treatment conditions of the two groups were not comparable. If lithium is an effective antimanic agent, some of the lithium group were therefore receiving early treatment for mania. It is also probable that this was accompanied by other efforts to prevent relapse in these patients, such as increased social support. (p. 571)

Finally, most of the early investigations based on experimental paradigms similar to that of the Prien et al. study involved the use of patients who had had multiple previous manic episodes and who had already demonstrated positive therapeutic response to lithium. Often they are described as having been "stabilized" on lithium before being subjected to experimental manipulations (e.g., being discontinued from lithium). Two troubling issues emerge. First, patients who have had a large number of manic episodes may constitute an extreme category of bipolars and therefore not be suitably representative. Second, if the patients in these studies had already been "stabilized" on lithium, they could be a selective "responder" sample. There is no dependable way of ascertaining how many patients were in the original pool from which the responders emerged. This means that relapse rates cited for those taken off lithium could very well be deceptively favorable because they discount the unknown numbers of patients who originally responded to lithium only minimally.

Parenthetically, if the patients in the early investigations were, indeed, relatively more seriously disturbed than the average bipolar, this would artificially inflate the placebo relapse rates. Suppes, Baldessarini, Faedda, and Tohen (1991) commented:

Prien et al. found a 68% risk of relapse in . . . placebo-treated patients within a year. However, such rates . . . in placebo trials may reflect the study of relatively ill patients . . . many of whom were specifically selected for having had relatively frequent episodes or were recovering from an acute episode of mania. In short, this experience with relapse rates in placebo-treated bipolar patients should not be accepted as representing the natural history of recurrences in typical untreated patients over prolonged follow-up. (p. 1086)

Our skepticism about the hyperpositive reports that emerged from the early investigations of lithium was affirmed by later findings. In a meta-analysis, Baker (1994) examined all of the available studies carried out since 1985 that concerned the comparative effects on bipolar patients of discontinuing their lithium (going on a placebo) or remaining on lithium. His search of the literature yielded 19 studies (with a total of 546 patients). In essence, he found overall that patients who remained on lithium relapsed significantly less often than those who shifted to placebo. However, the average difference was only 16% (37.5 vs. 53.5).[12] This stands in contrast to the claims of earlier studies that the superiority of lithium continuation was on the order of multiple times higher.[13]

One of Baker's particularly striking findings was that rate of lithium withdrawal was a significant element in the relapse rate. He encountered several studies in which it was possible to ascertain the differential impact of fast versus slow withdrawal. Fast withdrawal was accomplished roughly within a 2-week period; and slow withdrawal meant taking longer than 2 weeks or in one instance simply involved a large reduction in dosage. Baker summarized the pooled data from these studies as follows: "Of those in the rapid withdrawal condition, 46 out of 74 (62%) suffered relapse compared to 23 out of 78 (29%) of those who withdrew gradually or had their lithium reduced" (p. 191).

The 29% relapse rate of those who were withdrawn from lithium gradually compares quite favorably with numerous reports of modal relapse rates of patients who were not taken off lithium.[14] This is an extraordinarily important finding. It suggests that it was not so much being taken off lithium that produced relapse as the shock of doing so suddenly. One could interpret this at a psychological level as meaning that the speed of the change was so great that it undermined existing self-anchors and security defenses. Apparently, when the change was more gradual, there was an opportunity to adapt fairly successfully. Himmelhoch (1994) offers a more physiologically phrased possible explanation of what occurs with a sudden decrease of lithium dosage: "Manic relapse is readily triggered, probably by the release of supersensitized receptors or membrane pathways" (p. 245). Possibly both levels of explanation are cogent. It should also be noted that Baldessarini and Viguera (1995) present data indicating that abrupt withdrawal of antipsychotics from schizophrenics significantly increases relapse rates compared with more gradual withdrawal.

In contrast to the somewhat modest outcome results depicted by Baker, a meta-analysis (based on 10 studies) presented by Davis, Wang, and Janicak (1993) reported that the relapse rate for patients on maintenance lithium

---

[12] It was also true that by the end of 18 months there was little or no difference between lithium continuers and discontinuers in the percentage who "survived" without relapse.
[13] One study claimed the risk of relapse was 28 times higher per month for discontinuers compared with continuers.
[14] It is difficult to ascertain what is a proper statement of the efficacy of lithium in treating acute manic symptoms. One finds citations ranging from 32% to 90% (e.g., Chou, 1991; Tryer, 1985; Vestergaard, 1992).

was 30%, whereas for those on placebo it was 85%. This is a difference of 55%. The Baker difference was only 16%. Why do the two analyses differ so starkly? One of the major possibilities is that the Baker meta-analysis was based only on studies completed after 1985; whereas Davis et al. provide no information concerning the source of the 10 studies involving bipolars they appraised. If the Davis et al. analysis included the hyperpositive findings of the flawed 1970 studies, one can see why such a large lithium-placebo difference would emerge. Also, the Davis et al. analysis seems to be totally unaware of the mediating factor relating to the speed with which patients are taken off lithium and assigned to placebo. There is no way of knowing what percentage of the patients covered by their meta-analysis had been shifted in less than or more than 2 weeks from lithium to placebo. In any case, the contradiction between the two meta-analyses leaves one with a sense of uncertainty. Such uncertainty highlights a point that we have made repeatedly—The data relating to the therapeutic efficacy of psychotropic drugs are often fragile and difficult to interpret.

Relatedly, Moncrieff (1995), after reviewing a number of the major controlled studies dealing with lithium prophylaxis, decided that their designs were often seriously flawed. He concluded: "Unfortunately, after scrutinizing the evidence, it seems that lithium might not be the successful prophylactic that was hoped for. Psychiatrists should, therefore, reappraise the current consensus on the long-term treatment of manic-depressive disorder" (p. 572).

The doubts raised here about the therapeutic power of lithium are mirrored in a number of publications that have scrutinized the effectiveness of lithium in actual routine clinical settings. Symonds and Williams (1981) reported that the readmission rate for mania in England had increased even though there was an overall larger number of prescriptions for lithium on record. Several studies involving multiple clinical sites in England and the United States (Harrow, Goldberg, Grossman, & Meltzer, 1990; Mander, 1986; Marker & Mander, 1989) essentially found that bipolar patients treated with lithium do not really fare better than those who do not receive lithium. One of the largest and best controlled of the studies involved 73 patients (Harrow et al., 1990). The investigators concluded as follows:[15]

> Manic patients taking lithium carbonate did not show better outcomes than those not taking lithium carbonate. The results suggest (1) many hospitalized manic patients have a severe, recurrent, and pernicious disorder; and

---

[15] The question has been raised in such studies whether the maximum power of lithium was mobilized in view of possible failure of patients to take their lithium consistently.

(2) in routine clinical practice, lithium carbonate treatment is an effective prophylaxis for fewer than the 70% to 80% of manic patients previously reported. (p. 665)[16]

Similar doubts can be detected in an overview by Thase and Kupfer (1996) of mood disorder research:

> More recent studies underscore the limitations of lithium salts for acute-phase treatment of mania. . . . Whereas success rates of 80% to 90% were once expected . . . lithium response rates of only 40% to 50% are now common. . . . Lithium efficacy for prophylaxis against mania also appears to be significantly lower now than in previous decades; 40% to 60% recurrence rates are now typical. (pp. 652, 653)

It should be added, though, that occasional reports (cited by F. K. Goodwin & Jamison, 1990) depict high positive therapeutic results for lithium prophylaxis in some clinical settings. It is not clear why such contradictory findings exist, but F. K. Goodwin and Jamison (1990) suggest, "Disparities in patient characteristics probably explain some of the discrepancy in findings" (p. 695).

As earlier indicated, dissatisfaction with lithium has also expressed itself in an active search for alternative therapeutic drugs (e.g., Chou, 1991; Prien & Gelenberg, 1989; Sachs, 1989). The suggested alternatives have variously included neuroleptics, anticonvulsants, and calcium channel blockers. Intermittent attempts have been made to compare the therapeutic efficacies of such agents with lithium. There are too few well-controlled studies to arrive at confident conclusions. However, some agents (e.g., carbamazepine) may possibly turn out to be roughly equivalent to lithium in therapeutic impact (Dardennes, Even, Bange, & Heim, 1995).

The history of the research relating to lithium follows a familiar pattern. Once again, there is a cycle of exaggerated initial results (fostered by

---

[16] Maj, Pirozzi, and Kemali (1991) reported, on the basis of an unusually lengthy follow-up (5 years) of 50 bipolar patients: "Overall, only 36% were still successfully treated with lithium carbonate prophylaxis . . . . These data suggest that the impact of lithium carbonate prophylaxis on the long-term course of bipolar affective disorder in ordinary clinical conditions is less dramatic than currently believed" (p. 772). Relatedly, Tohen, Waternaux, and Tsuang (1990) reported that in a naturalistic study involving a 4-year follow-up period, only 28% of the bipolars being treated (largely with lithium), were still in remission at the 4-year end point. Further, Solomon, Keitner, Miller, Shea, and Keller (1995) concluded after a literature review: "A substantial percentage of patients ultimately fails lithium prophylaxis . . . studies show . . . findings with failure rates extending as high as 42% to 64%" (p. 6).

enthusiasm and rents in the double-blind design); then, increasingly more conservative reports concerning the magnitude of the difference in efficacy between active drug and placebo; growing disappointment among clinicians with their everyday results; and heightened efforts to find alternative treatments that will compensate for what the original magic bullet no longer achieves.

REFERENCES

Amenson, C. S., & Lewinsohn, P. M. (1981). An investigation into the observed sex difference in prevalence of unipolar depression. *Journal of Abnormal Psychology, 90,* 1–13.

American College of Neuropsychopharmacology Task Force. (1993). Suicidal behavior and psychotropic medication. *Neuropsychopharmacology, 8,* 177–182.

American Psychiatric Association. (1980). *Diagnostic and statistical manual of mental disorders* (3rd ed.). Washington, DC: Author.

American Psychiatric Association. (1993). Practice guideline for major depressive disorder in adults. *American Journal of Psychiatry, 150*(Suppl. 4), 1–26.

American Psychiatric Association (APA) Task Force. (1985). Tricyclic antidepressants—Blood level measurements and clinical outcome. *American Journal of Psychiatry, 142,* 155–162.

Anderson, I. M., & Tomenson, B. M. (1994). The efficacy of selective serotonin reuptake inhibitors in depression: A meta-analysis of studies against tricyclic antidepressants. *Journal of Psychopharmacology, 4,* 238–249.

Anderson, I. M., & Tomenson, B. M. (1995). Treatment discontinuation with selective serotonin reuptake inhibitors compared with tricyclic antidepressants: A meta-analysis. *British Medical Journal, 310,* 1433–1438.

Anstay, K., & Brodaty, H. (1995). Antidepressants and the elderly: Double-blind trials 1987–1992. *International Journal of Geriatric Psychiatry, 10,* 265–279.

Antonuccio, D. O. (1995). Psychotherapy for depression: No stronger medicine. *American Psychologist, 50,* 450–451.

Antonuccio, D. O., Danton, W. G., & DeNelsky, G. Y. (1995). Psychotherapy versus medication for depression: Challenging the conventional wisdom with data. *Professional Psychology: Research and Practice, 26,* 574–585.

Arya, D. K. (1994). Extrapyramidal symptoms with selective serotonin reuptake inhibitors. *British Journal of Psychiatry, 165,* 728–733.

Atkinson, R. M., & Ditman, K. S. (1965). Tranylcypromine: A review. *Clinical Pharmacology and Therapeutics, 6,* 631–655.

Baastrup, P. C., Poulsen, J. C., Schou, M., Thomsen, K., & Amdisen, A. (1970, August 15). Prophylactic lithium: Double blind discontinuation in manic-depressive and recurrent-depressive disorders. *Lancet, ii,* 326–330.

Baker, J. P. (1994). Outcomes of lithium discontinuation: A meta-analysis. *Lithium, 5,* 187–192.

Baldessarini, R. J. (1989). Current status of antidepressants: Clinical pharmacology and therapy. *Journal of Clinical Psychiatry, 50,* 117–126.

Baldessarini, R. J., & Viguera, A. C. (1995). Neuroleptic withdrawal in schizophrenic patients. *Archives of General Psychiatry, 52,* 189–192.

Balon, R., Yeragani, V. K., Pohl, R., & Ramesh, C. (1993). Sexual dysfunction during antidepressant treatment. *Journal of Clinical Psychiatry, 54,* 209–212.

Beasley, C. M., Dornseif, B. E., Bosonworth, J. C., Sayler, M. E., Rampey, A. H., Heiligenstein, J. H., Thompson, V. L., Murphy, D. J., & Masica, D. N. (1992). Fluoxetine and suicide: A meta-analysis of controlled trials of treatment for depression. *International Clinical Psychopharmacology, 6*(Suppl. 6), 35–57.

Bech, P. (1993). Acute therapy of depression. *Journal of Clinical Psychiatry, 54,* 18–27.

Beck, A. T. (1967). *Depression: Causes and treatment.* Philadelphia: University of Pennsylvania Press.

Beck, A. T., Hollon, S. D., Young, Y. E., Bedrosian, R. C., & Budenz, D. (1985). Treatment of depression with cognitive therapy and amitriptyline. *Archives of General Psychiatry, 42,* 142–148.

Beck, A. T., Ward, C. H., Mendelson, M., Mock, J., & Erbaugh, J. (1961). An inventory for measuring depression. *Archives of General Psychiatry, 4,* 561–571.

Bellack, A. S., Hersen, M., & Himmelhoch, J. (1981). Social skills training compared with pharmacotherapy and psychotherapy in the treatment of unipolar depression. *American Journal of Psychiatry, 138,* 1562–1567.

Belsher, G., & Costello, C. G. (1988). Relapse after recovering from unipolar depression: A critical review. *Psychological Bulletin, 104,* 84–96.

Beutler, L. E., Scogin, F., Kirkish, P., Schretlen, D., Corbishley, A., Hamblin, D., Meredith, K., Potter, R., Bamford, C. R., & Levenson, A. I. (1987). Group cognitive therapy and alprazolam in the treatment of depression in older adults. *Journal of Consulting and Clinical Psychology, 55,* 550–556.

Bialik, R. J., Ravindran, A. V., Bakish, D., & Lapierre, Y. D. (1995). A comparison of placebo responders and nonresponders in subgroups of depressive disorders. *Journal of Psychiatry and Neuroscience, 20,* 265–270.

Bielski, R. J., & Friedel, R. O. (1976). Prediction of tricyclic antidepressant response. *Archives of General Psychiatry, 33,* 1479–1489.

Black, D. W., & Winokur, G. (1990). Suicide and psychiatric diagnosis. In S. J. Blumenthal & D. J. Kupfer (Eds.), *Suicide over the life cycle: Risk factors, assessment, and treatment of suicidal patients* (pp. 135–153). Washington, DC: American Psychiatric Press.

Blackburn, I. M., Bishop, S., Glen, A. I. M., Whalley, L. J., & Christie, J. E. (1981). The efficacy of cognitive therapy in depression: A treatment trial using cognitive therapy and pharmacotherapy, each alone and in combination. *British Journal of Psychiatry, 139,* 181–189.

Blackburn, I. M., Eunson, K. M., & Bishop, S. (1986). A two-year naturalistic follow-up of depressed patients treated with cognitive therapy, pharmacotherapy and a combination of both. *Journal of Affective Disorders, 10,* 67–75.

Blackwell, B. (1982). Antidepressant drugs: Side effects and compliance. *Journal of Clinical Psychiatry, 43,* 14–18.

Blehar, M. C., Weissman, M. M., Gershon, E. S., & Hirschfeld, R. M. A. (1988). Family and genetic studies of affective disorders. *Archives of General Psychiatry, 45,* 289–292.

Breggin, P. R. (1991). *Toxic psychiatry*. New York: St. Martin's Press.

Brown, W. A. (1994a). Placebo as a treatment for depression. *Neuropsychopharmacology, 10*, 265–269.

Brown, W. A. (1994b). Reply to commentaries. *Neuropsychopharmacology, 10*, 287–288.

Brown, W. A., Johnson, M. F., & Chen, M. G. (1992). Clinical features of depressed patients who do and do not improve with placebo. *Psychiatry Research, 41*, 203–214.

Brugha, T. S., Bebbington, P. E., MacCarthy, B., Sturt, E., & Wykes, T. (1992). Antidepressants may not assist recovery in practice: A naturalistic prospective survey. *Acta Psychiatrica Scandinavica, 86*, 5–11.

Buchholtz-Hansen, P. E., Wang, A. G., Kragh-Sorensen, P., and the Danish University Antidepressant Group (1993). Mortality in major affective disorder: Relationship to subtype of depression. *Acta Psychiatrica Scandinavica, 87*, 329–335.

Buda, M., & Tsuang, M. T. (1990). The epidemiology of suicide: Implications for clinical practice. In S. J. Blumenthal & D. J. Kupfer (Eds.), *Suicide over the life cycle: risk factors, assessment, and treatment of suicidal patients* (pp. 17–37). Washington, DC: American Psychiatric Press.

Cade, F. (1949). Lithium salts in the treatment of psychotic excitement. *Medical Journal of Australia, 2*, 349–352.

Chou, J. C. Y. (1991). Recent advances in treatment of acute mania. *Journal of Clinical Psychopharmacology, 11*, 3–21.

Clarkin, J. F., Pilkonis, P. A., & Magruder, K. M. (1996). Psychotherapy of depression. *Archives of General Psychiatry, 53*, 717–723.

Cole, J. O. (1964). Therapeutic efficacy of antidepressant drugs. A review. *Journal of the American Medical Association, 190*, 124–131.

Conte, H. R., Plutchik, R., Wild, K. V., & Karasu, T. B. (1986). Combined psychotherapy and pharmacotherapy with treatment of depression. A systematic analysis of the evidence. *Archives of General Psychiatry, 43*, 471–479.

Coppen, A., Noguera, R., Bailey, J., Burns, B. H., Swani, M. S., Hare, E. H., Gardner, R., & Maggs, R. (1971, August 7). Prophylactic lithium in affective disorders. *Lancet, ii*, 275–279.

Cowley, G., Springen, K., Leonard, E. A., Robins, K., & Gordon, J. (1990, March). The promise of Prozac. *Newsweek*, 38–41.

Damluji, N. F., & Ferguson, J. M. (1988). Paradoxical worsening of depressive symptomatology caused by antidepressants. *Journal of Clinical Psychopharmacology, 5*, 347–349.

Dardennes, R., Even, C., Bange, F., & Heim, A. (1995). Comparison of carbamazepine and lithium in the prophylaxis of bipolar disorders. *British Journal of Psychiatry, 166*, 378–381.

Dasgupta, K. (1990). Additional cases of suicidal ideation associated with fluoxetine. *American Journal of Psychiatry, 147*, 1570.

Davis, J. (1965). Efficacy of tranquilizing and antidepressant drugs. *Archives of General Psychiatry, 13*, 552–572.

Davis, J., Klerman, G., & Schildkraut, J. (1968). Drugs used in the treatment of depression. In D. H. Efron (Ed.), *Psychopharmacology: A review of progress* (1957–1967) (pp. 719–747). Public Health Service Publication No. 1,836.

Davis, J. M., Wang, Z., & Janicak, P. G. (1993). A quantitative analysis of clinical drug trials for the treatment of affective disorders. *Psychopharmacology Bulletin, 29,* 175–181.

Depression Guideline Panel. (1993). *Depression in primary care: Vol. 2. Treatment of major depression* (Clinical Practice Guideline No. 5, AHCPR Publication No. 93-0551). Rockville, MD: Department of Health and Human Services, Public Health Service, Agency for Health Care Policy and Research.

DePue, R. A., & Iacono, W. G. (1989). Neurobehavioral aspects of affective disorders. In M. R. Rosenzweig & L. W. Porter (Eds.), *Annual review of psychology* (Vol. 40, pp. 457–492). Palo Alto, CA: Annual Reviews.

DeRubeis, R. J. (1983, December). *The cognitive-pharmacotherapy project: Study design, outcome, and clinical follow-up.* Paper presented at the meeting of the American Association of Behavior Therapy, Washington, DC.

Dewan, M. J., & Koss, M. (1989). The clinical impact of the side effects of psychotropic drugs. In S. Fisher & R. P. Greenberg (Eds.), *The limits of biological treatments for psychological distress: Comparisons with psychotherapy and placebo* (pp. 189–234). Hillsdale, NJ: Erlbaum.

Dewan, M. J., & Koss, M. (1995). The clinical impact of reported variance in potency of antipsychotic agents. *Acta Scandinavica Psychiatrica, 91,* 229–232.

Diekstra, R. F. W. (1989). Suicide and attempted suicide: An international perspective. *Acta Psychiatrica Scandinavica, 80*(Suppl. 354), 1–24.

DiMascio, A., Weissman, M. M., Prusoff, B. A., Neu, C., Zwilling, M., & Klerman, G. L. (1979). Differential symptom reduction by drugs and psychotherapy in acute depression. *Archives of General Psychiatry, 36,* 1450–1456.

Dobson, K. S. (1989). A meta-analysis of the efficacy of cognitive therapy for depression. *Journal of Consulting and Clinical Psychology, 57,* 414–419.

Dunlop, S. R., Dornseif, B. E., Wernicke, J. F., & Potvin, J. H. (1990). Pattern analysis shows beneficial effect of fluoxetine treatment in mild depression. *Psychopharmacology Bulletin, 26,* 173–180.

Dunner, D. L. (1994). Commentary on "Placebo as treatment for depression." *Neuropsychopharmacology, 10,* 273–274.

Dunner, D. L., Stallone, F., & Fieve, R. R. (1976). Lithium carbonate and affective disorders. *Archives of General Psychiatry, 33,* 117–120.

Edwards, B. C., Lambert, M. J., Moran, P. W., McCully, T., Smith, K. C., & Ellingson, A. G. (1984). A meta-analytic comparison of the Beck Depression Inventory and the Hamilton Rating Scale for Depression as measures of treatment outcome. *British Journal of Clinical Psychology, 23,* 93–99.

Edwards, J. G. (1992). Selective serotonin reuptake inhibitors: A modest though welcome advance in the treatment of depression. *British Medical Journal, 304,* 1644–1646.

Edwards, J. G. (1995). Drug choice in depression: Selective serotonin reuptake inhibitors or tricyclic antidepressants. *CNS Drugs, 4,* 141–159.

Elkin, I., Gibbons, R. D., Shea, M. T., & Shaw, B. F. (1996). Science is not a trial (but it can sometimes be a tribulation). *Journal of Consulting and Clinical Psychology, 64,* 92–103.

Elkin, I., Gibbons, R. D., Shea, M. T., Sotsky, S. M., Watkins, J. T., Pilkonis, P. A., & Hedeker, D. (1995). Initial severity and differential treatment outcome in the National Institute of Mental Health Treatment of Depression Collaborative Research Program. *Journal of Consulting and Clinical Psychology, 63,* 841–847.

Elkin, I., Shea, T., Watkins, J. T., Imber, S. D., Sotsky, S. M., Collins, J. F., Glass, D. R., Pilkonis, P. A., Leber, W. R., Docherty, J. P., Fiester, S. J., & Parloff, M. B. (1989). National Institute of Mental Health Treatment of Depression Collaborative Research Program: General effectiveness of treatments. *Archives of General Psychiatry, 46,* 971–982.

Engelhardt, D. M., & Margolis, R. (1967). Drug identity, doctor conviction & outcome. In H. Brill, J. Cole, P. Deniker, H. Hippius, & P. B. Bradley (Eds.), *Neuropsychopharmacology* (pp. 543–544). Amsterdam: Excerpta Medica Foundation.

Evans, M. D., Hollon, S. D., DeRubeis, R. J., Piasecki, J. M., Grove, W. M., Garvey, M. J., & Tuason, V. B. (1992). Differential relapse following cognitive therapy and pharmacotherapy for depression. *Archives of General Psychiatry, 49,* 802–808.

Fava, M., & Kaji, J. (1994). Continuation and maintenance treatments of major depressive disorder. *Psychiatric Annals, 24,* 281–290.

Feighner, J. P., Aden, G. C., Fabre, L. F., Rickels, K., & Smith, W. T. (1983). Comparison of alprazolam, imipramine, and placebo in the treatment of depression. *Journal of the American Medical Association, 249,* 3057–3064.

Feinberg, M. (1992). Comment: Subtypes of depression and response to treatment. *Journal of Consulting and Clinical Psychology, 60,* 670–674.

Fisher, S. (1986). *Development and structure of the body image* (Vols. 1 & 2). Hillsdale, NJ: Erlbaum.

Fisher, S., & Greenberg, R. P. (1989). *The limits of biological treatments for psychological distress: Comparisons with psychotherapy and placebo.* Hillsdale, NJ: Erlbaum.

Fisher, S., & Greenberg, R. P. (1993). How sound is the double-blind design for evaluating psychotropic drugs? *Journal of Nervous and Mental Disease, 181,* 345–350.

Frank, E., Karp, J. F., & Rush, A. J. (1993). Efficacy of treatments for major depression. *Psychopharmacology Bulletin, 29,* 457–475.

Frank, E., Kupfer, D. J., Perel, J. M., Cornes, C., Jarrett, D. B., Malinger, A. G., Thase, M. E., McEachran, A. B., & Grochocinski, V. J. (1990). Three-year outcomes for maintenance therapies in recurrent depression. *Archives of General Psychiatry, 47,* 1093–1099.

Friedel, R. O. (1982). The relationship of therapeutic response to antidepressant plasma levels: An update. *Journal of Clinical Psychiatry, 43,* 37–42.

Friedel, R. O. (1983). Clinical predictors of treatment response: An update. In J. M. Davis & J. W. Maas (Eds.), *The affective disorders* (pp. 379–384). Washington, DC: American Psychiatric Press.

Friedman, A. S., Granick, S., Cohen, H. W., & Cowitz, B. (1966). Imipramine (tofranil) vs. placebo in hospitalized psychotic depressives: A comparison of patients' self-ratings, psychiatrists' ratings and psychological test scores. *Journal of Psychiatric Research, 4,* 13–36.

Gaffan, E. A., Tsaousis, I., & Kemp-Wheeler, S. M. (1995). Researcher allegiance and meta-analysis: The case of cognitive therapy for depression. *Journal of Consulting and Clinical Psychology, 63,* 966–980.

Gallagher, D. E., & Thompson, L. W. (1983). Effectiveness of psychotherapy for both endogenous and nonendogenous depression in older adult outpatients. *Journal of Gerontology, 38,* 707–712.

Gatz, M., Pedersen, N. S., Plomin, R., Nesselroade, J. R., & McClearn, G. E. (1992). Importance of shared genes and shared environments for symptoms of depression in older adults. *Journal of Abnormal Psychology, 101,* 701–708.

Gerson, S. C., Plotkin, D. A., & Jarvik, L. F. (1988). Antidepressant drug studies, 1964 to 1986: Empirical evidence for aging patients. *Journal of Clinical Psychopharmacology, 8,* 311–322.

Gitlin, M. J. (1994). Psychotropic medications and their effects on sexual function: Diagnosis, biology, and treatment approaches. *Journal of Clinical Psychiatry, 55,* 406–413.

Glassman, A. H. (1994). Antidepressant plasma levels revisited. *International Clinical Psychopharmacology, 9*(Suppl. 2), 25–30.

Glassman, A. H., Perel, J. M., Shostak, M., Kantor, S. J., & Fleiss, J. L. (1977). Clinical implications of imipramine plasma levels for depressive illness. *Archives of General Psychiatry, 34,* 197–204.

Goodwin, F. K., & Jamison, K. R. (1990). *Manic-depressive illness.* New York: Oxford University Press.

Goodwin, G. M. (1995). Lithium revisited. A reply. *British Journal of Psychiatry, 167,* 573–574.

Gram, L. F. (1994). Fluoxetine. *New England Journal of Medicine, 331,* 1354–1361.

Greenberg, R. P., Bornstein, R. F., Greenberg, M. D., & Fisher, S. (1992a). A meta-analysis of antidepressant outcome under "blinder" conditions. *Journal of Consulting and Clinical Psychology, 60,* 664–669.

Greenberg, R. P., Bornstein, R. F., Greenberg, M. D., & Fisher, S. (1992b). As for the kings: A reply with regard to depression subtypes and antidepressant response. *Journal of Consulting and Clinical Psychology, 60,* 675–677.

Greenberg, R. P., Bornstein, R. F., Zborowski, M. J., Fisher, S., & Greenberg, M. D. (1994). A meta-analysis of fluoxetine outcome in the treatment of depression. *Journal of Nervous and Mental Disease, 182,* 547–551.

Greenberg, R. P., & Fisher, S. (1989). Examining antidepressant effectiveness: Findings, ambiguities, and some vexing puzzles. In S. Fisher & R. P. Greenberg (Eds.), *The limits of biological treatments for psychological distress: Comparisons with psychotherapy and placebo* (pp. 1–37). Hillsdale, NJ: Erlbaum.

Greenberg, R. P., & Fisher, S. (1994). Seeing through the double-masked design: A commentary. *Controlled Clinical Trials, 15,* 244–246.

Greenberg, R. P., Fisher, S., & Riter, J. A. (1995). Placebo washout is not a meaningful part of antidepressant drug trials. *Perceptual and Motor Skills, 81,* 688–690.

Greenblatt, M., Grosser, G. H., & Wechsler, H. (1964). Differential response of hospitalized depressed patients to somatic therapy. *American Journal of Psychiatry, 120,* 935–943.

Hall, R. C., Popkin, M. K., Devaul, R. A., Fallaice, L. A., & Stickney, S. K. (1978). Physical illness presenting as psychiatric disease. *Archives of General Psychiatry, 35,* 1315–1320.

Hamilton, M. (1960). A rating scale for depression. *Journal of Neurology, Neurosurgery, and Psychiatry, 23,* 56–62.

Harrison, G. (1994). New or old antidepressants? New is better. *British Medical Journal, 309,* 1280–1281.

Harrow, M., Goldberg, J. F., Grossman, L. S., & Meltzer, H. Y. (1990). Outcome in manic disorders. *Archives of General Psychiatry, 47,* 665–671.

Henker, B., Whalen, C. K., & Collins, B. E. (1979). Double-blind and triple-blind assessments of medication and placebo responses in hyperactive children. *Journal of Abnormal Child Psychiatry, 7,* 1–13.

Himmelhoch, J. M. (1994). On the failure to recognize lithium failure. *Psychiatric Annals, 24,* 241–250.

Hirschfeld, R. M., & Goodwin, F. K. (1988). Mood disorders. In J. A. Talbott, R. F. Hales, & S. C. Yudofsky (Eds.), *The American Psychiatric Press textbook of psychiatry* (pp. 403–443). Washington, DC: American Psychiatric Press.

Hirschfeld, R. M., & Davidson, L. (1988). Risk factors for suicide. In A. J. Frances & R. E. Hales (Eds.), *Psychiatry update: American Psychiatric Association annual review* (Vol. 7, pp. 307–333). Washington, DC: American Psychiatric Press.

Hollon, S. D., & DeRubeis, R. J. (1981). Placebo-psychotherapy combinations: Inappropriate representations of psychotherapy in drug-psychotherapy comparative trials. *Psychological Bulletin, 90,* 467–477.

Hollon, S. D., DeRubeis, R. J., Evans, M. D., Wiemer, M. D., Garvey, M. J., Grove, W. M., & Tuason, V. B. (1992). Cognitive therapy and pharmacotherapy for depression: Singly and in combination. *Archives of General Psychiatry, 49,* 774–781.

Hollon, S. D., Evans, M., & DeRubeis, R. (1990). Cognitive mediation of relapse prevention following treatment for depression: Implication of differential risk. In R. Ingram (Ed.), *Contemporary psychological approaches to depression* (pp. 117–136). New York: Guilford Press.

Hollon, S. D., Shelton, R. C., & Loosen, P. T. (1991). Cognitive therapy and pharmacotherapy for depression. *Journal of Consulting and Clinical Psychology, 59,* 88–89.

Hotopf, M., Lewis, G., & Normand, C. (1996). Are SSRIs a cost-effective alternative to tricyclics? *British Journal of Psychiatry, 168,* 404–409.

Hsu, J. Y., & Shen, W. T. (1995). Male sexual side effects associated with antidepressants: A descriptive clinical study of 32 patients. *International Journal of Psychiatry, 25,* 191–201.

Jacobsen, F. M. (1994). SSRI-induced sexual dysfunction. *American Society of Clinical Psychopharmacology Progress Notes, 5,* 1–4.

Jacobson, N. S., & Hollon, S. D. (1996a). Cognitive-behavior treatment versus pharmacotherapy: Now that the jury's returned its verdict, it's time to present the rest of the evidence. *Journal of Consulting and Clinical Psychology, 64,* 74–80.

Jacobson, N. S., & Hollon, S. D. (1996b). Prospects for future comparisons between drugs and psychotherapy: Lessons from the CBT-Versus-Pharmacotherapy exchange. *Journal of Consulting and Clinical Psychology, 64,* 104–108.

Jani, N. N., & Wise, T. N. (1988). Antidepressants and inhibited female orgasm: A literature review. *Journal of Sex and Marital Therapy, 14,* 279–284.

Jick, S. S., Dean, A. D., & Jick, H. (1995). Antidepressants and suicide. *British Medical Journal, 310,* 215–218.

Jonsson, B., & Bebbington, P. E. (1994). What price depression? The cost of depression and the cost-effectiveness of pharmacologic treatment. *British Journal of Psychiatry, 164,* 665–673.

Kaplan, H. I., & Sadock, B. J. (1989). *Comprehensive textbook of psychiatry* (5th ed.). Baltimore: Williams & Wilkins.

Kapur, S., Mieczkowski, T., & Mann, J. J. (1992). Antidepressant medications and the relative risk of suicide attempt and suicide. *Journal of the American Medical Association, 268,* 3441–3445.

Kasper, S., Fuger, J., & Moller, H. J. (1992). Comparative efficacy of antidepressants. *Drugs, 43,* 11–23.

Kathol, R. G., & Henn, F. A. (1983). Tricyclics—The most common agent used in potentially lethal overdoses. *Journal of Nervous and Mental Disease, 71,* 250–252.

Katschnig, H., Nutzinger, D., & Schanda, H. (1986). Validating depressive subtypes. In H. Hippius, G. L. Klerman, & N. Matussek (Eds.), *New results in depression research* (pp. 36–44). Berlin: Springer-Verlag.

Kelly, M. W., Perry, P. J., Holstead, S. C., & Garvey, M. J. (1989). Serum fluoxetine and norfluoxetine concentrations and antidepressant response. *Therapy Drug Monitor, 11,* 165–170.

Kessler, R. C., McGonagle, K. A., Zhao, S., Nelson, C. B., Hughes, M., Eshleman, S., Wittchen, H., & Kendler, K. S. (1994). Lifetime and 12-month prevalence of *DSM-III-R* psychiatric disorders in the United States. *Archives of General Psychiatry, 51,* 8–19.

King, R. A., Riddle, M. A., Chappell, P. B., Hardin, M. T., Anderson, G. M., Lombroso, P., & Scahill, L. (1991). Emergence of self-destructive phenomena in children and adolescents during fluoxetine treatment. *Journal of the American Academy of Child and Adolescent Psychiatry, 30,* 179–186.

Klein, D. F. (1994). Identified placebo treatment? *Neuropsychopharmacology, 10,* 271–272.

Klein, D. F. (1996). Preventing hung juries about therapy studies. *Journal of Consulting and Clinical Psychology, 64,* 81–87.

Klein, D. F., & Davis, J. M. (1969). *Diagnosis and drug treatment of psychiatric disorders.* Baltimore: Williams & Wilkins.

Klein, D. F., Gittleman, R., Quitkin, F., & Rifkin, A. (1980). *Diagnosis and drug treatment of psychiatric disorders: Adults and children* (2nd ed.). Baltimore: Williams & Wilkins.

Klerman, G. L. (1986). Scientific and ethical considerations in the use of placebo controls in clinical trials in psychopharmacology. *Psychopharmacology Bulletin, 22,* 25–29.

Klerman, G. L., & Cole, J. O. (1965). Clinical pharmacology of imipramine and related antidepressant compounds. *Pharmacological Reviews, 17,* 101–141.

Kocsis, J. H., Hanin, I., Bowden, C., & Brunswick, D. (1986). Imipramine and amitriptyline plasma concentrations and clinical response in major depression. *British Journal of Psychiatry, 148,* 52–57.

Koranyi, E. D. (1979). Morbidity and rate of undiagnosed physical illnesses in a psychiatric clinic population. *Archives of General Psychiatry, 36,* 414–419.

Kovacs, M., Rush, A. J., Beck, A. T., & Hollon, D. (1981). Depressed outpatients treated with cognitive therapy or pharmacotherapy. A one-year follow-up. *Archives of General Psychiatry, 38,* 33–39.

Krupnick, J. L., Sotsky, S. M., Simmens, S., Moyer, J., Elkin, I., Watkins, J., & Pilkonis, P. A. (1996). The role of the therapeutic alliance in psychotherapy and pharmacotherapy outcome: Findings in the National Institute of Mental Health Treatment of Depression Collaborative Research Program. *Journal of Consulting and Clinical Psychology, 64,* 532–539.

Kupfer, D. J., Frank, E., Perel, J. M., Cornes, C., Mallinger, A. G., Thase, M. E., McEachran, A. B., & Grochocinski, V. J. (1992). Five-year outcome for maintenance therapies in recurrent depression. *Archives of General Psychiatry, 49,* 769–773.

Lambert, M. J., Hatch, D. R., Kingston, M. D., & Edwards, B. C. (1986). Zung, Beck, and Hamilton rating scales as measures of treatment outcome: A meta-analytic comparison. *Journal of Consulting and Clinical Psychology, 54,* 54–59.

Lasagna, L. (1955). The controlled clinical trial: Theory and practice. *Journal of Chronic Disease, 1,* 353–367.

Letemendia, F. J. J., & Harris, A. D. (1959). The influence of side effects on the reporting of symptoms. *Psychopharmacologia, 1,* 39–47.

Lewis, D. J. (1934). Melancholia: A clinical survey of depressive states. *Journal of Mental Science, 80,* 277–378.

Lin, K. M., Poland, R. E., & Nakasaki, G. (1993). *Psychopharmacology and psychobiology of ethnicity.* Washington, DC: American Psychiatric Press.

Maj, M., Pirozzi, R., & Kemali, D. (1991). Long-term outcome of lithium prophylaxis in bipolar patients. *Archives of General Psychiatry, 48,* 772.

Mander, A. J. (1986). Is lithium justified after one manic episode? *Acta Psychiatrica Scandinavica, 73,* 60–67.

Marini, J. L., Sheard, M. H., Bridges, C. I., & Wagner, E., Jr. (1976). An evaluation of the double-blind design in a study comparing lithium carbonate with placebo. *Acta Psychiatrica Scandinavica, 53,* 343–354.

Markar, H. R., & Mander, J. (1989). Efficacy of lithium prophylaxis in clinical practice. *British Journal of Psychiatry, 155,* 496–500.

Masand, P., Gupta, S., & Dewan, M. (1991). Suicidal ideation related to fluoxetine treatment. *New England Journal of Medicine, 324,* 420.

McKnight, D. L., Nelson-Gray, R. D., & Barnhill, J. (1992). Dexamethasone suppression test and response to cognitive therapy and antidepressant medication. *Behavior Therapy, 1,* 99–111.

McLean, P. D., & Hakstian, A. R. (1979). Clinical depression: Comparative efficacy of outpatient treatments. *Journal of Consulting and Clinical Psychology, 47,* 818–836.

McLean, P. D., & Taylor, S. (1992). Severity of unipolar depression and choice of treatment. *Behaviour Research and Therapy, 30,* 443–451.

McNair, D. M. (1974). Self-evaluations of antidepressants. *Psychopharmacologia, 37,* 281–301.

McNally, R. J. (1996). Methodological controversies in the treatment of panic disorder. *Journal of Consulting and Clinical Psychology, 64,* 88–91.

Miller, I. W., Norman, W. H., Keitner, G. I., Bishop, S. B., & Dow, M. G. (1989). Cognitive-behavioral treatment of depressed inpatients. *Behavior Therapy, 20,* 25–47.

Moller, S. E., Reisby, N., Elley, J., Krautwald, O., Ortmann, J., & Larsen, O. B. (1985). Biochemical and diagnostic classification and serum drug levels: Relation to antidepressive effect of imipramine. *Neuropsychobiology, 13,* 160–166.

Moncrieff, J. (1995). A re-examination of the placebo-controlled trials of lithium prophylaxis in manic-depressive disorder. *British Journal of Psychiatry, 167,* 569–573.

Montgomery, S. A. (1993). Suicide prevention and serotonergic drugs. *International Clinical Psychopharmacology, 8*(Suppl. 2), 83–85.

Montgomery, S. A., Henry, J., McDonald, G., Dinan, T., Lader, M., Hindmarch, I., Clare, A., & Nutt, D. (1994). Selective serotonin reuptake inhibitors meta-analysis of discontinuation rates. *International Clinical Psychopharmacology, 9,* 47–53.

Montgomery, S. A., & Kasper, S. (1995). Comparison of compliance between serotonin reuptake inhibitors and tricyclic antidepressants: A meta-analysis. *International Clinical Psychopharmacology, 9*(Suppl. 4), 33–40.

Montgomery, S. A., & Pinder, R. M. (1987). Do some antidepressants promote suicide? *Psychopharmacology, 92,* 265–266.

Morris, J., & Beck, A. (1974). The efficacy of antidepressant drugs. A review of research (1958–1972). *Archives of General Psychiatry, 30,* 667–674.

Muijen, M., Roy, D., Silverstone, T., Mehmet, A., & Christie, M. (1988). A comparative clinical trial of fluoxetine, mianserin, and placebo in depressed outpatients. *Acta Psychiatrica Scandinavica, 78,* 384–390.

Muñoz, R. F., Hollon, S. D., McGrath, E., Rehm, L. P., & VandenBos, G. R. (1994). On the AHCPR depression in primary care guidelines: Further considerations for practitioners. *American Psychologist, 49,* 42–61.

Murphy, G. E., Simons, A. D., Wetzel, R. D., & Lustman, P. J. (1984). Cognitive therapy and pharmacotherapy: Singly and together in the treatment of depression. *Archives of General Psychiatry, 41,* 33–41.

Murray, E. J. (1989). Measurement issues in the evaluation of pharmacological therapy. In S. Fisher & R. P. Greenberg (Eds.), *The limits of biological treatments for psychological distress: Comparisons with psychotherapy and placebo* (pp. 39–67). Hillsdale, NJ: Erlbaum.

Narrow, W. E., Regier, D. A., Rae, D. S., Manderscheid, R. W., & Locke, B. Z. (1993). Use of services by persons with mental and addictive disorders: Findings from the National Institute of Mental Health Epidemiological Catchment Area Program. *Archives of General Psychiatry, 50*, 95–107.

Nelson, J. C. (1994). Are the SSRIs really better tolerated than the TCAs for treatment of major depression? *Psychiatric Annals, 24*, 628–631.

Nierenberg, A. A. (1994). The treatment of severe depression: Is there an efficacy gap between SSRI and TCA antidepressant generations? *Journal of Clinical Psychiatry, 55*(Suppl. A), 55–59.

Ogles, B. M., Lambert, M. J., & Sawyer, J. D. (1995). Clinical significance of the National Institute of Mental Health Treatment of Depression Collaborative Research Program data. *Journal of Consulting and Clinical Psychology, 63*, 321–326.

Oliver, J. M., & Simmons, M. E. (1985). Affective disorders and depression as measured by the diagnostic interview schedule and the Beck Depression Inventory in an unselected adult population. *Journal of Clinical Psychology, 41*, 469–477.

Ostrow, D. (1985). The new generation antidepressants: Promising innovation or disappointments? *Journal of Clinical Psychiatry, 46*, 25–30.

Owens, D. (1994). Benefits of new drugs are exaggerated. *British Medical Journal, 309*, 1281–1282.

Oxtoby, A., Jones, A., & Robinson, M. (1989). Is your "double-blind" design truly double-blind? *British Journal of Psychiatry, 155*, 700–701.

Paykel, E. S., & Priest, R. G. (1992). Recognition and management of depression in general practice consensus statement. *British Medical Journal, 305*, 1198–1202.

Persons, J. B., Thase, M. E., & Crits-Christoph, P. (1996). The role of psychotherapy in the treatment of depression: Review of two practice guidelines. *Archives of General Psychiatry, 53*, 283–290.

Philipp, M., & Maier, W. (1985). Operational diagnosis of endogenous depression: 1. Comparisons with clinical diagnosis. *Pharmacopsychiatry, 18*, 112–113.

Pies, R. (1995). One foot on the bandwagon? *Journal of Clinical Psychopharmacology, 15*, 303–305.

Pollack, M. H., Reiter, S., & Hammerness, P. (1992). Genitourinary and sexual adverse effects of psychotropic medication. *International Journal of Psychiatry in Medicine, 22*, 305–327.

Preskorn, S. H., Silkey, B., Beber, J., & Dorey, C. (1991). Antidepressant response and plasma concentrations of fluoxetine. *Annals of Clinical Psychiatry, 3*, 147–151.

Prien, R. F., Caffey, E. M., & Klett, J. (1973). Prophylactic efficacy of lithium carbonate in manic-depressive illness. *Archives of General Psychiatry, 28*, 337–341.

Prien, R. F., & Gelenberg, A. J. (1989). Alternatives to lithium for preventive treatment of bipolar disorder. *American Journal of Psychiatry, 146*, 840–848.

Prien, R. F., & Kupfer, D. J. (1986). Continuation drug therapy for major depressive episodes: How long should it be maintained? *American Journal of Psychiatry, 143*, 18–23.

Prusoff, B. A., Weissman, M. M., Klerman, G. L., & Rounsaville B. J. (1980). Research Diagnostic Criteria subtypes of depression: Their role as predictors of differential response to psychotherapy and drug treatment. *Archives of General Psychiatry, 37,* 796–801.

Quality Assurance Project. (1983). A treatment outline for depressive disorders. *Australian and New Zealand Journal of Psychiatry, 17,* 129–146.

Quitkin, F. M. (1985). The importance of dosage in prescribing antidepressants. *British Journal of Psychiatry, 147,* 593–597.

Quitkin, F. M., Rabkin, J. G., Ross, D., & McGrath, P. J. (1984). Duration of antidepressant drug treatment: What is an adequate trial? *Archives of General Psychiatry, 41,* 238–245.

Rabkin, J. G., Markowitz, J. S., Stewart, J., McGrath, P., Harrison, W., Quitkin, F. M., & Klein, D. S. (1986). How blind is blind? Assessment of patient and doctor medication guesses in a placebo-controlled trial of imipramine and phenelzine. *Psychiatric Research, 19,* 75–86.

Reimherr, F. W., Ward, M. F., & Byerley, W. F. (1989). The introductory placebo washout: A retrospective evaluation. *Psychiatry Research, 30,* 191–199.

Reisby, N., Gram, L. F., Beck, P., Nagy, A., Petesen, G. O., Ortmann, J., Ibsen, I., Dencker, S. J., Jacobsen, O., Krautwald, O., Sondergaard, I., & Christiansen, J. (1977). Imipramine: Clinical effects and pharmacokinetic variability. *Psychopharmacology, 54,* 263–272.

Reynolds, C. F., Frank, E., Perel, J. M., Imber, S. D., Cornes, C., Morycz, R. K., Mazumdar, S., Miller, M. D., Pollock, B. G., Rifai, A. H., Stack, J. A., George, C. J., Houck, P. R., & Kupfer, D. J. (1992). Combined pharmacotherapy and psychotherapy in the acute and continuation treatment of elderly patients with recurrent major depression: A preliminary report. *American Journal of Psychiatry, 149,* 1687–1692.

Rickels, K., & Case, W. G. (1982). Trazodone in depressed outpatients. *American Journal of Psychiatry, 139,* 803–806.

Rickels, K., Cattell, R. B., Weiss, C., Gray, B., Yee, R., Mallin, A., & Aaron, H. G. (1966). Controlled psychopharmacological research in private psychiatric practice. *Psychopharmacologia, 9,* 288–306.

Rickels, K., Raab, E., & Carranza, J. (1965). Doctor medication guesses: An indication of clinical improvement in double-blind studies. *Journal of New Drugs, 5,* 67–71.

Roberts, A. H. (1995). The powerful placebo revisited: Magnitude of nonspecific effects. *Mind Body Medicine, 1,* 35–43.

Robinson, L. A., Berman, J. S., & Neimeyer, R. A. (1990). Psychotherapy for the treatment of depression: A comprehensive review of controlled outcome research. *Psychological Bulletin, 108,* 30–49.

Rogers, S. C., & Clay, P. M. (1975). A statistical review of controlled trials of imipramine and placebo in the treatment of depressive illnesses. *British Journal of Psychiatry, 127,* 599–603.

Ross, M., & Olson, J. M. (1981). An expectancy-attribution model of the effects of placebos. *Psychology Review, 88,* 408–437.

Roth, D., Bielski, R., Jones, M., Parker, W., & Osborn, G. (1982). A comparison of self-control therapy and combined self-control therapy and antidepressant medication in the treatment of depression. *Behavior Therapy, 13,* 133–144.

Rush, A. J. (1994). Placebo responsiveness does not imply that placebo is a sufficient treatment. *Neuropharmacology, 10,* 281–283.

Rush, A. J., Beck, A. T., Kovacs, M., & Hollon, S. (1977). Comparative efficacy of cognitive therapy and pharmacotherapy in the treatment of depressed outpatients. *Cognitive Therapeutic Research, 1,* 17–37.

Rush, A. J., & Watkins, J. T. (1981). Group versus individual cognitive therapy: A pilot study. *Cognitive Therapy and Research, 5,* 95–103.

Sachs, G. S. (1989). Bipolar affective disorder. *Journal of Clinical Psychiatry, 50,* 31–47.

Schatzberg, A. F., & Rothschild, A. J. (1992). Psychotic (delusional) major depression: Should it be included as a distinct syndrome in *DSM-IV? American Journal of Psychiatry, 149,* 733–745.

Schildkraut, J. J., Green, A. I., & Mooney, J. J. (1989). Mood disorders: Biochemical aspects. In H. I. Kaplan & B. J. Sadock (Eds.), *Comprehensive textbook of psychiatry* (pp. 868–879). Baltimore: Williams & Wilkins.

Schumer, F. (1989, December). Bye-bye, blues: A new wonder drug for depression. *New York Magazine,* 46–50.

Shea, M. T. (1994). Commentary on "Placebo as a treatment for depression."*Neuropsychopharmacology, 10,* 285–286.

Shea, M. T., Elkin, I., Imber, S. D., Sotsky, S. M., Watkins, J. T., Collins, J. F., Pilkonis, P. A., Beckham, E., Glass, D. R., Dolan, R. T., & Parloff, M. B. (1992). Course of depressive symptoms over follow-up: Findings from the National Institute of Mental Health Treatment of Depression Collaborative Research Program. *Archives of General Psychiatry, 49,* 782–787.

Simons, A. D., Murphy, G. E., Levine, J. L., & Wetzel, R. D. (1986). Cognitive therapy and pharmacotherapy for depression: Sustained improvement over one year. *Archives of General Psychiatry, 43,* 43–48.

Simons, A. D., & Thase, M. E. (1992). Biological markers, treatment outcome, and 1-year follow-up of endogenous depression: Electroencephalographic sleep studies and response to cognitive therapy. *Journal of Consulting and Clinical Psychology, 60,* 392–401.

Simpson, G. H., Edmond, H. P., & White, K. (1983). Plasma drug levels and clinical response to antidepressants. *Journal of Clinical Psychiatry, 44,* 27–34.

Simpson, G. M., Lee, J. H., Cuculic, A., & Kellner, R. (1976). Two doses of imipramine in hospitalized endogenous and neurotic depressives. *Archives of General Psychiatry, 33,* 1093–1102.

Smith, A., Traganza, E., & Harrison, G. (1969). Studies on the effectiveness of antidepressant drugs. *Psychopharmacology Bulletin, 5,* 1–53.

Smith, M. L., Glass, G. V., & Miller, T. I. (1980). *The benefits of psychotherapy.* Baltimore: Johns Hopkins University Press.

Solomon, D. A., Keitner, G. I., Miller, I. W., Shea, M. T., & Keller, M. B. (1995). Course of illness and maintenance treatments for patients with bipolar disorder. *Journal of Clinical Psychiatry, 56,* 5–13.

Song, F., Freemantle, N., Sheldon, T. A., House, A., Watson, P., Long, A., & Mason, J. (1993). Selective serotonin reuptake inhibitors: Meta-analysis of efficacy and acceptability. *British Medical Journal, 306,* 683–687.

Sotsky, S. M., Glass, D. R., Shea, M. T., Pilkonis, P. A., Collins, J. F., Elkin, I., Watkins, J. T., Imber, S. D., Leber, W. R., Moyer, J., & Oliveri, M. E. (1991). Patient predictors of response to psychotherapy and pharmacotherapy. Findings in the NIMH Treatment of Depression Collaborative Research Program. *American Journal of Psychiatry, 148,* 997–1008.

Stallone, F., Mendlewicz, J., & Fieve, R. R. (1975). Double-blind procedure: An assessment in a study of lithium prophylaxis. *Psychological Medicine, 5,* 78–82.

Stallone, F., Shelley, E., Mendlewicz, J., & Fieve, R. R. (1973). The use of lithium in affective disorders: 3. A double-blind study of prophylaxis in bipolar illness. *American Journal of Psychiatry, 130,* 1006–1010.

Steinbrueck, S. M., Maxwell, S. E., & Howard, G. S. (1983). A meta-analysis of psychotherapy and drug therapy in the treatment of unipolar depression with adults. *Journal of Consulting and Clinical Psychology, 51,* 856–863.

Suppes, T., Baldessarini, R. J., Faedda, G. L., & Tohen, M. (1991). Risk of recurrence following discontinuation of lithium treatment in bipolar disorder. *Archives of General Psychiatry, 48,* 1082–1088.

Symonds, R. L., & Williams, P. (1981). Lithium and the changing incidence of mania. *Psychological Medicine, 11,* 193–196.

Teasdale, J. D., Fennell, M. J. V., Hibbert, G. A., & Amies P. L. (1984). Cognitive therapy for major depressive disorder in primary care. *British Journal of Psychiatry, 144,* 400–406.

Teicher, M. H., Glod, C., & Cole, J. O. (1990). Emergence of intense suicidal preoccupation during fluoxetine treatment. *American Journal of Psychiatry, 147,* 207–210.

Thase, M. E. (1983). Cognitive and behavioral treatments for depression: A review for recent developments. In F. J. Ayd, I. J. Taylor, & B. T. Taylor (Eds.), *Affective disorders reassessed* (pp. 234–243). Baltimore: Ayd Medical Communications.

Thase, M. E., Greenhouse, J., Frank, E., Reynolds C. F., III, Pilkonis, P. A., Hurley, K., Grochocinski, V. J., & Kupfer, D. J. (1994). Correlates of remission of major depression during standardized trials of psychotherapy, pharmacotherapy, or their combination: Results from the Pittsburgh 600 [Abstract]. *Psychopharmacology Bulletin, 30,* 642.

Thase, M. E., & Kupfer, D. J. (1996). Recent developments in the pharmacotherapy of mood disorders. *Journal of Consulting and Clinical Psychology, 64,* 646–659.

Thase, M. E., & Simons, A. D. (1992). Cognitive behavior therapy and relapse of nonbipolar depression: Parallels with pharmacotherapy. *Psychopharmacology Bulletin, 28,* 117–122.

Thase, M. E., & Sullivan, L. R. (1995). Relapse and recurrence of depression: A practical approach for prevention. *CNS Drugs, 4,* 261–277.

Thomson, R. (1982). Side effects and placebo amplification. *British Journal of Psychiatry, 140,* 64–68.

Tohen, M., Waternaux, C. M., & Tsuang, M. T. (1990). Outcome in mania. *Archives of General Psychiatry, 47,* 1106–1111.

Trivedi, M. H., & Rush, J. (1994). Does a placebo run-in or a placebo treatment cell affect the efficacy of antidepressant medications? *Neuropsychopharmacology, 11,* 33–43.

Tryer, S. P. (1985). Lithium in the treatment of mania. *Journal of Affective Disorders, 8,* 251–257.

Vestergaard, P. (1992). Treatment and prevention of mania: A Scandinavian perspective. *Neuropsychopharmacology, 7,* 249–259.

Wakelin, J. S. (1988). The role of serotonin in depression and suicide: Do serotonin reuptake inhibitors provide a key? *Advances in Biological Psychiatry, 17,* 70–83.

Watt, D. C., Crammer, J. L., & Elkes, A. (1972). Metabolism, anticholinergic effects, and the therapeutic outcome of desmethylimipramine in depressive illness. *Psychological Medicine, 2,* 397–405.

Wechsler, H., Grosser, G. H., & Greenblatt, M. (1965). Research evaluating antidepressant medications on hospitalized mental patients: A survey of published reports during a 5-year period. *Journal of Nervous and Mental Disease, 141,* 231–239.

Weissman, M. M., Klerman, G. L., Prusoff, B. A., Sholomskas, D., & Padian, N. (1981). Depressed outpatients: Results one year after treatment with drugs and/or interpersonal psychotherapy. *Archives of General Psychiatry, 38,* 51–55.

Weissman, M. M., Prusoff, B. A., DiMascio, A., Neu, C., Goklaney, M., & Klerman, G. L. (1979). The efficacy of drugs and psychotherapy in the treatment of acute depressive episodes. *American Journal of Psychiatry, 136,* 555–558.

Wernicke, J. F., Dunlop, S. R., Dornseif, B. E., Bosomworth, J. C., & Humbert, M. (1988). Low-dose fluoxetine therapy for depression. *Psychopharmacology Bulletin, 24,* 183–188.

Wernicke, J. F., Dunlop, S. R., Dornseif, B. E., & Zerbe, R. L. (1987). Fixed-dose fluoxetine therapy for depression. *Psychopharmacology Bulletin, 23,* 164–168.

Wexler, B. E., & Cicchetti, D. V. (1992). The outpatient treatment of depression: Implications of outcome research for clinical practice. *Journal of Nervous and Mental Disease, 180,* 277–286.

Wilson, P. H. (1982). Combined pharmacological and behavioral treatment of depression. *Behavior Research and Therapy, 20,* 173–184.

Workman, E. A., & Short, D. D. (1993). Atypical antidepressants versus imipramine in the treatment of major depression: A meta-analysis. *Journal of Clinical Psychiatry, 54,* 5–12.

Zimmerman, M., Coryell, W., & Pfohl, B. (1986). Melancholic subtyping: A qualitative or quantitative distinction? *American Journal of Psychiatry, 143,* 98–100.

Zimmerman, M., & Spitzer, R. L. (1989). Melancholia: From *DSM-III* to *DSM-III-R*. *American Journal of Psychiatry, 146,* 20–28.

CHAPTER 5

A Critique of the Use of Neuroleptic Drugs in Psychiatry

DAVID COHEN

O ver the past 45 years, neuroleptic (NLP), or antipsychotic, drugs have been prescribed to tens of millions of individuals diagnosed as suffering from various functional and organic psychotic disorders. NLPs are the mainstay of treatment for schizophrenic patients. They are also prescribed to more than 20% of nursing home residents and individuals with developmental disabilities (Ray et al., 1993). By the mid-1980s, 19 million outpatient NLP prescriptions were written annually in the United States (Wysosky & Baum, 1989). Yet, NLPs—which include risperidone (Risperdal®), haloperidol (Haldol®), chlorpromazine (Thorazine®), thioridazine (Mellaril®), thiothixene (Navane®), clozapine (Clozaril®), and a dozen other drugs—remain among the least prescribed psychotropics.

Those who ingest NLPs rarely request them and generally dislike them very much (Wallace, 1994). The popular expressions "chemical strait-jacket" and "zombie effect" well describe NLPs' unique psychomotor subduing effect, used until the mid-1980s in the former Soviet Union to disable imprisoned political dissidents. Among the different classes of psychotropics, NLPs probably produce the most substantial iatrogenic morbidity (Dewan & Koss, 1989), such as the frequently irreversible tardive dyskinesia (TD) or sometimes fatal neuroleptic malignant syndrome. Several civil suits have been filed against psychiatrists for damages suffered as a result of TD (Simon, 1992), and the American Psychiatric

173

Association (APA) issued three cautionary reports about TD between 1979 and 1992, asking psychiatrists to use NLPs prudently. In 1990, congressional legislation limited and regulated the use of NLPs in nursing homes (Semla, Palla, Poddig, & Brauner, 1994).

Nevertheless, most clinicians today consider NLPs indispensable to treat psychotic disorders and it is very likely that a person diagnosed with schizophrenia will receive these drugs for months, years, or indefinitely. At the same time, there are numerous indications that NLPs remain unsatisfying to clinicians and insufficient for their main clinical purpose. Although lip service continues to be paid to the extraordinary antipsychotic properties of a course of acute treatment with NLPs, in recent practice in the United States over 80% of short-term hospital patients prescribed NLPs also have received other powerful central nervous system depressants, notably anticonvulsants and lithium (Baldessarini, Kando, & Centorrino, 1995).

The official date of the introduction in psychiatry of NLPs—1952—also marks the beginning of modern biological psychiatry.[1] No class of drugs before or since has provided such impetus to clinical and experimental investigation in psychiatry or triggered such far-reaching changes in the organization of mental health services. Today, the near-universal consensus on NLPs is that they are "antipsychotics," uniquely and specifically suited to treat schizophrenia: "Conventional neuroleptic agents have, since the mid-1950s, proven to be the most consistently effective compounds in the treatment of acute and chronic schizophrenic patients" (Wirshing, Marder, Van Putten, & Ames, 1995, p. 1259). The consensus is said to rest on solid scientific and clinical justifications: "The antipsychotic efficacy of neuroleptics has been confirmed in numerous studies based on a meticulous method. It is only antipsychotic medication that enables many patients to benefit from [other interventions]" (Windgassen, 1992, p. 405).

This view deliberately ignores much conflicting evidence, to be presented here. Worse, it implies that to question the usefulness of NLPs may relegate one to the fringe of scientific credibility (see accounts by Karon, 1989; Mosher & Burti, 1989; Ross & Pam, 1995). This may discourage critical inquiry by researchers and clinicians embarking on their careers (Kemker & Khadivi, 1995). Just as damaging, the prevailing consensus is acultural, failing to explain why NLPs are conceptualized quite differently in Europe than in America. Nor can it account for replicated findings from

---

[1] Earlier dates have been proposed: 1931, when the purified extract of rauwolfia serpentina, later known as reserpine, was tested on inmates of Indian insane asylums (Frankenburg, 1994); 1943, when Albert Hoffman discovered the hallucinogenic effects of LSD (Strassman, 1995); 1949, when William Cade hypothesized and then described the sedating effects of lithium salts on psychotic patients.

the World Health Organization cross-cultural schizophrenia studies showing that patients from developing countries, where only 16% were prescribed NLPs most or all of the time, had a significantly better outcome than patients from developed countries, with 61% on NLPs (de Girolamo, 1996; Jablensky, 1987).

The current consensus is also ahistorical, blind to serious doubts raised periodically about the enterprise of NLP drug treatment. The doubts are distracted away by "pragmatic" concerns about the control of "dangerous mental patients" (Klitzman, 1995), by the "unfeasibility" of nondrug alternatives requiring changes in philosophies and methods of service delivery, or by new "discoveries" confirming that treatment success only requires newer, better drugs (Kerwin, 1994). Invariably, the compromise is disillusioning because it fails to come to terms with the basic deficiencies of NLP treatment of seriously disturbed persons.

For example, after the first APA report on TD estimated that 20% of psychiatric patients showed "more than minimal signs of the disorder" (Baldessarini et al., 1979), the positive consensus about NLPs began to strain. After a few isolated reports the previous decade in the United States describing profound iatrogenesis, the "behavioral toxicity" of NLPs came to be squarely discussed by the APA and by leading clinical psychopharmacologists (e.g., APA, 1985, 1992; Gualtieri & Sprague, 1984; Van Putten & Marder, 1987). Few clinicians could feel unperturbed by the suggestion that NLPs had created, in the words of one well-known critic, "an epidemic of neurologic disease . . . among the worst medically-induced disasters in history" (Breggin, 1983, p. 109)—an opinion echoed in the pages of the *American Journal of Psychiatry* (Appelbaum, Schaffner, & Meisel, 1985). Even Pierre Deniker (1986), who introduced chlorpromazine in psychiatry with Jean Delay, published an article entitled "Are the Antipsychotic Drugs to Be Withdrawn?" (Deniker answered his question in the negative.)

Early in the 1990s, the doubts gave way to optimism about the treatment of schizophrenia, due to the marketing of new or formerly shelved compounds such as risperidone and clozapine, or the expected introduction of other "atypical" NLPs (olanzapine, remoxipride, sertindole, etc.). These are stated to be equal or superior to the older (conventional or classical) NLPs, especially for "neuroleptic nonresponsive" patients, but to produce fewer toxic effects. The latter are of extreme importance. In Wirshing et al.'s (1995) assessment of NLPs quoted earlier, immediately after the glowing evaluation of antipsychotic effectiveness, a number of caveats appear:

> This efficacy [of conventional NLP agents], though, has come at the cost of a number of untoward neurological side effects. Prominent among these are disturbances of the extrapyramidal system including dystonia, tremor,

akinesia, bradykinesia, rigidity, akathisia, and a variety of tardive dyskinetic (TD) syndromes. These side effects have been linked to notorious patient noncompliance and iatrogenic morbidity. Additionally, conventional
neuroleptics have been shown to be only partially effective at ameliorating
the psychosis which contributes to persistent disability, subjective distress,
and family burden. Finally, a substantial minority of patients derive little if
any benefit from drug treatment. (p. 1259)

When risperidone was introduced in North America, its advertisement in
the April 1994 issue of the *American Journal of Psychiatry* stated, "Incidence and severity of extrapyramidal symptoms (EPS) were similar to
placebo." Almost identical statements have been made for soon to be introduced NLPs such as olanzapine and sertindole (Neergard, 1996). Such
pronouncements may have a powerful impact. It matters little that later
evaluations of the new drugs in ordinary clinical settings with ordinary
patients may greatly modify the original enthusiastic assessments. For example, within one year of its introduction, risperidone—only the second
NLP approved by the Food and Drug Administration in 20 years—became
the second most used NLP in some hospitals. In one institution, Carter
et al. (1995) found that its use spread far beyond the population of adult
schizophrenics, the only one for whom efficacy data were available. In fact,
the cost of risperidone alone exceeded the amount spent on *all* NLPs during
the preceeding year. However, in that ordinary setting, risperidone did not
show less toxicity than haloperidol, and the mean drug dose at which toxic
effects appeared was distinctly lower than that suggested by data from
premarketing clinical trials. With each passing year, risperidone presents
itself as less and less "atypical": As of this writing, several published reports have implicated this drug in the production of quintessential neuroleptic effects such as TD and neuroleptic malignant syndrome (Buzan,
1996; Dave, 1995; Singer, Richards, & Boland, 1995; Woerner, Sheitman,
Lieberman, & Kane, 1995). Yet, less than three years after its market approval and with no published data on long-term effects, risperidone became in October 1996 the most widely prescribed NLP in the United States
(Neergard, 1996).

   The reception given clozapine—the first atypical NLP, from the benzodiazepine family, introduced in North America in 1990—is equally informative. Modestly used in Europe since the early 1960s, clozapine had its
use greatly restricted after about 20 people died from it, due to agranulocytosis (sharp drop in white blood cells) in 1975 in Finland and Switzerland (Kerwin, 1994). Healy (1993) notes that "With the problems of
launching clozapine in the US and the UK owing to its toxicity, company-
sponsored research has focused on a treatment-resistance indication,"

although previous studies from Europe showed that the drug's efficacy for schizophrenia "has been no more and no less than that of other neuroleptic agents" (p. 25). Clozapine was also described as being free of EPS: Its advertisement in the January 1990 issue of the *American Journal of Psychiatry* contains the following headline: "Hope continues with a virtual absence of certain acute extrapyramidal symptoms." Some researchers stated simply that clozapine "does not cause extrapyramidal effects" (Schwartz & Brotman, 1992, p. 981). By 1993, however, as D. Cohen (1994a) reviewed, clozapine had been associated—in over a dozen open and blind studies—with tremor, akathisia, tardive dyskinesia, neuroleptic malignant syndrome, as well as other typical NLP effects. Relative to other NLPs, the frequency of clozapine-induced EPS was typically lower, but the findings were unmistakably clear. Yet, even after these reports appeared, one could read in no less a publication than *The New England Journal of Medicine:* "Unlike classic neuroleptic agents, *clozapine is not associated with the development of acute extrapyramidal symptoms* [italics added]" (Alvir, Lieberman, Safferman, Schwimmer, & Schaff, 1993, p. 162).

Skelton, Pepe, and Pineo (1995) undertook a meta-analysis of 11 studies to derive a quantitative estimate of the magnitude of clozapine's effect on patient symptoms, relative to other NLPs. In eight studies that used the Brief Psychiatric Rating Scale (BPRS) to rate psychopathology, the average symptom score was improved by 26 percentile points. Skelton et al. state that this suggests that "the comparative effect of clozapine over other antipsychotic medications may be regarded as moderate to large" (p. 276), but one should accept this finding with caution. One difficulty may arise because BPRS symptom ratings often correlate positively with EPS (Baldessarini, Cohen, & Teicher, 1988; D. Cohen, 1989; Halstead, Barnes, & Speller, 1994). For example, elevated scores on BPRS items such as "tension/anxiety" and "emotional withdrawal" may actually reflect EPS such as akathisia and parkinsonism. Given that EPS would probably have been lower in patients on clozapine, this could result in improved BPRS scores for these patients compared with patients on conventional NLPs. Also, although observer expectancies and "unblinding" in clinical trials may have a powerful impact on drug effect ratings (Double, 1995; Greenberg, Bornstein, Greenberg, & Fisher, 1992; White, Kando, Park, Waternaux, & Brown, 1992), only a single study described how observers were kept unaware of patients' treatment conditions. Finally, in only 2 of 11 studies were patients studied more than 2 months. Of course, these methodological features are not limited to the literature on clozapine.

Yet, the much-publicized introduction of "new, improved" drugs creates the impression that there is unequivocal *progress* in treating psychosis. This in turn reinforces the dominant biopsychiatric idea that "schizophrenia" represents a genetically predisposed, environmentally triggered, neurodevelopmental brain disease which, at this state of our knowledge, best responds to chemical intervention.[2] According to Mitchell (1993), "Forty years after the discovery of chlorpromazine finds us with the enthusiasm of the introduction of clozapine. At the same time, however, it is sobering to reflect on how little we have learned of the aetiology of the functional psychoses" (p. 344). Indeed, no biological dimension specific to schizophrenia has yet been charted (Chua & McKenna, 1995; Pam, 1995).

From where does the continued use of NLPs derive legitimacy? Possibly the first reason may be the natural desire to bring under quick control the seemingly inexplicable, disturbed, and disturbing behavior and moods displayed by a psychotic individual. Yet, the use of NLPs extends far beyond this limited indication, commonly encompassing lifelong medication for individuals who have been hospitalized on more than two or three occasions and raising questions about the extent to which chronicity in schizophrenia results from a system of "care" in which all interventions remain secondary to ensuring that the schizophrenic takes his or her medication. According to Kuhn (1970), the inertia of a scientific system is such that it can remain in a dominant position even after it is seen as *generating* the problems which necessitate alternative formulations. Support for an inefficient system comes mostly from extrascientific factors, which Karon (1989) hinted at in his conclusion of a detailed review of medication versus psychotherapy studies: "Political and economic factors and a concentration on short-term cost-effectiveness, rather than the scientific findings, currently seem to dictate [drug treatment of schizophrenia]" (p. 146). According to Ross (1995), several psychological strategies help erroneous logic keep hold in biological psychiatry: "The conceptual system of biological psychiatry is organized [such that the] tautologies, positive feedback loops, closure to alternative hypotheses, pervasive overgeneralization, use of dissociation to eliminate cognitive dissonance, and other structural and functional properties of the system maintain it in a dysfunctional homeostasis" (p. 127).

This appraisal of NLPs begins with early descriptions of their effects on psychiatric patients. These reports were stated in graphic terms that have virtually disappeared from the contemporary literature and focused on psychic indifference and abnormal movements, viewed as the sine qua non of NLPs' therapeutic action. By the late 1970s, despite the absence of any new or pertinent experimental, clinical, or epidemiological evidence,

---

[2] For different views on the nature of schizophrenia, see Boyle (1990), Carson (1991), Sarbin (1990), and Wiener (1991), among others.

most researchers in North America (but not in Europe) appeared to have rejected this view.

PSYCHIC INDIFFERENCE: THE FIRST CLINICAL EFFECT OF NEUROLEPTICS

Accounts and reminiscences of pioneers of clinical psychopharmacology suggest that NLPs gained favor in the hospital psychiatry of the 1950s because of the drugs' outstanding ability to stupefy agitated inmates as well or better than electric shock, insulin coma, and lobotomy (D. Cohen, in press). Most contemporary writers fail to appreciate that NLPs were entirely tried, evaluated, and found to be beneficial *within the institution,* where they coexisted harmoniously with convulsive treatments for a full decade, until society began to turn to noninstitutional solutions to manage the problems posed by dependent psychiatric populations (Gronfein, 1985).

Heinz Lehmann (1989, 1993), the first North American to publish an article on administering chlorpromazine (CPZ) to psychiatric patients (Lehmann & Hanrahan, 1954), reminds us that in the 1940s, "Our two major therapies were insulin-induced hypoglycemic coma and electroconvulsive shock therapies (ECT) for schizophrenia and affective disorders. . . . Paraldehyde and the barbiturates were about our only means to quell agitation and violence in addition to physical seclusion and restraint. . . . 70% to 80% of [patients] relapsed" (1993, p. 294). Lehmann therefore experimented with procedures "that would be impossible to repeat today" (p. 295). He describes "brain biopsies" done on randomly selected patients; "carbon dioxide treatment"; the use of "very large doses of caffeine" in stuporous catatonic schizophrenics, "of course with no results"; nitrous oxide "to the point where there was complete loss of consciousness"; injections of sulphur in oil and typhoid antitoxin, both of which only produced high fevers; injections of "turpentine into the abdominal muscles which produced—and was supposed to produce—a huge sterile abscess and marked leucocytosis" (1989, p. 263); etc. Lehmann's account illustrates the notion that, in devising experiments for their forgotten and socially devalued wards, asylum doctors had little incentive to choose treatments causing least harm.

The treatment of psychiatric patients with CPZ used alone, at Ste-Anne Hospital in Paris, was first reported by Delay and Deniker in May 1952. However, the very first psychiatric use of CPZ alone occurred on November 9, 1951, when Leon Chertok injected an unspecified intravenous dose of the drug into Cornelia Quarti, a 28-year old psychiatrist, and voice-recorded her comments (Chertok, 1982). Previously, Laborit (1967) had reproduced Quarti's own written account. Some excerpts:

I begin to feel that I am getting weaker and weaker, it is very difficult and harrowing. At 12h10, one of the assistants tries to . . . hypnotize me. I gather all my energies to shout at him (so it seems to me): "No, you are bothering me." In fact, [judging from the voice recording, I] transmitted a weak and monotonous voice. . . . At 13h . . . the painful feeling of imminent death gives way to a euphoric calm. I still feel I am dying, but this leaves me indifferent. . . . At 15h, . . . my speech has become painful, dysarthric, I can't find my words. . . . In the evening, I am still very tired and must stay in bed . . . The speech difficulty continues. . . . The lassitude and speech disorders persist for a few days to disappear progressively. (pp. 7168–7169)

In the first British report on CPZ in psychiatry, Anton-Stephens (1954) identified psychic indifference as "perhaps the characteristic response to chlorpromazine. Patients responding well to the drug have developed an attitude of indifference both to their surroundings and their symptoms best summarized by the current phrase 'couldn't care less'" (p. 544). Inevitably, these effects led the original investigators of CPZ to make formal connections with lobotomy or leucotomy, which produced a "frontal lobe syndrome" characterized by apathy, loss of initiative, indifference to environmental and bodily stimuli and impairment of sophisticated intellectual functions such as the ability to plan ahead (Stuss & Benson, 1986).

Freyhan (1955) explained that "the first hypothesis advanced by French authors for the action of chlorpromazine . . . assumed a synaptic interception between the cortex and the diencephalon, resulting in suppression of excitations. This 'chemical lobotomy' theory . . . has since appeared in various reports" (p. 72). Lehmann (1989) actually acknowledged that the idea to administer CPZ came to him because he thought the new drug might produce the effects of lobotomy: "I thought [CPZ] was just another non-barbiturate sedative. But there was a certain statement [in the new literature by Delay and Deniker]: it acted like a 'chemical lobotomy,' which puzzled me, and I said to myself, there is something more to it" (p. 264). In his second article on CPZ, Lehmann (1955) observed, "Chlorpromazine is of value in the treatment of pain associated with terminal carcinoma. The effect in these cases is probably similar to that observed following a frontal lobotomy" (p. 94). Anton-Stephens (1954), referring to two patients who, upon receiving the drug, became "mute," "dazed," and "incontinent," but "showed no concern over this," wrote: "The picture they presented and that sometimes encountered following a pre-frontal leucotomy was independently made by several observers" (p. 549). In a paper on parkinsonian symptoms produced by CPZ, the French psychiatrists Letailleur, Morin, and Monnerie (1956) suggested these symptoms amounted to "functional lobotomy" (p. 806). Hans Steck (1956), a noted Swiss neuropsychiatrist, was more explicit. Discussing motor disorders arising during CPZ treatment, he concluded as follows:

Here again it seems important in order to localize the [effects of] neuroleptics to highlight the common traits and the distinctive traits of the effect of
leucotomy and the action of Chlorpromazine. In both cases we witness the
appearance of passivity, a reduction of psychic tension, stimulation and
initiative . . . But this occurs with leucotomy with no one ever having described a parkinsonian syndrome, whereas with the new treatment it appears almost obligatory. (p. 789)

NEUROLEPTIC EFFECTS AND EXTRAPYRAMIDAL SYMPTOMS: FIRST IMPRESSIONS

The "almost obligatory" parkinsonian syndrome and other motor disorders arising during NLP treatment were first reported by Steck (1954). He
noted parkinsonism and akathisia in 37% of 299 patients treated with CPZ
or reserpine. At Vermont State Hospital, Brooks (cited in Goldman, 1955,
p. 51) estimated that "all patients who are on large doses of Thorazine—for
any length of time show signs of basal ganglion dysfunction." Similarly, at
Pilgrim State Hospital, New York, Pleasure stated, "Probably two-thirds of
our patients showed some degree of Parkinson-like symptoms" (cited in
Goldman, 1955, p. 55). Lehmann (1989) remembers that when he first no-
ticed CPZ-treated patients with typical symptoms of Parkinson's disease,
". . . it did not seem possible because at that time there was no such thing as
drug-induced Parkinsonism; there were no models known in animals or
humans of induced Parkinsonism, known only were the post-encephalitic
or the spontaneous, idiopathic Parkinsonism, yet this looked very much
like it" (1989, p. 265).

Steck (1954) was the first to note the similarities between the drug-
induced effects and encephalitis lethargica (EL) or von Economo's disease,
which he knew well. An epidemic of EL, thought to be of viral origin, swept
through Europe from the mid-1910s to late 1920s, killing hundreds of thousands of people and leaving others afflicted with permanent parkinsonism
and dementia.[3] Steck pointed to the initial sedation produced by CPZ and

---

[3] Boyle (1990, especially pp. 65–71) argues that the populations studied by Emil Kraepelin
(who coined "dementia praecox") and Eugen Bleuler (who coined "schizophrenia") in the
late 1800s and the populations studied by von Economo (who authored the classic description of encephalitis lethargica) in the early 1900s had many striking similarities. According to Boyle, although encephalitis lethargica had not yet been identified, "there are at
least good circumstantial grounds for supposing that [Kraepelin and Bleuler] were for the
most part dealing with the consequences of some forms of encephalitic infection and that
at least a sizeable minority of their patients would later have been diagnosed as cases of
post-encephalitic Parkinsonism" (p. 69). As these neurological diseases became rarer and
as psychiatry and neurology evolved into two separate disciplines, the referents of
"schizophrenia" changed until that diagnosis "came to be applied to a population who
bore only a slight, and possibly superficial, resemblance to Kraepelin's and Bleuler's"

reserpine and the initial lethargy of the encephalitis, followed in both cases by a parkinsonian syndrome, except that the new drugs seemed to "speed up" the process observed in cases of EL. He suggested that the upper brain stem and extrapyramidal system, where EL had been shown to produce its pathology, were the new drugs' site of action. In Germany, Haase (1958, 1961) reported similar findings dating from 1954. Just like Steck, he likened the drug effects to a "speeded-up film version" (tempo cinématographique accéléré) of EL.

Delay and Deniker also made connections between the drug effects and the encephalitis. Deniker (1989) recounts that he and his colleague were asked by the French military to explain the occurrence of "dyskinetic episodes" among soldiers undergoing disembarkation exercises (and receiving prochlorperazine as an antiemetic):

> . . . Delay and I found the explanation. He remembered that similar episodes had been observed during epidemics of encephalitis lethargica following the first World War, and I actually found a number of references thereto in the literature. . . . *All the side effects of neuroleptics had already been described between 1920 and 1935 as a sequelae of encephalitis. . . . With this medication one obtained with progressive doses all the syndromes of encephalitis from the initial akinesia without hypertonias up to a hyperkineto-hypertonic syndrome which preceded the tardive dyskinesias* [italics added]. Moreover, corresponding to each neurologic syndrome there were particular psychological changes, independent of the prior mental state of the patient: for example, indifference with akinesia, mental depression with Parkinsonism, impatience with the hyperkinesias. (Deniker, 1989, p. 255)

Delay and Deniker therefore formally proposed in 1957 the word "neuroleptic" ("which takes hold of the nerve") to formally define CPZ and related compounds. It included five characteristics: (a) creation of a special state of psychic indifference, characterized by a hypersomnia reversible with ordinary stimuli, reduction of spontaneous and provoked motor activity, inhibition of conditioned reflexes and of learning; (b) efficacy in sedating excitation, agitation, manic states and agressive and impulsive outbursts; (c) gradual reduction of acute and chronic psychotic disorders; (d) production of extrapyramidal and vegetative syndromes (paroxystic dyskinesias, parkinsonian syndrome and pathology of the postencephalitic parkinsonism kind: akinesia, hyperkinesia, hypertonia; modification of

---

p. 70). This occurred because the "validity" of schizophrenia was taken for granted, and because a shift to *behavioral* diagnostic criteria did not seem problematic to a profession "claiming jurisdiction over both disturbing behaviour and disturbing neurology" (p. 70). Boyle's thesis could explain why Kraepelin and Bleuler described cases that resemble TD, more than half a century before NLPs were introduced.

thermal regulation, of pulse, of blood pressure, of secretions, of metabolism); (e) dominant subcortical effects, accounting for the preceding neurological effects (see Delay & Deniker, 1961).

This definition helped crystallize a consensus that had formed soon after the introduction of CPZ, and which probably found its clearest expression in Denber (1959): "The ability to induce an extrapyramidal action is a *sine qua non* of therapeutic effectiveness" (p. 61). As a result, some psychiatrists wondered "whether we should consider deliberately producing basal ganglion symptoms in patients [in order to] produce a higher improvement rate" (Ayd, cited in Goldman, 1955, p. 57). Other clinicians, such as Flügel (1956), wrote: "We busied ourselves to produce these states [of parkinsonism and psychic disinterest] systematically through continuous treatment with Reserpine and Chlorpromazine. . . . Approximately half the patients [were] completely immobile. One could move them about like puppets" (pp. 790–791).

Were long-term negative effects considered? Steck (1956) asked "whether we were making our patients run the risk of contracting a severe illness, a chronic and incurable parkinsonism" (p. 787). Because of instances where EPS had disappeared after NLP withdrawal, Steck felt that the risk was minor—although early on, he and several others described cases of attenuated or full-blown extrapyramidal syndromes persisting in patients one full year after the cessation of NLP treatment (Delay, Deniker, Bourguignon, & Lempérière, 1956; Ey, Faure, & Rappard, 1956; Schöneker, 1957).

Interestingly, antipsychotic attributes of NLPs were third on Delay and Deniker's list. It is easy to imagine that once the psychotic individual became indifferent, verbally and physically withdrawn, and less excited, the "psychosis" would also be seen as "gradually reduced." As Lehmann (1993) writes, early clinicians did not impute antipsychotic properties to NLPs until several years after the drugs were in use: "Even in my correspondence with other clinicians in the United States working with the phenothiazines neither I, nor they, dared to attribute specific antipsychotic effects to these new drugs. In 1956, . . . I introduced the term 'antipsychotic' apologetically, and more as a metaphor than a designation" (p. 300).

I have cited extensively from the early clinical literature on NLPs to suggest that most contemporary writers display a blind spot about NLP toxicity. Recent textbooks of psychopharmacology and countless studies of the NLP treatment of schizophrenia might not contain a single mention of psychic indifference, the outstanding NLP effect. Suggestions that NLP effects mimic those of a serious infectious neurological disease or that NLP treatment and lobotomy may produce similar effects are rarer still, if nonexistent. Proceedings from the First International Meeting on the

Neuroleptic-induced Deficit Syndrome (NIDS) (Lader & Lewander, 1994) provide a telling example. Although NIDS appears clinically indistinguishable from the frontal lobe syndrome produced by lobotomy and characterized by apathy, disinterest, and lack of initiative, none of the published papers from this 1993 symposium mention lobotomy or encephalitis lethargica, including the one paper (Lewander, 1994) purporting to review Delay and Deniker's observations of CPZ-induced sedation, apathy, and indifference.

This blind spot also means that contemporary researchers erroneously report various NLP-induced phenomena as new clinical observations. For example, in tying particular mental states to particular abnormal involuntary movements, Delay and Deniker spelled out a full theory of the behavioral toxicity[4] of NLPs, 30 years before Van Putten and Marder (1987) published an article on that topic (also omitting to mention Delay or Deniker). Several papers have rediscovered that NLPs regularly induce dysphoric mental states, singly or jointly with EPS such as akathisia and dystonia (Halstead et al., 1994; Lewander, 1994; Newcomer et al., 1994; Thornton & McKenna, 1994; Young, Stewart, & Fenton, 1994). Thornton and McKenna (1994) actually emphasize similarities with postencephalitic parkinsonism; not to suggest that NLPs mimic that disease but, in a leap of unjustified biological reductionism, to advance that all "psychiatric" phenomena are really "neurological" phenomena.

Breggin (1983, 1993) stands out among contemporary writers for his use of early clinical observations to understand the nature of NLP action. He has suggested that psychic indifference reveals NLP-induced "deactivation," which "designates a continuum of phenomena variously described as disinterest, indifference, diminished concern, blunting, lack of spontaneity, reduced emotional reactivity, reduced motivation or will, apathy, and, in the extreme, a rousable stupor" (1993, p. 9). According to Breggin,

---

[4]Lehmann (1979) defined behavioral toxicity as the harmful modifications of behavior resulting from specific or nonspecific drug action. Summerfield (1978) dates first mention of the concept to 1956, as a result of attempts to minimize undesirable effects of the newly discovered NLPs. Although Summerfield does not otherwise discuss NLPs, he provides valuable insights to understand and evaluate NLPs' characteristic psychological effects:

Among the first effects [of drug-induced toxicity] are visible changes in behaviour. A very serious consequence is loss of self-critical monitoring of whatever one may be doing . . . impaired in the particularly dangerous way that the person concerned is unaware of the process of behavioural deterioration to which he or she is being subjected. . . . (H)igh-level psychological functions may be the first to go under the stress of poisons and pollutants. . . . Only therefore by looking for impairments of functions immediately dependent upon the highest levels for their control and coordination might any adverse effect be detectable at all. It is a profound conceptual issue that has spent more time in oblivion than in recognition. (pp. 336–337)

deactivation is the essence of what is termed the "antipsychotic effect" (and of the lobotomy effect). Reviewing clinical and physiological parallels between NLP effects and characteristic symptoms of encephalitis lethargica, Breggin (1993) notes insightfully that, aside from previous NLP exposure, nothing could differentiate an acute, severe attack of encephalitis from an attack of NLP malignant syndrome. This suggests clear lines of investigation, especially since the ultimate neurocognitive sequela of the encephalitis was dementia. After a flurry of articles in the 1980s (see section on Tardive Dementia and Tardive Psychosis), the issue of whether NLPs produce dementia after prolonged use or as a further deterioration of TD has mostly faded from discussion. However, this may be the start of another cycle of official discontent with NLPs. In several published reactions to a review (Hegarty, Baldessarini, Tohen, Waternaux, & Oepen, 1994) finding that outcome in schizophrenia is not better now than it was early in the century, it is suggested that NLPs may be responsible, by producing or worsening negative symptoms, deficit syndromes, and Alzheimer-type cerebral pathology (Dean, 1995; Oken & McGeer, 1995; Warner, 1995). More recently, in a longitudinal study of 71 subjects with dementia, McShane, Keene, Gedling, Fairburn, Jacoby, and Hope (1997) found that the mean decline in cognitive score in the subjects who took NLPs was twice that of the patients who did not. Furthermore, in the former subjects, the start of NLP treatment coincided with faster cognitive decline: the median rate of decline was 5 points per year before treatment and 11 points per year after that.

APPRAISING CURRENT USE OF NEUROLEPTICS

The following sections provide a review covering current use of NLPs. When considering one topic, such as dosage, it becomes necessary also to discuss EPS, therapeutic effectiveness, response rate, clinical practice styles, and so forth. Some repetitions are thus unavoidable. The remainder of this chapter focuses on a few topics that cover a broad sample of the literature and highlight key problematic areas.

THE QUESTION OF DOSE

After one is reasonably convinced that a drug should be prescribed to treat an undesirable condition, the first issue to consider is determining the appropriate dose. Today, the results of dose-response studies in humans and animals are available prior to the marketing of a given medication and dosage recommendations within generally narrow ranges are made to physicians by drug manufacturers.

However, after more than 40 years of research and clinical experience with NLPs, NLP dosages are not well mapped nor are patients' drug responses predictable. Furthermore, although NLP use is associated with several *dose-dependent* toxic effects, the minimum effective dosages of various NLPs are unknown. The phrase "minimum effective dosage" is that which the most authoritative NLP prescription guidelines recommend that clinicians prescribe in long-term NLP treatment (APA, 1992, p. 251). These guidelines—which focus on minimizing the risk of TD—are not universally accepted and have no *official* standing. As late as 1995, McIntyre and Simpson could write, "It would be helpful for practitioners if there were some sort of protocol to guide one through neuroleptic use" (p. 135).

The confusion over NLP dosage, in theory and in practice, highlights several of the general problems plaguing the overall use of NLPs. An obvious difficulty is that although dozens of studies specify a dosage range below which no "therapeutic" response is observed and above which toxicity appears unacceptable (to clinicians) and/or therapeutic efficacy does not increase, this range is rarely respected in clinical practice. The scientific consensus during the current decade holds that dosing above 10 mg/day of haloperidol (HPL) equivalents improves neither the speed nor the degree of therapeutic response in the vast majority of cases (Baldessarini et al., 1988; Dewan & Koss, 1995; McIntyre & Simpson, 1995). Data from controlled clinical trials, reinforced by comprehensive meta-analyses and continually endorsed by leading clinical psychopharmacologists, indicates that a dose between 3 and 7 mg/day of HPL equivalents suffices to maintain the full desired "antipsychotic" effect (Bollini, Pampallona, Orza, Adams, & Chalmers, 1994; Hogarty, 1993; McEvoy, Hogarty, & Steingard, 1991).

Yet, the majority of studies of prescription practices show mean daily doses far exceeding the range's upper limit (see, e.g., Peralta, Cuesta, Caro, & Martinez-Larrea, 1994; Reardon, Rifkin, Schwartz, Myerson, & Siris, 1989; Segal, Cohen, & Marder, 1992; Volavka et al., 1990). This "tendency for psychiatrists everywhere to use higher doses of antipsychotics than necessary . . . is true even more so in the United States than elsewhere" (McIntyre & Simpson, 1995, p. 135). Baldessarini et al. (1995) report a contrary finding from a Boston-area private teaching hospital: mean doses in 1993 were just under 5 mg/day in HPL equivalents. These investigators observed similar dosages at the same hospital in 1989 and believe their findings reflect a downward trend characterizing this decade. However, until confirming evidence is available, the findings may be considered an anomaly. Although clozapine was prescribed at a mean dose of 331 mg/day in that Boston study, it was prescribed the same year at a mean dose of 591 mg/day in a New York City hospital (Pollack et al.,

1995). This interstate variation in the dosing of clozapine—an NLP whose potential to induce the sometimes fatal agranulocytosis appears dose-dependent and whose prescription legally requires extremely close monitoring—suggests strongly that even wider variations still exist with respect to other, more widely used NLPs. One simply needs to compare daily doses from any number of published studies selected at random in the psychiatric literature or from surveys of practicing psychiatrists. D. Cohen and Bisson (1997) surveyed 350 Canadian psychiatrists; less than 2% indicated that a 20 mg/day dose of HPL for maintenance treatment for an adult or elderly chronic patient was too high or excessive. Meise, Kurz, and Fleishhacker (1994) surveyed Austrian psychiatrists and found a 50-fold difference between the lowest and highest recommended doses for NLP maintenance treatment (40 to 2,000 mg/day in CPZ equivalents).

Daily doses above 1 or 2 gm of CPZ equivalent are rarer nowadays, although it has been frequently observed that "high-potency" NLPs (such as haloperidol and fluphenazine) are prescribed in higher CPZ-equivalent doses than "low-potency" NLPs (such as CPZ and thioridazine). In CPZ-equivalents, Baldessarini, Katz, and Cotton (1984) found a high- to low-potency dose ratio of 3.5:1 in a sample of 110 Boston-area patients; Segal et al. (1992) reported a 5.3:1 ratio among a sample of 243 California sheltered-care residents. Many explanations have been given for this phenomenon, including clinicians' preference for managing adverse effects typical of high-dose, high-potency treatment (i.e., EPS) rather than toxic systemic syndromes produced by high-dose low-potency NLPs; ease of increasing high-potency doses if patients show little improvement. Dewan and Koss (1995) offered another explanation: large variance in the NLP equivalencies found in psychiatric manuals! These authors compared equivalency tables in a dozen manuals and found significant disagreement on the clinical equivalence of some NLPs, with up to 500% variance reported in texts. Most affected were the high-potency drugs. For example, two texts stated that 100 mg of CPZ were equivalent to 1 mg of HPL and two texts to 5 mg of HPL. Thus, "[an acutely psychotic] patient could be prescribed 5 mg of haloperidol daily or 25 mg daily by two different physicians who each thinks he is prescribing the appropriate minimum" (p. 231).

Classifying NLPs according to "potency" and determining their clinical equivalence with respect to a standard drug or each other is a mostly North American custom. Dewan and Koss (1995) can only include American texts in their review. In France the idea of high- and low-potency NLPs or of clinically equivalent doses of chemically different NLPs has no currency. It is not mentioned in the latest edition of that country's authoritative psychopharmacology manual (Ginestet & Kapsambelis, 1996), which still manages to describe seven different ways to classify NLPs. Generally, French authors believe that each NLP has a unique profile of up to six main clinical effects, even that different doses of the same NLP will produce quite different profiles. How seriously this notion is taken in American psychiatry is illustrated in a comment by Johns, Mayerhoff, Lieberman, and Kane (1990): "On a clinical level, there is certainly some feeling, based largely on anecdotal evidence, that some patients do better on one drug than another." Johns et al. do acknowledge, "Remarkably, there are very few reports in the literature that address this issue in a systematic fashion" (p. 58).

As mentioned, another difficulty related to NLP dosage is predicting clinical response to various fixed doses. More often than not, typical NLP effects will be more visible to outside observers at "moderate" or "higher" dosages. Yet one would expect that the field would have gone substantially beyond such a commonsense notion, given the energies, talents, and sums invested in NLP psychopharmacology since the 1950s. For example, in a study by Rifkin, Doddi, Karajgi, Borenstein, and Wachspress (1991), newly admitted inpatients with a diagnosis of schizophrenia were randomly assigned to receive either 10, 30, or 80 mg/day of HPL (at the time of the study, 20–25 mg/day was considered a "standard dose"). Subjects were then evaluated under double-blind conditions for 6 weeks. At the end of this period, no differences in clinical condition—and no differences in EPS—were noted between the three groups. More recently, Stone, Garver, Griffith, Hirschowitz, and Bennett (1995) also found no differences in clinical response between 4, 10, and 40 mg/day of HPL administered over a 2-week period. To be sure, other studies arrive at different results. Van Putten, Marder, and Mintz (1990) compared 5, 10, and 20 mg/day of HPL in the treatment of acute psychosis, finding an advantage for 20 mg at 1 week, but a clear deterioration because of "psychotoxicity" at 2 weeks, with 10 mg more effective overall and 5 mg effective for some patients. Stone and Garver (1996) insist that, given the state of knowledge, studies are needed to test the effectiveness of doses of HPL including 0 and 1 mg/day.

Minimum effective NLP dosages have not yet been determined, nor have investigators been able to demonstrate, even with the most sophisticated fixed-level blood studies, the existence of therapeutic plasma levels of NLPs (Kane, 1989; Simpson & Yadalam, 1985; Stone & Garver, 1996). Waddington, Weller, Crow, and Hirsch (1992) stated, "There is renewed appreciation of our previous failure to establish, even at this late stage in their evolution, the optimal usage of existing typical neuroleptic drugs and of the potential benefit still to be gained therefrom" (p. 994). Bitter,

Volavka, and Scheurer (1991) more directly summarized the state of the art of NLP dosing: "Despite intensive research and after almost four decades of neuroleptic treatment we still do not know the minimum effective dose of any neuroleptic" (p. 32).

If prescribing high doses of NLPs does not lead to improved clinical results, yet clinicians persist in prescribing high doses, one may turn one's attention to extraclinical influences on the prescribing situation. Referring to American high dosing, McIntyre and Simpson (1995) believe that it results partly from "the wave of managed health care engulfing psychiatry" and pressures from "third-party payers to do more and to do it faster. Psychiatrists . . . may find themselves changing their clinical techniques in order to accommodate these demands" (p. 135). Undoubtedly important, these recent economic pressures cannot account for the high-dosing phenomenon, which well antedates them.[5]

The inability to determine minimal dosages or to prescribe within dosage ranges recommended in the research literature raises fundamental questions about the ability of clinicians and researchers to make sense of their observations (an ability which may be mostly context-dependent). For example, Pollack et al. (1995) observed that, after 12 weeks of treatment, Austrian psychiatrists prescribed clozapine to their patients at a mean dose of 153 mg/day, compared with 458 mg/day for American psychiatrists. Yet, symptom ratings—similar at baseline for both groups of patients—had decreased significantly more in absolute and relative terms in the Austrian cohort by the 6th week and stayed lower through the 12 weeks of the study. Despite the sizable body of findings showing diminishing return with increasing dosage, the association of greater benefit with lower dose was characterized by Pollack et al. as "surprising," an "anomaly" (p. 315). Such "resistance" indicates that actual, observed clinical results weigh less in NLP use and evaluation than ingrained practice habits. More important, it suggests that the treatment zeitgeist may actively bias clinicians in favor of NLPs, influencing them to disregard essential information

---

[5] According to Deniker (1990), "As early as 1956, the question of why dosages were higher in America than in Europe was posed. Denber was appointed by New York State and by [Smith Kline & French] Company to investigate the reason. The answer was simple: American psychiatrists were more hurried than their European colleagues" (p. 84). Just how hurried the former were is indicated in this comment by Kinross-Wright, a Houston psychiatrist, who was asked during the first major symposium on CPZ in the United States, in 1955, why he used doses as high as 4,000 mg a day: "Well, the reason we haven't given more than 4,000 mg (actually, it is 4,800 mg now) is because we don't like to subject patients to more than 40 tablets a day. We think that is just about the limit. The reason we go so high is that in our intensive scheme of treatment we just keep pushing up the dosage until the patient shows definite signs of clinical improvement" (cited in *Chlorpromazine and Mental Health*, 1955, p. 68).

with critical bearing on their own prescribing behavior, their patients' clinical outcomes, and their judgment on the overall value of NLPs. This is also evident in the literature touching on the effectiveness of NLPs.

The Effectiveness of NLPs in the Acute and Long-Term Treatment of Schizophrenic Disorders

Zito and Provenzano (1995) distinguish between the *efficacy* and the *effectiveness* of drug therapies. The first refers to "the health outcomes of a drug when it is used under ideal conditions," in a well-controlled environment, with compliant and homogeneous subjects. The second refers to "how well a drug works under usual practice conditions" (p. 737), administered by different types of clinicians in a spectrum of settings, to a heterogeneous population often receiving other drugs. In theory, this distinction is useful and partially explains wide differences in reported outcomes and direct costs of certain drug treatments (Carter et al., 1995). In practice, both types of evaluations are difficult to distinguish. A random-assignment, double-blind study may be conducted with a heterogeneous, noncompliant population. Or, a new drug may be tested in an open trial in an ordinary clinical setting, but the extra care and enthusiasm of the researchers may make the conditions "ideal" (for patients). True efficacy studies might only refer to some premarketing drug trials that aim to meet regulatory requirements. As a rule, for recently introduced drugs, more efficacy studies are available. In any case, most reviews mix efficacy and effectiveness studies together. In this chapter, the term *effectiveness* will refer to both types of evaluations.

An Early NLP-Placebo Comparison

Two reports of placebo substitution of NLPs and antiparkinsonians raise intriguing, still unresolved questions bearing directly on the issue of effectiveness. During nine months of 1959, in a ward housing 68 chronic patients, French psychiatrist Serge Follin replaced the CPZ liquid preparations with an identical-looking placebo (Follin, Chanoit, Pilon, & Huchon, 1961). Aside from the hospital director, neither personnel nor patients were informed. The patients had been treated for a minimum of six months and a maximum of three years, at daily doses ranging from 150 to 700 mg. Although 29 of the patients were excluded from the analysis (they changed wards or received other treatments and no further information about them is provided), the results are still astonishing: Ward life remained completely unchanged and no one saw through the trick. Instances of patient misbehavior were neither less nor more common than before the placebo substitution. Various increases and decreases of placebo doses were made by unknowing ward physicians: clinical notes show that insomniac patients were able to sleep when the dose was increased while others who appeared sedated became more agitated when doses were decreased. After nine months, the authors tallied their results: 22 patients (56.5%) rated as definitely improved (including 11 discharged), 15 (38.5%) rated as unchanged, two (5%) rated as worsened.

A second experiment is recounted by Lemoine (1995). In the early 1980s, also in France, worried about the indiscriminate prescription of antiparkinsonians to patients receiving NLPs in his hospital, Lemoine replaced, after one month of baseline observation, the antiparkinsonian drugs with identical-looking placebo gelules in one half (randomly chosen) of the ward patients. Only the ward director and the hospital pharmacist were aware of the subterfuge. None of the placebo-treated patients showed any appearance or worsening of abnormal movements. More to the point, medical personnel noted clinical improvement in patients on placebo, who then received lower NLP doses. Lemoine phrased his astonishment thus: "Without his [antiparkinsonian drug], a patient was improved and reduced his use of neuroleptics!" (1995, p. 174).

Because of current requirements for informed consent in research, it would be difficult to carry out such experiments today. Strictly speaking, the studies tell us more about the power of placebo than the effectiveness of NLPs or the confounding effects of antiparkinsonians. However, it is regrettable that such studies were not analyzed in greater detail or that systematic efforts are not made to replicate them with a view to augmenting placebo effectiveness—results might go a long way in dispelling much of the aura surrounding the efficacy of NLPs or, at the very least, in establishing more precise indications for these drugs.

EFFECTIVENESS STUDIES

To evaluate the effectiveness of NLP treatment of schizophrenia, studies since the 1950s have measured how often patients on medication and patients not on medication experience a relapse. Generally, two groups of comparable patients, one administered NLPs and the other a placebo, are followed for a determined period (usually 2 to 6 months, occasionally 12 months, very rarely up to 24 months) following release from an index hospitalization or psychotic episode. Effectiveness is evaluated by estimating, by means of appropriate statistical tests, whether the proportions of patients who relapse in each group differ significantly. There is no uniform way to define relapse: It may operationalized as a return to active medication, rehospitalization (if patients are living in the community), an exacerbation of symptoms that would qualify as an active episode of schizophrenia, a set increase (sometimes over a set period) in psychotic symptoms as measured by a known rating scale, and so on. Although during the past decade the latter criterion is often used, there are no systematic reviews that have attempted to uncover differences in outcome of NLP treatment depending on definitions of relapse.

Approximately 1,300 NLP effectiveness studies have been published since the mid-1950s (Keck, Cohen, Baldessarini, & McElroy, 1989). The overall rate of effectiveness reported (see reviews by Baldessarini, 1985a; J. M. Davis, 1975) is similar to the rate recently estimated by J. M. Davis et al. (1993) from 35 random-assignment, double-blind studies involving 3,720 patients: "Patients on placebo relapse at a rate of 55%, whereas only 21% of schizophrenic patients relapse when they are on maintenance therapy" (p. 24). Subtracting from the placebo rate the 21% of patients who presumably would relapse even if they were on drugs, we obtain the "net" effectiveness rate of 34%. Put another way, for only one in three patients on NLPs who do not relapse during a set study period, NLP treatment appears to be the determining factor.

Numerous factors, internal and external to the individual, can be expected to trigger, provoke, or influence a relapse (or, inversely, a state of "clinical stability"). Almost by definition, these factors will vary among individuals, which also helps to explain the large variations in relapse rates observed within and across individual studies. But even the 34% net effectiveness rate, which is by no means insignificant—given the disturbing impact of psychosis on the individual and his or her social network—does not give an accurate picture of the NLPs' role in helping the schizophrenic function better in society. Until a decade or so ago, most formal evaluations of NLP effectiveness focused on symptom reduction and relapse prevention, not on improved social functioning or integration (Barnes, Milavic, Curson, & Platt, 1983). Symptoms and rehospitalization are relatively easy to measure, but do not reveal how patients really fare overall and over time, in social and vocational spheres. With the advent of "care in the community," researchers have had to broaden outcome measures to include social functioning and quality of life (Diamond, 1985). Yet, according to Meltzer (1992), "There are no studies that demonstrate the outcome of neuroleptic treatment in schizophrenia using all these criteria" (p. 516).

A search of articles published between 1989 and 1993 with the keyword "quality of life" located over 1,200 studies, only three of which dealt with NLPs (see D. Cohen, 1994b). These and earlier studies confirmed the conclusion by Diamond (1985): Although NLPs show some ability to prevent relapse in schizophrenia, they have no direct positive effect on social functioning. Whether on NLPs or on placebo, patients who do *not* relapse have very similar social functioning. In addition, NLP doses (and medication regimen) typically used in the 1980s exerted a negative impact on social integration (D. Cohen, 1989; Hogarty et al., 1988; Kreisman et al., 1988). In all likelihood, this negative impact results from NLPs' tendency to produce or accentuate social withdrawal or negative symptoms and to interfere with learning and with the ability to apply skills learned during the medicated state to nonmedicated states (Brenner et al., 1994; Lehmann, 1979; Lidz, 1993).

The lack of interest in seriously evaluating medicated patients' quality of life was noted by Awad and Hogan (1994). They attributed this to disagreement on a definition of quality of life, lack of a conceptual model for quality of life on NLPs, and scarcity of reliable and valid measures for the concept, though dozens of sophisticated rating scales exist, able to incorporate quantitative and qualitative evaluations of numerous objective and subjective dimensions. Awad and Hogan nevertheless point to what appears as the key explanation: ". . . uncritical rejection by clinicians of reports from their schizophrenic patients regarding their feelings about medication. . . . As psychiatry and psychiatric research has become markedly preoccupied with the 'objective,' a gradual disregard of the subjective dimension of our patients' experiences has followed" (p. 31). This disregard for schizophrenic patients' accounts of their subjective experience is based on the notion that these accounts are unreliable since patients suffer from disturbed thinking and communication. This notion, however, receives no support from the few studies that have attempted to validate subjective impressions of patients with other key informants such as relatives, friends, and clinicians (see, e.g., Epstein, Hall, Tognetti, Son, & Conant, 1989; Kreisman et al., 1988).

Closely related to the issue of quality of life on NLPs is that of negative subjective responses to NLPs. Despite evidence linking the emergence of such responses with poor treatment outcome several weeks and months later (see review by Awad & Hogan, 1994), this area of research, with rare exceptions, has been systematically avoided in the contemporary literature. Patients' negative subjective reactions to NLPs, especially at the initiation of treatment, are one of the most observable aspects of the NLP clinical experience. Scientific neglect of this ubiquitous NLP treatment feature, as well as of an intuitively and objectively important factor bearing on NLP effectiveness, parallels the adoption of clinical strategies aiming to ensure strict compliance with NLP treatment to decrease risk of relapse. Researchers and clinicians may be missing the point entirely for large subgroups of patients.

A meta-analysis of 368 schizophrenia outcome studies from 1895 to 1992 by Hegarty et al. (1994) reveals the relatively limited impact of NLPs as it highlights researcher bias in data analysis. In this study, cohorts from the first two decades of NLP use do show greater improvement (clinical or social) than cohorts from previous decades, especially the 1910s and 1920s. However, even in cohorts diagnosed with stricter Kraepelinian criteria (associated with lower improvement rates through-out the century), the differences between NLP treatment and convulsive treatments (electroshock, insulin coma, metrazol coma) are not impres-sive: 31% improvement rate for the former, 27% for the latter, compared with a 22.5% improvement rate for "nonspecific" treatments, defined as "placebo trials, psychotherapy, hydrotherapy, fever therapy, and nonneu-rological surgery" (p. 1411). When all cohorts are considered, improve-ment rates for NLP and convulsive treatments are also very similar: 46% and 42%, respectively. Nevertheless, the authors *exclude* convulsive treat-ment from their multiple regression model to establish predictors of im-provement. Of note, improvement declined after the 1970s, reaching the rate of 36% in the 20 NLP outcome studies published since 1986, "a level that is statistically indistinguishable from that found in the first half of the century" (p. 1412). Attempting to salvage the reputation of NLPs, Hegarty et al. conclude their review with this sentence: "In addition to an effect of broad versus narrow diagnosis, the results of this study support a favorable impact of modern treatment, *particularly the use of neuroleptic agents* [italics added]" (1994, p. 1415). Had the researchers not omitted con-vulsive therapy from the independent variables in the regression equation, the conclusion would be unsupportable. That such an incomprehensible—or ingenious—strategy in data analysis is allowed to pass through the re-view process of one of the most prestigious psychiatric journals indicates the strikingly prodrug bias in the field today. Furthermore, since the au-thors define "modern treatment" as NLP *and* convulsive therapies, one is led, again, to ponder precisely what was considered so radically innovative about NLPs when these agents were first evaluated in contexts where the use of convulsive therapies was also widespread.

The results of an unusual study raise other questions concerning the ef-fectiveness of NLPs. Keck et al. (1989) tried to define the onset and time course of antipsychotic effects of NLPs. Out of more than 1,300 published studies, they excluded open trials, studies of chronically psychotic pa-tients, and studies not using a placebo or non-NLP sedative as a control. Astonishingly, this left only five reports. In the three studies of NLP ver-sus placebo, and the two of NLP versus sedative:

> [T]he same overall degree of improvement was observed during treatment . . . within each of the markedly different time intervals stud-ied. Furthermore, when a neuroleptic was compared to a sedative—di-azepam or opium powder—the sedative demonstrated efficacy similar to that of the neuroleptic during the first day and through 4 weeks of treat-ment. (pp. 1290–1291)

Commenting on these results, an admittedly baffled psychiatrist wondered:

> Has our clinical judgment about the efficacy of antipsychotics been a fixed, encapsulated, delusional perception . . . ? If there is no difference in outcome in a month, how about 2 months, or 6, or a year, or a lifetime? Do sedatives prevent relapse as well as antipsychotics do? Are we back to square 1 in antipsychotic psychopharmacology? (Turns, 1990, p. 1576)

To summarize the preceding reports on NLPs:

- The ability of NLPs to reduce "relapse" in schizophrenia affects only one in three medicated patients.
- Chronic NLP use depresses social functioning.
- Researchers have systematically avoided studying the role played by patients' subjective responses to NLPs.
- The overall usefulness of NLPs in the treatment of schizophrenia—conceived as a broad, episodic impairment of various social-interpersonal-cognitive abilities—is far from established.

"Nonresponse" to Neuroleptic Treatment

Since the 1989 introduction in North America of clozapine, a drug marketed specifically for "neuroleptic nonresponders," much discussion has focused on this particular group of schizophrenic patients. In 1990, the APA Press published *The Neuroleptic Nonresponsive Patient* (Angrist & Schulz, 1990), perhaps the first book on the subject in nearly 40 years of NLP use. Despite the limited effectiveness of NLPs, previous discussions of NLP nonresponse were rare. The renewed interest in the issue, according to Johns et al. (1990), results from "increasing pressure to shorten the length of hospital stays" (p. 53).

"Response" to NLPs and "effectiveness" of NLPs may be linked conceptually and empirically, but the latter notion typically refers to NLPs' ability to delay relapse, whereas the former refers to NLPs' ability to bring psychotic symptoms under control within a few weeks' time. According to Karon (1989), both "common clinical experience" and "the usual inference from placebo trials" suggest "that medication is useful in the short run in improving immediate clinical status for most schizophrenic patients" (p. 108). Recently, though, some reports estimate a 25% nonresponse rate (e.g., Liberman et al., 1994) and informed observers have suspected that the rate is much higher (Easton & Link, 1986/1987).

What is the rate of nonresponse to NLP treatment for acute episodes of schizophrenia or psychotic symptoms? One answer is found in the results of a study conducted by Johns et al. (1990). The researchers first administered a "standard dose" of 20 mg/day of fluphenazine to 29 "acutely exacerbated, hospitalized chronic schizophrenic patients," and obtained a response rate of 37%. Although this seemed "surprisingly low" to the researchers, "review of an earlier pilot study undertaken with 31 schizophrenic inpatients at [their] institution revealed an almost identical response rate (35%) to the same treatment condition" (p. 62). The authors summarize their findings as follows:

> The most striking feature of these preliminary data is the poor response of . . . patients to a standard course of treatment with neuroleptics. Only one-third of such patients responded well to an initial 4-week course of neuroleptic treatment; continued neuroleptic treatment for an additional 4 weeks regardless of whether the neuroleptic class or dose was changed or held steady, resulted in almost no further improvement in clinical condition. (p. 63)

Because of the small sample size, the authors termed their findings "speculative at best" (p. 63). However, additional data from this ongoing study has been published, with the sample size increased to 156 "acutely ill schizophrenic, schizoaffective, and schizophreniform" hospitalized patients (Kinon et al., 1993). Of the 115 patients who completed the first 4-week phase of the study, 68% were rated as nonresponders. Of the latter who went on to randomized treatment (lower dose, higher dose, or other NLP), "only 4 of 47 subjects (9%) subsequently responded" (p. 309). Despite their surprise with the 63% nonresponse rate in 1990, the authors characterize the 68% nonresponse rate in 1993 as "consistent with a range in previous reports" (p. 310). No data are given on the 41 subjects who did not complete the study; it is not known if they too might be rated as nonresponders and further deflate the dismal response rate.

Systematic studies focusing on nonresponse are scarce, making it difficult to assess how often this occurs in typical practice. Yet, despite NLPs' unique capacities to diminish spontaneous movement or excitation (Clinton, Sterner, Stelmachers, & Ruiz, 1987; Ellison & Pfaelzer, 1995), one senses that nonresponse is quite common. Meltzer's (1992) review of treatment strategies for NLP nonresponders estimates that up to 45% of patients do not respond to NLPs or develop such severe drug-induced behavioral toxicity that treatment cannot be continued after a few weeks. Collins, Hogan, and Awad (1992) rated 50% of all schizophrenic patients hospitalized for more than 6 months in Ontario's largest psychiatric hospital as nonresponders (these patients were nevertheless maintained on daily NLP doses as high as acute patients).

Another indication of high rates of NLP nonresponse—or response so evaluated in current contexts of shorter hospitalization—may be found in rates of polypharmacy with central nervous system (CNS) depressants. Baldessarini et al. (1995) examined pharmacy records of all cases of inpatients treated with a NLP in mid-1993 at their hospital and compared them with a sample of similar cases from 1989. In the interval, length of hospitalization for these patients had decreased markedly, from an average of 73.1 days to 18.5 days. There was no increase in daily NLP dose, but the use of adjunctive anticonvulsants had doubled to 84% of patients in 1993. A "potent benzodiazepine" was prescribed to 81% of patients (unchanged from 1989), lithium was given to 70% (increased from 50% in 1989). Overall, 84% of patients on NLPs received another CNS depressant, 45% two or more (no figures were given for anticholinergic drugs). Separating from this chemical soup the specific impact of NLPs on patients' outcomes may be an impossible task.

NEUROLEPTIC WITHDRAWAL

Faced with NLPs' limited effectiveness and substantial handicaps (see following section), researchers have begun to study the impact of withdrawing the drugs from medicated patients. The issue of NLP withdrawal drew national attention following an article in the *New York Times* (Hilts, 1994) reporting on official blame leveled at University of California researchers for failing to get "proper consent" from schizophrenic patients "in an experiment in which they were taken off their medication and allowed to suffer severe relapses" (p. A1). The researchers were aiming to find out "if some schizophrenics might do better without medication" (p. B10). Although the subjects signed documents stating that they understood the consequences of withdrawal, the severity of some reactions—one subject committed suicide, another threatened to kill his parents—angered patients' families. Many reasons exist to withdraw NLPs from "responding" or "nonresponding" patients under well-monitored conditions. However, there is little psychiatric tradition in initiating and supervising *patient-centered* drug withdrawal to minimize predictable withdrawal reactions.

Support for the foregoing assertion—and further glimpses into the confusion surrounding researchers' judgment of NLP effectiveness—is found in data from the first systematic review of the literature on NLP withdrawal in schizophrenic patients (Gilbert, Harris, McAdams, & Jeste, 1995). Gilbert et al. located 66 English and foreign-language publications (1958 to 1993, involving over 4,000 patients) reporting new data on NLP withdrawal in a minimum of 10 subjects with a diagnosis of schizophrenia or schizoaffective disorder. They found the overall relapse rate of withdrawn patients to be 46.6% for a mean length of follow-up of 7 months. In 29 studies, NLP withdrawal groups were matched to NLP maintenance groups: after a mean follow-up of 10 months, relapse rate was 53.2% in the former and 15.6% in the latter. This obvious and significant difference, highlighted in the review's text and abstract, nevertheless vanishes under a closer look. Unless a patient is the victim of acute drug-induced toxicity, there exist few good reasons to withdraw a psychotropic drug abruptly. Yet, in 42 of 60 studies (70%) where information about the length of NLP taper was given, NLP treatment "was withdrawn acutely over 1 day" (1995, p. 175).

In their published commentary on this review, Baldessarini and Viguera (1995) re-analyzed the data in 46 studies (33 with abrupt discontinuation—less than two weeks, usually one day—and 13 involving longer discontinuation). They found that "the proportion of patients relapsing per month was threefold greater after abrupt discontinuation of treatment [14.5% vs. 5.3%, $p = .008$]" (p. 191). Surprisingly, Gilbert et al. (1995) report only NLP withdrawal itself and length of follow-up to be significantly associated with the relapse rates. Nevertheless, as Baldessarini and Viguera show, it appears that *gradual* NLP taper might almost erase any differences in relapse rates between withdrawal and maintenance groups.

In their own reply commentary, Jeste, Gilbert, McAdams, and Harris (1995) acknowledge, "Baldessarini and Viguera make an excellent point regarding the relapse rate being three times greater following abrupt withdrawal compared with gradual discontinuation" (p. 211), yet they remain silent on any implications for their results. Here are the implications: *Gradual NLP withdrawal is associated with the same relapse rate as continued NLP treatment.* At the very least, one must endorse Gilbert et al.'s conclusion, which again highlights the little progress made these past four decades in the wise use of NLPs: "There is a critical need . . . to identify patients who do not need long-term neuroleptic maintenance therapy and to optimize strategies for neuroleptic taper that minimize the danger of relapse" (1995, p. 186).

Baldessarini and Viguera's (1995) reanalysis of the Gilbert et al. (1995) data raise other intriguing questions about the extent and nature of NLP iatrogenesis. They show the risk of relapse appears nonlinearly distributed over time, with most of the excess risk after stopping treatment arising early, within the first three months. Baldessarini and Viguera cite almost identical findings from studies of lithium withdrawal in bipolar patients. They suggest, "The state following the interruption of maintenance treatment may not be clinically or psychobiologically identical to that reflected in the natural history of the untreated illness" (p. 190). They propose the existence of an "iatrogenic-pharmacologic stress effect" operating after drug withdrawal, "particularly abrupt interruption." They conclude, "An excess of relapse following *rapid* drug withdrawal may inflate drug vs. no-drug comparisons . . ." (p. 191, italics added).

Many of the studies in the Gilbert et al. (1995) review were probably not designed to study withdrawal; thus withdrawal conditions may not have been carefully planned. Yet, despite its obviously confounding effects, *abrupt* withdrawal is used by van Kammen et al. (1995) to test behavioral and biochemical indicators of schizophrenia relapse. Van Kammen's team is described by Zubin, Steinhauer, and Condray (1992) as using "one of the most closely controlled approaches to studying relapse after withdrawal of medication" (p. 15). In this study of 88 men with a diagnosis of chronic schizophrenia of several years' duration and maintained on HPL, "identical-looking placebo capsules replaced the haloperidol capsules overnight . . ." (van Kammen et al., 1995, p. 674). After six weeks, 60% of patients were classified as relapsing, a rate van Kammen et al. suggest appears "higher than those usually reported" (p. 676). The investigators tested three regression models to predict relapse, but there is no telling how the various independent variables might differ if NLP withdrawal were more gradual. It is reasonable to expect that chemical ratings of neurotransmitter levels and behavioral ratings of psychosis, depression, and anxiety would vary depending on the speed of NLP withdrawal. The researchers went to considerable trouble to collect their data (for example, using lumbar punctures to obtain cerebrospinal fluid from subjects). Their article appears five months after the Gilbert et al. (1995) review of NLP withdrawal studies and the commentary by Baldessarini and Viguera (1995), in the same journal, but nowhere do van Kammen et al. discuss the possible impact on relapse rates and relapse architecture of abrupt NLP withdrawal.

Liberman et al. (1994) describe careful NLP withdrawal, with consequent positive results. Thirteen "treatment-refractory schizophrenic patients" receiving over 50 mg/day of HPL and continually hospitalized for a mean of five years had their NLP dose reduced every 5 weeks by 15 mg/day, as long as the patient was rated unchanged or improved. If the patient was rated slightly worse, the dose was held steady for another 5 weeks, and if rated much worse, the dose was increased to the previous increment. After 5 weeks at their "optimal" dose, the patients received "individualized behavioral analysis and therapy" for target problems such as agitation, assaultiveness, incoherence. Eleven of 13 patients tolerated a mean NLP dose reduction of 88% (most patients still received a benzodiazepine). This "produced improvements in positive symptoms, depression, anxiety, and side effects, and the addition of intensive behavior therapy yielded improvements in functional behavioral and negative symptoms" (p. 758). For 20 weeks, one patient was "remarkably improved at a dose of 0 mg" (p. 757). For 9 patients, the clinical status reached on the "optimal" dose was sustained for a minimum of 1 year of follow-up. Caldwell (1994) provides illuminating case studies of two "extraordinarily violent" individuals in maximum security hospital units who showed dramatic improvements following drug discontinuation and the application of a "social constructionist" treatment approach. Caldwell pointedly recognizes, "Within the conventional thinking of the mental health field, such so-called miracle cures are simply not believable" (1994, p. 600).

PSYCHOSOCIAL ALTERNATIVES TO NEUROLEPTIC TREATMENT

Several studies comparing psychotherapeutic treatment of schizophrenic patients with NLP drug treatment have been published. The most careful and detailed review of the six major American controlled studies (carried out from 1959 to 1981) was done by Karon (1989). He noted at the outset the prevailing opinion by the end of the 1960s, to the effect that treatment of schizophrenia without medication was unjustifiable. During the 1970s, a few studies modified this opinion to suggest that social treatment improved patients' quality of life and clinical outcome and should be combined with maintenance drug therapy. This opinion, with slight modification and refinement of the psychosocial interventions such that these are seen as important but insufficient ingredients in a comprehensive treatment program, prevails today. For example, in one study (Kleinman, Schacter, Jeffries, & Goldhamer, 1993) the written information on risks and benefits of NLP medication given patients to obtain their informed consent included the statement, "Psychotherapy and social therapy are other forms of treatment used to help patients with schizophrenia, but neither is as effective as neuroleptic medication in preventing relapse" (*Risks and benefits,* no date). This opinion, however, cannot be supported by the available evidence.

Karon (1989) discussed several problems explaining the lack of positive results for psychotherapy found in some of the controlled studies: (a) using unwilling, uninterested, or inexperienced therapists and supervisors, (b) using therapists unfamiliar with patients from lower socioeconomic classes or nonwhite ethnic groups, (c) examining patients on the day of termination of psychotherapy, discharge, and other irregular intervals, (d) not measuring thought disorder carefully, (e) taking ward behavior, not real-world functioning, as a key outcome measure, (f) not following patients in the long-term, or (g) all of the preceding. Despite these strategies, most studies reviewed showed psychotherapy to be at least as effective as NLPs.

The Soteria studies (Matthews, Roper, Mosher, & Menn, 1979; Mosher & Menn, 1978) were mentioned but not reviewed by Karon. These studies, conducted in San Jose, California, between 1971 and 1983, established conclusively that an intensive interpersonal intervention with newly diagnosed schizophrenic patients within a "therapeutic community" context—and staffed by nonmedical, nonprofessional personnel—could substantially reduce the use of NLPs. Treatment outcome was predominantly positive for approximately 200 acute schizophrenic patients maintained on very low dosage or no NLPs. After 6 weeks, no significant differences in psychopathology levels were observed between 28 index patients treated without drugs at Soteria and 11 hospitalized control patients receiving an average daily dose of 700 mg of chlorpromazine equivalent. At 2-year follow-up, however, the Soteria patients had better levels of social adjustment and occupation, had experienced their psychosis in a less distressing manner, and incurred lower treatment costs. These findings were not subject to systematic replication until the establishment of Soteria Berne in Switzerland in 1984. The treatment program in the latter project, run in a 12-room house accommodating six to eight patients and two staff, was quite similar to that used in the original Soteria, except for a greater reliance on low-dose, targeted medication as well as the systematic use of medical personnel.

Ciompi et al. (1992) reported data on 51 patients treated for at least 10 days and discharged from Soteria Berne between 1984 and 1990, including outcome comparisons over a 2-year period between the first 14 index and 14 matched control patients (hospitalized in four different psychiatric clinics and hospitals). Twenty (39%) of the 51 Soteria received no NLPs during their entire stay, and the rest received "low" doses (about 170 mg/day of chlorpromazine equivalent) for approximately two-thirds of their stay. In 61% of the index cases, the immediate global outcome was rated as "good" or "fairly good," and in 35% as "rather poor" or "poor." Patients receiving no medication demonstrated significantly better clinical results. Matched-pair comparisons were made by matching index and control patients with respect to age, sex, and the two most relevant predictors of outcome, premorbid social adjustment and prevailing positive or negative symptoms. No significant differences were found in seven out of a total of nine outcome and progression variables (including psychopathology, housing arrangements, job situation, social autonomy, and relapse rate). The only significant differences found were for mean daily NLP dose and total cumulative NLP dose. However, treatment costs were significantly higher for the Soteria patients, probably because of the long postdischarge, rehabilitation phase of the Soteria program. While not definitive, these findings confirm those of Mosher and Menn (1978) and Matthews et al. (1979), strongly suggesting that important subgroups of newly diagnosed schizophrenic patients may be helped with no or little use of NLPs.

NEUROLEPTIC-INDUCED BEHAVIORAL TOXICITY

Neuroleptics' near-sacred reputation as "antipsychotics" is only equaled by their record as one of the most behaviorally toxic classes of psychotropic drugs. In two studies including 2,700 NLP-treated patients (Dencker, Ahlfors, Bech, Elgen, & Lingjaerde, 1986; Segal et al., 1992), patients themselves most frequently report dry mouth, loss of sex drive, agitation, weight gain or loss, sleepiness, diarrhea or constipation, depression or lethargy, vertigo, and general physical weakness. The intensity of the effect matters probably more than its simple occurrence but we lack knowledge on the impact of subtle but persistent drug-induced dysfunction.

The most widely acknowledged yet least scientifically studied effects of NLPs are the lethargy and negative symptoms they induce in patients. Recent descriptions of these effects are given by Wallace (1994), who summarized topics discussed by thousands of callers to SANELINE, a telephone helpline for people diagnosed or coping with severe mental disorders. After queries for actual psychological or medical help, the second most common reason for calling SANELINE is worries about medication.

> What we have found is that most people with schizophrenia dislike taking the drugs they are being prescribed. . . . [T]he negative parts [of the side effects] are perceived as quite often worse than the illness itself. . . . [I]n the anonymity of phone calls to SANELINE, even the most deluded person is often extraordinarily articulate and lucid on the subject of their medication. . . . "When I take my medication, I feel as though I am walking with lead in my shoes" one young man told me on the telephone. Another told the volunteer who took his call "I feel emptied out, devoid of ideas." Another young man sent us a poem in which he compares the effects of the drugs with drowning—"I was always under the water gasping for air and sunshine," he writes. . . . Almost all of our callers report sensations of being separated from the outside world by a glass screen, that their senses are numbed, their willpower drained and their lives meaningless. It is these insidious effects that appear to trouble our callers much more than the dramatic physical ones, such as muscular spasms. (pp. 34–35)

Acute manifestations of EPS are occasionally reported present in 90% of NLP-treated patients (Casey, 1989, 1991). It is beyond the scope of this critical review to describe EPS in detail (see Kane & Lieberman, 1992a; Keshavan & Kennedy, 1992). Nor will there be a discussion of neuroleptic malignant syndrome, an explosive toxic reaction affecting 0.5% to 2% of NLP users, with a reported fatality rate of 5% to 30% (Addonizio, Susman, & Roth, 1987). Topics touched on here will include some problems EPS pose for patients and clinicians, professional-clinical reactions to EPS, prevention of tardive dyskinesia, and controversies surrounding ominous long-term NLP effects such as tardive psychosis and tardive dementia. The backdrop for this discussion is the commonly held notion that the advantages of NLP treatment outweigh its drawbacks.

REIFYING "SIDE EFFECTS": OBSTACLE TO REALISTIC ASSESSMENT OF
NEUROLEPTIC EFFECTS

The psychiatric literature distinguishes between "main" and "side" effects of psychotropic drugs. The first are "therapeutic" effects, the second are "toxic" (or "adverse") effects. What actually distinguishes a main effect from a side effect is not the action of the chemical substance but rather the *intent* of the prescriber: a "side" effect may be just as frequent as, or more common than, a "main" effect (see Dewan & Koss, 1989, p. 216), but it is unwanted. However, for a given individual (patient or clinician) at a given time, one drug effect may be desirable and another undesirable, or both sought simultaneously. At what point does NLP-induced sedation and indifference (valued during the acute psychotic episode) become "akinetic depression" or, later, "NLP-induced deficit syndrome" (condemned as a major chronic treatment complication)? When does "effective reduction of psychomotor excitation" become "NLP-induced parkinsonism"? When does "reducing the flow of unfiltered external stimuli" become "intense distress with one's discomfort" (in severe akathisia)? Individual patient differences aside, the drug's range of actions does not commonly vary, but these will be categorized according to the requirements of the social-interpersonal-clinical situation. If this analysis has merit, the distinction between "therapeutic" and "adverse" effects has been reified by clinicians and researchers, operating in a zeitgeist of propsychotropic drug bias.[6]

As a class of psychotropics originally named because their neurological toxicity coincided with the sought-after goals of treatment, NLPs exemplify the preceding point. Furthermore, the clinical reality of inextricable link between "therapeutic" and "toxic" has probable biochemical parallels. In 1963, Carlsson (1975) suggested that NLPs blocked striatal dopaminergic (DA) receptors. It was later shown that an NLP's ability to occupy 65% to 80% of D_2 receptor sites correlated with its "antipsychotic potency." The DA hypothesis of NLP action—not fully satisfactory to explain most observations but still dominant (see Kahn & Davis, 1995)—thus attributes NLPs' "therapeutic" effects to D_2 receptor blocking. Yet that is precisely the same mechanism invoked to account for EPS and, with alterations in the DA and other neurotransmitter systems after prolonged blockade, for TD. The ongoing discovery since the 1970s of several families of DA receptors and the observation that NLPs such as clozapine have lesser affinity for D_2 receptor blockade and lower frequency of EPS, led to the current belief that particular biochemical actions (i.e., blockade of D_3 and D_4 receptors and/or receptors from other neurotransmitter systems) can produce "main" effects

---

[6] Of course, similar considerations apply to other types of drugs (see Montagne, 1988).

without producing "side" effects. Based on what we know about the brain and its nearly infinite yet integrated complexity, such a belief may be illusory, reminding one of the futile search for nearly 60 years now, of "anxyolitic" molecules not inducing dependence or sedation.

Do NLPs produce distinct desired effects (antipsychotic) *in addition* to distinct undesired effects (adverse) or do they produce a *global neurological syndrome* that can be evaluated in some contexts and over time as partially or fully beneficial? In the case of illicit psychotropics (which many users actually report *liking*), researchers have no difficulty conceptualizing desired effects as in fact part of a spectrum of psychological and neurological toxicity. In the case of NLPs (which most users actually report *disliking*), there is strong resistance to this idea. This suggests that a naive realism pervades psychopharmacological research.

NEUROLEPTIC-INDUCED EXTRAPYRAMIDAL SYMPTOMS (EPS)

The main types of EPS include parkinsonism, dystonia, akathisia, and dyskinesia. In a clinical context showing enthusiasm toward NLPs, and without the standardized rating scales developed the following decade, Ayd (1961) observed a global incidence of 39% among nearly 4,000 NLP-treated patients. Twenty years later, Ayd (1983) estimated a 61.9% incidence.

Among EPS' most disturbing characteristics is that they resemble typical psychiatric symptoms (i.e., they add significantly to any preexisting emotional-mental problems and may not be recognized as drug-induced); they may remain resistant to chemical treatment; and they may become irreversible, even after complete cessation of NLPs. Each syndrome may occur alone, as a distinct entity, or concomitantly with other drug-induced syndromes. Each syndrome may appear any time during NLP treatment. Each is traditionally characterized as "acute" when it arises early in the course of treatment and "tardive" when it appears after months or years, but there exists no clear phenomenological distinction between the two forms. On a pharmacological level, however, early-appearing EPS are *always* lessened by reducing the NLP dose and sometimes by adding an antiparkinsonian (anticholinergic) drug, which partially and temporarily restores the dopamine-acetylcholine equilibrium upset by D_2 receptor blockade. Tardive EPS, on the other hand, are usually unaffected or worsened by a dose reduction. Similarly, EPS are reversible at the beginning, but may become irreversible later. There is no way to know this in advance—only discontinuation of NLPs will tell: Cases that resolve will be termed "reversible" and those that persist, "irreversible." At best, a tardive syndrome will show decrease of the symptoms over time and may be slightly relieved by symptomatic treatment.

The first symptoms of NLP-induced parkinsonism, also called pseudo-parkinsonism, are identical to those of idiopathic Parkinson's disease: reduced facial expression, reduced arm swing, general muscular rigidity, monotonous speech. This is often referred to as akinesia or hypokinesia. Postural instability, tremor of the extremities, and hypersalivation appear sometimes. As noted, the reduced motor and psychic spontaneity may be indistinguishable from negative or deficit signs of schizophrenia or from a postpsychotic depression: they are frequently unrecognized (Van Putten & Marder, 1987, p. 15).

Van Putten and May (1978) found that 30% of 94 chronic schizophrenic patients showed pure akinesia, 17% had akinesia and other EPS, 19% had EPS without akinesia, while 34% had no EPS. Parkinsonism typically appears between a few hours and 20 days after the start of NLP treatment and tends to disappear gradually after a few months (Herrington & Lader, 1981). In a small percentage of cases, it will reappear, persist, and worsen, months after the cessation of NLPs (Melamed, Achiron, Shapira, & Davidovicz, 1991).

Rifkin, Quitkin, and Klein (1975) described a 22-year-old NLP-treated man, whose anticholinergic drug was switched to placebo following his enrollment in a clinical study. Two weeks later, the man became quite depressed and suicidal as a result of his being completely unable to sustain conversations at social events. An hour after reinstitution of the anticholinergic, the symptoms were greatly reduced and disappeared in 24 hours. However, the parkinsonism persisted in the form of a rigid gait. Because of parkinsonism's frequency and resemblance to negative symptoms, such examples of complex NLP emotional-behavioral toxicity are doubtless more frequent than the number of published case studies would suggest.

DYSTONIAS

Dystonias are strange, uncoordinated movements produced by sustained muscular spasms, mostly affecting the head and neck, occasionally the extremities and the trunk. Forced opening of the mouth, protrusion and distortion of the tongue result in speech, swallowing, and breathing difficulties (laryngeal dystonia). The individual may show an empty, fixed stare, followed by vertical or lateral movements of the eyes (oculogyric crises). Or, the eyes may be forced tightly shut (blepharospasm). Possibly the most extensive descriptions of dystonia and tardive dystonia are by Burke et al. (1982) and Burke and Kang (1988).

Acute dystonias generally appear between 1 hour and 5 days after the start of NLPs, a dose increase or a sudden NLP change. Dewan and Koss (1989) report prevalences averaging 1% to 10%. Because dystonias often occur suddenly, are painful and bizarre, they frighten patients and families. This must be appreciated in light of the fact that younger patients, especially men, seem more predisposed (Klein, Gittelman, Quitkin, & Rifkin, 1980). NLPs such as haloperidol, molindone, and the piperazines are more likely to produce dystonic reactions than other drugs (Bezchlibnyk-Butler & Jeffries, 1996).

Contrary to the tardive dyskinesias, where older patients and women are at higher risk, young and old patients are equally at risk of developing tardive dystonia, with an estimated prevalence of 1% to 5%. Yadalam, Korn, and Simpson (1990) described four such cases, in three of which the abnormal movements interfered "with all daily activities" (p. 17).

AKATHISIA

Recognized today as the most frequent (5% to 76% incidence) and distressing EPS, akathisia was relatively ignored by researchers until recently (Sachdev & Loneragan, 1991). This may be partly because the problem is often subjective, described differently by patients: inability to sit still, a sense of gloom and anxiety originating in the abdomen, restless legs, and so forth (Lavin & Rifkin, 1992). In "mild" cases, the individual may show no visible movement (especially if there is a co-occurring akinesia) but nevertheless feel significant psychic agitation or muscular tension. When visible, the motor agitation typically takes the form of shifting weight from foot to foot or walking on the spot, inability to keep legs still, shifting of body position while sitting (Sachdev & Kruk, 1994). Akathisia usually appears within hours or days of the start of NLPs and is often mistaken for psychotic agitation; this may result in a NLP dose increase, which worsens the akathisia (Lavin & Rifkin, 1991). In one study (Hermesh, Shalev, & Munetz, 1985), akathisia was reported to contribute to 3.4% of emergency hospital admissions. In extreme cases, it has led to suicide and homicide (Van Putten & Marder, 1987).

Akathisia is frequently accompanied by a dysphoric mental state, described by some normal subjects as a "paralysis of will" (Belmaker & Wald, 1977). A medical student who received 1 mg of HPL described the sensation of an external force forcing him to move (Kendler, 1976). Vaughan, Oquendo, and Horwath (1991) described the case of a 34-year-old man on fluphenazine who developed a severe akathisia and attributed his agitation to an external force, described by Vaughan et al. as a "psychotic delusion." Manos, Gkiouzepas, and Logothetis (1981) described patients who experienced psychotic flare-ups, making statements such as "A woman tried to strangle me last night," "I burn inside," and "A pair of pliers squeezed my body and throat." However, the authors stressed that the symptoms were subjective accounts of objective manifestations of disturbing EPS. Commenting on these cases, Lavin and Rifkin (1991) believe, "It is likely that [they] occur more frequently than is usually recognized" (p. 1615).

Tardive akathisia—which resists any treatment and persists despite NLP discontinuation—represents a particularly troubling problem. Its prevalence has been estimated at 18% of patients referred to a TD evaluation clinic (R. J. Davis & Cummings, 1988), and 14% among 180 intellectually handicapped individuals treated with NLPs (Gualtieri, 1990). Gualtieri (1993) illustrates well a dilemma posed by chronic NLP use: after attempting and failing to discontinue NLPs (because of the acute behavioral and motor flare-ups) in a group of intellectually handicapped individuals with tardive akathisia, he concludes that these unfortunates are condemned to remain on the drugs because of NLP-induced toxicity.

TARDIVE DYSKINESIA

Bezchlibnyk-Butler and Jeffries (1996) estimate the risk of TD (in adult patients) as "38% after 5 yrs, 56% after 10 yrs" (p. 45). Most cases are of "mild" intensity. An undetermined proportion (5%–10%?) are very severe and incapacitating. Occasionally, some authors muse about the impact of factoring TD into the cost-benefit ratio of prolonged NLP treatment, but this has never been done seriously in the mainstream literature (but see Dewan & Koss, 1989). As will be discussed, significant resistance still exists today about its prevention.

The TD syndrome (which includes tardive dystonia and tardive akathisia) is a complex disorder that includes up to 25 different abnormal movements (Singh & Simpson, 1988). Movements and grimaces of mouth, tongue and lips predominate in about 80% of patients (Kane & Lieberman, 1992b). Tics and mannerisms are sometimes confounded with TD, especially among intellectually handicapped persons, and abnormal movements resembling TD were described in psychotic patients well before NLPs were introduced. Nevertheless, since the first reported cases, the prevalence of TD has grown significantly. In 1981, Jeste and Wyatt estimated a 13% prevalence rate, which had increased to 24% a decade later (Yassa & Jeste, 1992).

A recent study with 2,250 subjects shows how rates vary depending on the populations studied: 36% of chronic, hospitalized patients had signs of TD; among less frequently hospitalized patients, the rate was 13%; among those never exposed to NLPs, including elderly persons, the rate of spontaneous or senile dyskinesia varied between 0% and 2% (Woerner et al., 1991). Lower rates among chronically hospitalized patients in Italy and in China (see Yassa & Jeste, 1992) suggest that higher NLP doses used in North America help explain the scope of the problem here. There are remarkably few actual *number* estimates of TD victims. Dewan and Koss (1989) provide such an estimate, although based on extrapolations from a 1983 study of outpatient NLP use in the Unites States. Their best-case and worst-case scenarios result in the astounding range of 90,000 to 625,000 people who suffer *irreversible* TD in a given *year*.

In up to 85% of elderly patients with TD, there is complete unawareness of the movements (Myslobodsky, 1986). This anosognosia is typically found in syndromes of generalized brain dysfunction. Institutionalization, schizophrenia, psychic indifference produced by the NLPs, mental deterioration, and dementia (including NLP-induced tardive dementia), have been invoked, singly or together, as factors explaining it (Bourgeois, 1988).

Aside from NLP exposure, the only unanimously recognized risk factor is advanced age, which also increases the probability of TD persisting. Yassa, Nastase, Camille, and Belzile (1988) found that 41% of patients over 63 years developed TD after only 2 years of NLP treatment. Female gender is also consistently implicated. Individual studies suggest a dozen other factors, including previous EPS, diagnoses of affective disorders, cumulative NLP dose, concomitant use of antiparkinsonians, previous existing brain damage or use of convulsive treatments, frequent NLP holidays. All NLPs commonly used are likely to provoke TD, with fluphenazine sometimes said to pose a higher risk. Hill (1983) denounced the fact that, given ongoing use of NLPs, research priorities have not been directed at ruling out whether any particular NLPs pose higher risk.

After 5 years, in patients in whom NLPs are discontinued, the rate of spontaneous remission of TD ranges from 14% to 40% (Bezchlibnyk-Butler & Jeffreys, 1996; Casey, 1985; DeVeaugh-Geiss, 1988). In patients maintained on NLPs, however, results are less encouraging. Yassa et al. (1984) observed remission after 2 years in 16% of 55 TD patients; DeVeaugh-Geiss (1988) reported no improvement in 17 patients after 1 year; Bergen et al. (1989) reported improvement in only 11% of 101 patients after 5 years; Glazer, Morgenstern, and Doucette (1991) reported that 58% of 192 TD patients followed for 3 to 55 months showed a "chronic and persistent" pattern, the rest an "intermittent" pattern.

The main medical complications of TD include breathing problems (Turnier, Desrosiers, & Chouinard, 1988; Yassa & Lal, 1986), gait and posture problems (Lauterbach, Singh, Simpson, & Morrison, 1990), gastrointestinal dysfunction (Goldberg, Morris, & Lidofsky, 1990), as well as speech problems (Laporta, Archambault, Ross-Chouinard, & Chouinard, 1990). These appear to result directly from the abnormal movements affecting certain muscles. In the elderly, oesophegeal, diaphragm, and respiratory dyskinesia "may be fatal" (Turnier et al., 1988, p. 41).

COGNITIVE AND PSYCHOSOCIAL COMPLICATIONS OF TARDIVE DYSKINESIA

Most known motor disorders appear to produce a deterioration of cognitive functions. About 30 studies have assessed the cognitive functioning of patients with TD and have established that, in particular, various memory and nonverbal dysfunctions are associated with TD (H. Cohen & D. Cohen, 1993a, 1993b). The severity of cognitive deficits sometimes correlates positively with the severity of the movements. The main research questions center around determining whether these deficits predate the apparition of TD, result directly from presumed brain lesions caused by NLPs and underlying TD, result from the psychiatric disorder, or develop from an interaction of these or other factors. The primary impediment to answering these questions remains the unwillingness or inability of researchers—given the official view of NLPs as essential or lifesaving—to constitute and follow a sizable control group of unmedicated schizophrenic patients.

Psychosocial complications of TD have been documented, including suicidal thoughts, higher death rate, and vocational problems (Yassa, 1989). Although evidence remains mostly anecdotal, D. Cohen (1994b) noted that only one or two published studies have looked specifically at psychosocial dimensions of TD, and has suggested that TD is a socially stigmatized condition. For example, in the first complete description of TD, by Schöneker in 1957, the author wrote, "The repetitive mouth movements . . . were repugnant to people around [the patient]" (as cited in DeVeaugh-Geiss, 1982, p. 201). For Mosher and Burti (1989), "The dyskinesic is stigmatized by the impossible-to-hide, cosmetic disfigurement of tardive dyskinesia" (p. 3). According to Diamond (1985), "the movements tend to change the appearance of the patient and accentuate social distance" (p. 32). Among 22 patients interviewed by Yassa (1989), 12 complained of embarrassment caused by their abnormal movements and by reactions from people in public places.

TARDIVE DEMENTIA AND TARDIVE PSYCHOSIS

The issue of psychopathological symptoms appearing during prolonged NLP treatment was debated for some years in articles on "tardive dysmentia." Wilson et al. (1983) first proposed the term to describe certain behavioral changes seen in prolonged NLP treatment. These changes showed strong positive correlation with TD and were described as a "behavioral equivalent" of TD: loud voice, loquacity, incoherent speech, euphoria that could rapidly turn into hostility, autistic preoccupations punctuated with hyperactivity and intrusiveness. Like TD, this syndrome would result from a hyperactivity of the striatal DA system caused by chronic NLP antagonism. Mukherjee (1984) implicated schizophrenia as the cause of this dementia-like syndrome, but Jones (1985) felt that it was an iatrogenic complication of NLPs. In Myslobodsky's (1993) case descriptions, tardive dementia is presented as a behavioral and psychological disorder certainly associated with TD and characterized as "a paradoxical combination of apathy, irritability, and euphoria" (p. 89). Myslobodsky suggests that TD represents "larval dementia."

The concept of "subcortical dementia" (Cummings, 1990) may shed light on that of tardive dementia. The former refers to a slowing of cognitive and motor functions, impaired recall, emotional problems—especially depression and apathy—as well as deficits in so-called executive functions (primarily involving concept formation and the capacity to change mental set). Signs of subcortical dementia are notably visible in diseases of the extrapyramidal system (Parkinson's, Huntington's). Physiological, cognitive, and behavioral parallels between these two diseases and TD suggest that tardive dementia of the NLPs may be a variant of subcortical dementia (Breggin, 1990; Myslobodsky, Tomer, Holden, Kempler, & Sigal, 1985).

Supersensitivity or tardive psychosis has also been associated with chronic NLP treatment. Chouinard and Jones's (1980) diagnostic criteria include appearance after NLP reduction or withdrawal; mostly made up of positive schizophrenic symptoms; concomitant signs of DA supersensitivity, such as TD; association with central nervous system tolerance to NLPs, necessitating increased doses to maintain the antipsychotic effect. NLPs constitute the most effective "treatment" for the disorder, which exists on a severity continuum. The final phase of tardive psychosis is an irreversible, manifest psychosis that continues despite NLP treatment. This ominous entity remains controversial. For example, Chouinard, Annable, and Ross-Chouinard (1986) reported a 27% prevalence of "definite" cases among 224 chronic schizophrenics on NLPs, while Hunt, Singh, & Simpson (1988), only found 12 "probable" cases after a chart review of 256 patients.

The syndromes of tardive dementia and tardive psychosis illustrate the potentially complex and far-reaching nature of NLP effects. As for any drug effect, a good dose of skepticism is required to evaluate their validity. However, given what is known about the action of NLPs on the central nervous system and given their visible effects on mood and behavior, there is ample justification and evidence to entertain the hypothesis that these irreversible syndromes are consequences of NLP treatment. Yet, if previous professional reactions to TD are any indication, one should not expect researchers or policymakers to hastily tackle the prevention or implications of these other tardive NLP iatrogenic syndromes.

PROFESSIONAL RESISTANCE TO PREVENTING
NEUROLEPTIC IATROGENESIS

Despite TD's significance as a public health problem, psychiatrists in North America have resisted taking effective steps to deal with it. A gleaning of the relevant literature reveals three types of resistance: resistance to informing patients about TD, to changing prescription habits, and to acknowledging the noxious effects of NLPs.

D. Cohen and McCubbin (1990) found evidence of large NLP dose increases in the 1970s and 1980s and of nonrecognition or misdiagnosis of TD in clinical practice (see also Hansen, Brown, Weigel, & Casey, 1992). They saw no indication that the incidence of TD was about to decline. In addition, Wolf and Brown (1988) observed, "Few institutions have adopted the APA guidelines, and in those that have, many professionals try to circumvent them. Even when informed consent about psychiatric treatment is seriously pursued, patients are provided little information about side effects. When side effects are mentioned, tardive dyskinesia is frequently not among those named" (p. 24).

Nearly a decade later, Meltzer (cited in Gerlach & Peacock, 1995, p. 32s) pointedly asked: "How good a job are we really doing in making patients aware, at the onset of treatment with typical neuroleptics, that they are facing a 30% risk of irreversible tardive dyskinesia once it is established that they need prolonged treatment, or that there is an 80% risk over the course of time that they would have significant EPS?" Data from two recent surveys provide a depressing answer. Kennedy and Sanborn (1992) surveyed 520 state or county hospital psychiatrists in 35 American states. Almost half of respondents said they routinely fail to disclose to their patients on NLPs that they run any risk of developing TD. Given the sensitive topic of the survey, we can only speculate how many respondents would not so admit. For their part, Benjamin and Munetz (1994) surveyed directors of 160 Community Mental Health Centers in the United States about their TD screening practices. Only 41% reported having any monitoring system in place to detect the condition. Benjamin and Munetz conclude that their results are due to "the denial of tardive dyskinesia, plus the great fear that making its risk known will drive patients off their needed medication" (p. 346).

Resistance to viewing TD as a frank neurological disorder also appears strong. Although TD's precise physical correlates are still unknown, a syndrome of involuntary movements—especially when it assumes an irreversible form—can *strongly* be considered to have an *organic, structural* substrate. Here is a (moderately) clear expression of this idea (published in a European psychiatric journal): "[all EPS] entail the risk of becoming irreversible and may thus be an expression of the neuroleptic's ability to produce persisting central nervous system changes" (Gerlach & Peacock, 1995, p. 27s). However, because of NLPs' near-sacred standing in schizophrenia treatment, TD remains conceptualized as being not exactly what it looks like: a progressive, drug-induced brain syndrome with accompanying physical, behavioral, and cognitive complications (H. Cohen & D. Cohen, 1993).

Neuroleptic effects, like those of any other psychotropic, result from an interaction between the drug, the individual, and the context. This helps explain why abnormal movements characteristic of TD may change over time, be exacerbated during periods of stress, attenuated temporarily by efforts of concentration, be less bothersome to chronically institutionalized patients, and so forth. However, despite occasional findings of spontaneous or senile dyskinesia in unmedicated patients, the weight of the historical, epidemiological, and clinical evidence with humans, and of the experimental laboratory evidence with animals, points overwhelmingly in one direction: NLP drugs "cause" TD. Nevertheless, one may still observe that psychiatric researchers exaggerate the importance of any data that cast doubt on the causal connection or seize opportunities to exonerate NLPs and limit their own responsibility in the production of TD. An outstanding example appears in an article by Fenton, Wyatt, and McGlashan (1994). Having found the presence of oral-facial dyskinesias documented in the records of 15 of 100 presumably NLP-naive schizophrenic patients, the authors offer the following advice in an unprecedented conclusion titled "Medicolegal Caution": "Those physicians who find the case for a significant prevalence of spontaneous dyskinesia in schizophrenia compelling may find it prudent to inform patients and families that the progression of *schizophrenia* [italics added] . . . may be accompanied by the emergence of movement disorders" (p. 649). One looks in vain across the medical literature for similar prominently titled cautions advising physicians to inform patients and families of the prevalence of a vastly more compelling case, that of the emergence of movement disorders with the progression of *NLP treatment.*

CONCLUSION

This selective review of the literature suggests that the value of NLPs in the short- and long-term treatment of schizophrenia has been greatly exaggerated. Forty-five years of NLP use and evaluation have not produced a treatment scene suggesting the steady march of scientific or clinical progress. On the contrary, NLP drug treatment varies widely from country to country, decade to decade, even state to state or hospital to hospital.

Unquestionably, NLPs frequently exert a tranquillizing and subduing action on persons episodically manifesting agitated, aggressive, or disturbed behavior. This unique capacity to swiftly dampen patients' emotional reactivity should once and for all be recognized to account for NLPs' impact on acute psychosis. Yet, only a modestly critical look at the evidence on short-term response to NLPs will suggest that this often does not produce an abatement of psychosis. And in the long-run, this outstanding NLP effect probably does little to help persons diagnosed with schizophrenia remain stable enough to be rated as "improved"—whereas it is amply sufficient to produce disabling toxicity.

A probable response to this line of argument is that, despite obvious drawbacks, NLPs remain the most effective of all available alternatives in preventing relapse in schizophrenia. However, existing data on the effectiveness of psychotherapy or intensive interpersonal treatment in structured residential settings contradicts this. Systematic disregard for patients' own accounts of the benefits and disadvantages of NLP treatment also denigrates much scientific justification for continued drug treatment, given patients' near-unanimous dislike for NLPs. Finally, when social and interpersonal functioning are included as important outcome variables, the limitations of NLPs become even more evident and the systematic implementation and evaluation of nondrug treatment alternatives even more pressing.

Despite the extraordinary interest generated by the introduction and now widespread use of "atypical" NLPs, and of published findings of relatively greater efficacy and lesser toxicity, it is too early to tell whether these represent a true step forward or merely another false dawn. It may be that—whatever neurotransmitters may be targeted by a particular compound—rapid or effective control of spontaneous psychomotor activity can only be obtained for a "price" (i.e., behavioral or other toxicity). Any other expectation might be, simply, unrealistic. Furthermore, scientific inquiry and communication do not take place in a vacuum; the majority of individuals who conduct research in psychopharmacology operate within a profoundly prodrug context and have a direct stake in the maintenance of the scientific and clinical status quo. This long-standing positive bias in favor of NLPs is continually highlighted, as when published research findings pointing to blatant deficiencies, disadvantages, or ineffectiveness of NLPs remain unexamined or are simply glossed over, even by the very researchers who generate them.

In the field of psychopharmacology, concerned with drugs specifically designed or prescribed to alter the functioning of the central nervous system, the distinction between main and side effects may be no more than a once-heuristic concept to guide clinical practice. Yet, despite this

ubiquitous conceptual distinction and the development of tools to identify and map numerous undesirable cognitive, emotional, and physical effects of NLPs, their impact has been barely studied in relation to both
short- and long-term clinical and social outcome in schizophrenia. Combined with the lack of active interest in actual and potential tardive iatrogenesis from the NLPs—in the form of chronic deficit syndromes—the
state of research and practice seems even more unsatisfactory. Huge gaps
remain in our knowledge of NLP drugs; partially filling only some of
these gaps could profoundly alter the conventional view on the effectiveness of NLPs. The positive consensus about NLPs cannot resist a critical,
scientific appraisal.

REFERENCES

Addonizio, G., Susman, V. L., & Roth, S. D. (1987). Neuroleptic malignant syn-
drome: Review and analysis of 115 cases. *Biological Psychiatry, 22,* 1004–1020.
Alvir, J. M. J., Lieberman, J. A., Safferman, A. Z., Schwimmer, J. L., & Schaaf,
J. A. (1993). Clozapine-induced agranulocytosis: Incidence and risk factors
in the United States. *New England Journal of Medicine, 329,* 162–167.
American Psychiatric Association. (1985). APA statement on tardive dyskinesia.
Hospital and Community Psychiatry, 36, 902–903.
American Psychiatric Association. (1992). *Tardive dyskinesia: A task force report of
the American Psychiatric Association.* Washington, DC: Author.
Angrist, B., & Schulz, S. C. (Eds.). (1990). *The neuroleptic-nonresponsive patient:
Characterization and treatment.* Washington, DC: American Psychiatric Press.
Anton-Stephens, D. (1954). Preliminary observations on the psychiatric uses of
chlorpromazine (Largactil). *Journal of Mental Science, 100,* 543–557.
Appelbaum, P. S., Schaffner, K., & Meisel, A. (1985). Responsibility and compen-
sation for tardive dyskinesia. *American Journal of Psychiatry, 142,* 806–810.
Awad, A. G., & Hogan, T. P. (1994). Subjective response to neuroleptics and the
quality of life: Implications for treatment outcome. *Acta Psychiatrica Scandinav-
ica, 89*(Suppl. 380), 27–32.
Ayd, F. J. (1961). A survey of drug-induced extrapyramidal reactions. *Journal of
the American Medical Association, 175,* 1054–1060.
Ayd, F. J. (1983). Early-onset neuroleptic-induced extrapyramidal reactions: A
second survey 1961–1981. In J. T. Coyle & S. J. Enna (Eds.), *Neuroleptics:
Neurochemical, behavioral, and clinical perspectives* (pp. 75–92). New York:
Raven Press.
Baldessarini, R. J. (1985a). Chemotherapy in psychiatry: Principles and practices.
Cambridge, MA: Harvard University Press.
Baldessarini, R. J. (1985b). Drugs and the treatment of psychiatric disorders. In
A. G. Gilman, L. S. Goodman, T. W. Rall, & F. Murad (Eds.), *Goodman and
Gilman's The pharmacological basis of therapeutics* (7th ed., pp. 387–445). New
York: Macmillan.

Baldessarini, R. J., Cohen, B. M., & Teicher, M. H. (1988). Significance of neuroleptic dose and plasma level in the pharmacological treatment of the psychoses. *Archives of General Psychiatry, 45,* 79–91.

Baldessarini, R. J., Cole, J. O., Davis, J. M., Gardos, G., Preskorn, S. H., Simpson, G. M., & Tarsy, D. (1979). *Tardive dyskinesia: Report of the American Psychiatric Association Task Force on late neurological effects of antipsychotic drugs.* Washington, DC: American Psychiatric Association.

Baldessarini, R. J., Kando, J. C., & Centorrino, F. (1995). Hospital use of antipsychotic agents in 1989 and 1993: Stable dosing with decreased length of stay. *American Journal of Psychiatry, 152,* 1038–1044.

Baldessarini, R. J., Katz, B., & Cotton, P. (1984). Dissimilar dosing with high-potency and low-potency neuroleptics. *American Journal of Psychiatry, 141,* 748–752.

Baldessarini, R. J., & Viguera, A. C. (1995). Neuroleptic withdrawal in schizophrenic patients. *Archives of General Psychiatry, 52,* 189–192.

Barnes, T. R. E., Milavic, G., Curson, D. A., & Platt, S. D. (1983). Use of the Social Behavior Assessment Schedule (SBAS) in a trial of maintenance antipsychotic therapy in schizophrenic outpatients: Pimozide versus fluphenazine. *Social Psychiatry, 18,* 193–199.

Belmaker, R. H., & Wald, D. (1977). Haloperidol in normals. *British Journal of Psychiatry, 131,* 222–223.

Benjamin, S., & Munetz, M. R. (1994). CMHC practices related to tardive dyskinesia screening and informed consent for neuroleptic drugs. *Hospital and Community Psychiatry, 45,* 343–346.

Bergen, J. A., Eyland, E. A., Campbell J. A., Jenkings, P., Kellehear, K., Richards, A., & Beaumont, J. V. (1989). The course of tardive dyskinesia in patients on long-term neuroleptics. *British Journal of Psychiatry, 154,* 523–528.

Bezchlibnyk-Butler, K. Z., & Jeffries, J. J. (1996). *Clinical handbook of psychotropic drugs* (6th ed., rev.). Toronto: Hogrefe & Huber.

Bitter, I., Volavka, J., & Scheurer, J. (1991). The concept of the neuroleptic threshold: An update. *Journal of Clinical Psychopharmacology, 11,* 28–33.

Bollini, P., Pampallona, S., Orza, M. J., Adams, M. E., & Chalmers, T. C. (1994). Antipsychotic drugs: Is more worse? A meta-analysis of the published randomized control trials. *Psychological Medicine, 24,* 307–316.

Bourgeois, M. (1988). Les dyskinésies tardives des neuroleptiques en France [Neuroleptic-associated tardive dyskinesia in France]. *Encéphale, 14,* 195–201.

Boyle, M. (1990). *Schizophrenia: A scientific delusion?* New York: Routledge.

Breggin, P. R. (1983). *Psychiatric drugs: Hazards to the brain.* New York: Springer.

Breggin, P. R. (1990). Brain damage, dementia, and persistent cognitive dysfunction associated with neuroleptic drugs: Evidence, etiology, implications. *Journal of Mind and Behavior, 11,* 425–464.

Breggin, P. R. (1993). Parallels between lethargic encephalitis and neuroleptic effects: The production of dyskinesias and cognitive disorders. *Brain and Cognition, 23,* 8–23.

Brenner, H., Roder, V., Hodel, B., Kienzle, N., Reed, D., & Liberman, R. (1994). *Integrated psychological therapy for schizophrenic patients.* Seattle, WA: Hogrefe & Huber.

Brown, P., & Funk, S. C. (1986). Tardive dyskinesia: Professional barriers to the recognition of an iatrogenic disease. *Journal of Health and Social Behavior, 27,* 116–132.

Burke, R. E., Fahn, S. E., Jankovic, J., Marsden, C. D., Lang, A. E., Golomp, S., & Ilson, J. (1982). Tardive dystonia: Late onset and persistent dystonia caused by antipsychotic drugs. *Neurology, 32,* 1335–1346.

Burke, R. E., & Kang, U. J. (1988). Tardive dystonia: Clinical aspects and treatment. In J. Jankovic & E. Tolosa (Eds.), *Advances in neurology: Vol. 49. Facial dyskinesias* (pp. 199–210). New York: Raven Press.

Buzan, R. E. (1996). Risperidone-induced tardive dyskinesia [Letter to the editor]. *American Journal of Psychiatry, 153,* 734–735.

Caldwell, M. F. (1994). Applying social constructionism in the treatment of patients who are intractably aggressive. *Hospital and Community Psychiatry, 45,* 597–600.

Carlsson, A. (1975). Monoamine precursors and analogues. *Pharmacology & Therapeutics—Part B: General & Systematic Pharmacology, 1,* 381–392.

Carson, R. C. (1991). Tunnel vision and schizophrenia. In W. F. Flack, D. R. Miller, & M. Wiener (Eds.), *What is schizophrenia?* (pp. 245–250). New York: Springer-Verlag.

Carter, S. C., Mulsant, B. H., Sweet, R. A., Maxwell, R., Coley, K., Ganguli, R., & Branch, R. (1995). Risperidone use in a teaching hospital during its first year after market approval: Economic and clinical implications. *Psychopharmacology Bulletin, 31,* 719–726.

Casey, D. E. (1985). Tardive dyskinesia: Epidemiological factors as a guide for prevention and management. In D. Kemali & G. Racagni (Eds.), *Chronic treatments in neuropsychiatry* (pp. 15–24). New York: Raven Press.

Casey, D. E. (1989). Clozapine: Neuroleptic-induced EPS and tardive dyskinesia. *Psychopharmacology, 99*(Suppl.), S47–S53.

Casey, D. E. (1991). Neuroleptic-induced extrapyramidal syndromes and tardive dyskinesia. *Schizophrenia Research, 14,* 109–120.

Chertok, L. (1982). 30 ans après: La petite histoire de la découverte des neuroleptiques [Thirty years later: The untold story of the discovery of neuroleptics]. *Annales médico-psychologiques, 140,* 971–976.

Chlorpromazine and mental health. (1955). *Proceedings of the Symposium held under the auspices of Smith, Kline & French Laboratories, June 6, 1955, Warwick Hotel, Philadelphia.* Philadelphia: Lea & Febiger.

Chouinard, G. (1990, March). Facteurs qui influent sur l'évolution de la dyskinésie tardive—Etude de suivi sur dix années [Factors bearing on the course of tardive dyskinesia—A ten-year follow-up study]. *Canada's Mental Health,* p. 24.

Chouinard, G., Annable, L., & Ross-Chouinard, A. (1982). Fluphenazine enanthate and fluphenazine decanoate in the treatment of schizophrenic outpatients: Extrapyramidal symptoms and therapeutic effects. *American Journal of Psychiatry, 139,* 312–318.

Chouinard, G., Annable, L., & Ross-Chouinard, A. (1986). Supersensitivity psychosis and tardive dyskinesia: A survey in schizophrenic outpatients. *Psychopharmacology Bulletin, 22,* 891–896.

Chouinard, G., & Jones, B. D. (1980). Neuroleptic-induced supersensitivity psychosis: Clinical and pharmacological characteristics. *American Journal of Psychiatry, 137,* 16–21.

Chua, S. E., & McKenna, P. J. (1995). Schizophrenia—A brain disease? *British Journal of Psychiatry, 166,* 563–582.

Ciompi, L., Dauwalder, H.-P., Maier, C., Aebi, E., Trütsch, K., Kupper, Z., & Rutishauer, C. (1992). The pilot project 'Soteria Berne': Clinical experiences and results. *British Journal of Psychiatry, 161*(Suppl. 18), 145–153.

Clinton, J., Sterner, S., Stelmachers, Z., & Ruiz, E. (1987). Haloperidol for sedation of disruptive emergency patients. *Annals of Emergency Medicine, 16,* 319–322.

Cohen, B. M., Keck, P. E., Satlin, A., & Cole, J. O. (1991). Prevalence and severity of akathisia in patients on clozapine. *Biological Psychiatry, 29,* 1215–1219.

Cohen D. (1989). *Psychotropic drugs and the chronically mentally ill: A longitudinal study.* Unpublished doctoral dissertation, University of California, Berkeley.

Cohen, D. (1994a). Neuroleptic drug treatment of schizophrenia: The state of the confusion. *Journal of Mind and Behavior, 15,* 139–156.

Cohen, D. (1994b). Quelles sont les conséquences sociales et psychologiques en termes de qualité de vie des neuroleptiques et de leurs effets secondaires? [What are the social and psychological effects of neuroleptics and their side effects on quality of life?] In Fédération Française de Psychiatrie (Ed.), *Conférence de consensus: Stratégies thérapeutiques à long terme dans les psychoses schizophréniques. Textes des experts* (pp. 149–184). Paris: Frison-Roche.

Cohen, D. (in press). Psychiatrogenics: The introduction of chlorpromazine in psychiatry. *Review of Existential Psychology and Psychiatry.*

Cohen, D., & Bisson, J. (1997). Médication neuroleptique et risque de dyskinésie tardive: Une enquête auprès de psychiatres et d'omnipraticiens du Québec [Neuroleptic medication decisions and the risk of tardive dyskinesia: A survey of psychiatrists and general practitioners in Quebec]. *Santé mentale au Québec, 22,* 263–282.

Cohen, D., & McCubbin, M. (1990). The political economy of tardive dyskinesia: Asymmetries in power and responsibility. *Journal of Mind and Behavior, 11,* 465–488.

Cohen, H., & Cohen, D. (Eds.). (1993a). Tardive dyskinesia and cognitive deficits [Special issue]. *Brain and Cognition, 23,* 1–110.

Cohen, H., & Cohen, D. (1993b). What may be gained from neuropsychological investigations of tardive dyskinesia? *Brain and Cognition, 23,* 1–7.

Collins, E. J., Hogan, T. P., & Awad, A. G. (1992). The pharmacoepidemiology of treatment-refractory schizophrenia. *Canadian Journal of Psychiatry, 37,* 192–195.

Cummings, J. L. (1990). *Subcortical dementia.* New York: Oxford University Press.

Dave, M. (1995). Two cases of risperidone-induced neuroleptic malignant syndrome [letter to the editor]. *American Journal of Psychiatry, 152*, 1233–1234.

Davis, J. M., Kane, J. M., Marder, S. R., Brauder, B., Gierl, B., Schooler, N., Casey, D. E., & Hassan, M. (1993). Dose response of prophylactic antipsychotics. *Journal of Clinical Psychiatry, 54*(Suppl.), 24–30.

Davis, J. M. (1975). Overview: Maintenance therapy in psychiatry: 1. Schizophrenia. *American Journal of Psychiatry, 132*, 1237–1245.

Davis, R. J., & Cummings, G. L. (1988). Clinical variants of tardive dyskinesia. *Neuropsychiatry, Neuro-psychology, and Behavioral Neurology, 1*, 31–38.

Dean, C. E. (1995). Comment on "Schizophrenia: A 100-year retrospective" [letter to the editor]. *American Journal of Psychiatry, 152*, 1694.

de Girolamo, G. (1996). WHO studies on schizophrenia: An overview of the results and their implications for the understanding of the disorder. *The Psychotherapy Patient, 9*, 213–231.

Delay, J., & Deniker, P. (1952). Trente-huit cas de psychoses traitées par la cure prolongée et continue de 4560 RP [Thirty-eight cases of psychoses treated by long term and continuous administration of 4560 RP]. In *Congrès des Aliénistes et Neurologues de Langue Française*, C.R. (pp. 505–513). Paris: Masson Éditeur.

Delay, J., & Deniker, P. (1961). *Méthodes chimiothérapiques en psychiatrie* [Chemotherapeutic methods in psychiatry]. Paris: Masson.

Delay, J., Deniker, A., Bourguignon, A., & Lempérière, T. (1956). Complications d'allure extrapyramidale au cours des traitements par la chlorpromazine et la réserpine (Étude clinique et électromyographique) [Extrapyramidal-like complications during chlorpromazine and reserpine treatments—A clinical and electromyographic study]. In *Colloque international sur la chlorpromazine et les médicaments neuroleptiques en thérapeutique psychiatrique, Paris, 20, 21, 22 Octobre 1955* (pp. 793–798). Paris: G. Douin et Cie.

Denber, H. C. B. (1959). Side effects of phenothiazines. In N. S. Kline (Ed.), *Psychopharmacology frontiers* (pp. 61–62). Boston: Little, Brown.

Dencker, S. J., Ahlfors, U. G., Bech, P., Elgen, K., & Lingjaerde, O. (1986). Classification of side effects in psychopharmacology. *Pharmacopsychiatry, 19*, 40–42.

Deniker, P. (1986). Are the anti-psychotic drugs to be withdrawn? In C. Shagass, R. Josiassen, & W. Bridger (Eds.), *Biological psychiatry* (pp. 1–9). New York: Elsevier.

Deniker, P. (1989). From chlorpromazine to tardive dyskinesia (brief history of the neuroleptics). *Psychiatric Journal of the University of Ottawa, 14*, 253–259.

Deniker, P. (1990). The neuroleptics: A historical survey. *Acta Psychiatrica Scandinavica, 82*(Suppl. 358), 83–87.

DeVeaugh-Geiss, J. (Ed.). (1982). *Tardive dyskinesia and related movement disorders: The long-term effects of anti-psychotic drugs*. Boston: J. Wright/PSG.

DeVeaugh-Geiss, J. (1988). Clinical changes in tardive dyskinesia during long-term follow-up. In M. Wolf & A. Mosnaim (Eds.), *Tardive dyskinesia: Biological mechanisms and clinical aspects* (pp. 87–106). Washington, DC: American Psychiatric Press.

Dewan, M. J., & Koss, M. (1989). The clinical impact of the side effects of psychotropic drugs. In S. Fisher & R. P. Greenberg (Eds.), *The limits of biological treatments for psychological distress: Comparisons with psychotherapy and placebo* (pp. 189–234). Hillsdale, NJ: Erlbaum.

Dewan, M. J., & Koss, M. (1995). The clinical impact of reported variance in potency of antipsychotic agents. *Acta Psychiatrica Scandinavica, 91,* 229–232.

Diamond R. (1985). Drugs and the quality of life: The patient's point of view. *Journal of Clinical Psychiatry, 46,* 29–35.

Double, D. B. (1995). Unblinding in trials of the withdrawal of anticholinergic agents in patients maintained on neuroleptics. *Journal of Nervous and Mental Disease, 183,* 599–602.

Easton, K., & Link, I. (1986/1987). Do neuroleptics prevent relapse? Clinical observations in a psychosocial rehabilitation program. *Psychiatry Quarterly, 58,* 42–50.

Ellison, J. M., & Pfaelzer, C. (1995, Fall). Emergency pharmacotherapy: The evolving role of medications in the emergency department. *New Directions in Mental Health Services,* no. 67, 87–97.

Epstein, A. M., Hall, J. A., Tognetti, J., Son, L. H., & Conant, L. (1989). Using proxies to evaluate quality of life: Can they provide valid information about patients' health status and satisfaction with medical care? *Medical Care,* 27(Suppl.), S91–S98.

Ey, H., Faure, H., & Rappard, P. (1956). Les réactions d'intolérance vis-à-vis de la chlorpromazine [Intolerance reactions to chlorpromazine]. *Encéphale, 45,* 790–796.

Farde, L., Nordström, A. L., Wiesel, F.-A., Pauli, P., Halldin, C., & Sedvall, G. (1992). Positron emission tomographic analysis of central D1 and D2 dopamine receptor occupancy in patients treated with classical neuroleptics and clozapine. *Archives of General Psychiatry, 49,* 538–544.

Fenton, W. S., Wyatt, R. J., & McGlashan, T. H. (1994). Risk factors for spontaneous dyskinesia in schizophrenia. *Archives of General Psychiatry, 51,* 643–650.

Flügel, F. (1956). Thérapeutique par médication neuroleptique obtenue en réalisant systématiquement des états parkinsoniformes [Therapeutic intervention with neuroleptic medication obtained by systematically producing parkinsonian states]. In *Colloque international sur la chlorpromazine et les médicaments neuroleptiques en thérapeutique psychiatrique, Paris, 20, 21, 22 Octobre 1955* (pp. 790–792). Paris: G. Douin & Cie.

Follin, S., Chanoit, J.-C., Pilon, J.-P., Huchon, C. (1961). Le remplacement du largactil par des placebos dans un service psychiatrique [Replacing largactil by placebos in a psychiatric ward]. *Annales médico-psychologiques, 119,* 976–983.

Frankenburg, F. R. (1994). History of the development of antipsychotic medication. *Psychiatric Clinics of North America, 17,* 531–540.

Freyhan, F. (1955). The immediate and long range effects of chlorpromazine on the mental hospital. In *Chlorpromazine and mental health. Proceedings of the Symposium held under the auspices of Smith, Kline & French Laboratories, June 6, 1955, Warwick Hotel, Philadelphia* (pp. 71–98). Philadelphia: Lea & Febiger.

Gerlach, J., & Peacock, L. (1995). Intolerance to neuroleptic drugs: The art of avoiding extrapyramidal symptoms. *European Psychiatry, 10*(Suppl. 1), 27s–31s.

Gilbert, P. L., Harris, J., McAdams, L. A., & Jeste, D. V. (1995). Neuroleptic withdrawal in schizophrenic patients: A review of the literature. *Archives of General Psychiatry, 52,* 173–188.

Ginestet, D., & Kapsambelis, V. (1996). Neuroleptiques [Neuroleptics]. In D. Ginestet & V. Kapsambelis (Eds.), *Thérapeutique médicamenteuse des troubles psychiatriques de l'adulte* [Drug treatment of psychiatric disorders in adults] (pp. 44–69). Paris: Flammarion Médecine-Sciences.

Glazer, W. M., Morgenstern, H., & Doucette, J. T. (1991). Prediction of chronic persistent versus intermittent tardive dyskinesia: A retrospective follow-up study. *British Journal of Psychiatry, 158,* 822–828.

Goldberg, R. J., Morris, P. L. P., & Lidofksy, S. (1990). Tardive dyskinesia presenting as gastrointestinal disorder. *Journal of Clinical Psychiatry, 51,* 253–254.

Goldman, D. (1955). The effect of chlorpromazine on severe mental and emotional disturbance. In *Chlorpromazine and mental health. Proceedings of the Symposium held under the auspices of Smith, Kline & French Laboratories, June 6, 1955, Warwick Hotel, Philadelphia* (pp. 19–69). Philadelphia: Lea & Febiger.

Greenberg, R. P., Bornstein, R. F., Greenberg, M. D., & Fisher, S. (1992). A meta-analysis of antidepressant outcome under "blinder" conditions. *Journal of Consulting and Clinical Psychology, 60,* 664–669.

Gronfein, W. (1985). Psychotropic drugs and the origins of deinstitutionalization. *Social Problems, 32,* 437–454.

Gualtieri, C. T. (1990). *Neuropsychiatry and behavioral pharmacology.* Berlin: Springer-Verlag.

Gualtieri, C. T. (1993). The problem of tardive akathisia. *Brain and Cognition, 23,* 102–109.

Gualtieri, C. T., & Sprague, R. L. (1984). Preventing tardive dyskinesia and preventing tardive dyskinesia litigation. *Psychopharmacology Bulletin, 24,* 346–348.

Haase, H.-J. (1958). La valeur thérapeutique des symptômes extrapyramidaux dans le traitement à la chlorpromazine et réserpine [The therapeutic value of extrapyramidal symptoms in chlorpromazine and reserpine treatment]. *Encéphale, 48,* 519–532.

Haase, H.-J. (1961). Extrapyramidal modifications of fine movements—A "condition sine qua non" of the fundamental therapeutic action of neuroleptic drugs. *Canadian Journal of Biology, 20,* 425–449.

Halstead, S. M., Barnes, T. R. E., & Speller, J. C. (1994). Akathisia: Prevalence and associated dysphoria in an in-patient population with chronic schizophrenia. *British Journal of Psychiatry, 164,* 177–183.

Hansen, T. E., Brown, W. L., Weigel, R. M., & Casey, D. E. (1992). Underrecognition of tardive dyskinesia and drug-induced parkinsonism by psychiatric residents. *General Hospital Psychiatry, 14,* 340–344.

Healy, D. (1993). Psychopharmacology and the ethics of resource allocation. *British Journal of Psychiatry, 162,* 23–29.

Hegarty, J., Baldessarini, R. J., Tohen, M., Waternaux, C., & Oepen, G. (1994). One hundred years of schizophrenia: A meta-analysis of the outcome literature. *American Journal of Psychiatry, 151,* 1409–1416.

Hermesh, H., Shalev, A., & Munetz, H. (1985). Contribution of adverse drug reaction to admission rates in an acute psychiatric ward. *Acta Psychiatrica Scandinavica, 72,* 104–110.

Herrington, R., & Lader, M. (1981). Antipsychotic drugs. In H. M. van Praag (Ed.), *Handbook of biological psychiatry* (Vol. 5, pp. 73–104). New York: Marcel Dekker.

Hill, D. (1983). *The politics of schizophrenia.* Lanham, MD: University Press of America.

Hilts, P. J. (1994, March 10). Agency faults a U.C.L.A. study for suffering of mental patients. *The New York Times,* pp. A1, B10.

Hogarty, G. E. (1993). Prevention of relapse in chronic schizophrenic patients. *Journal of Clinical Psychiatry, 54*(Suppl.), 18–23.

Hogarty, G. E., McEvoy, J. P., Munetz, M., DiBarry, A. L., Bartone, P., Cather, R., Cooley, S. J., Ulrich, R. F., Carter, M., & Madonia, M. J. (1988). Dose of fluphenazine, familial expressed emotion, and outcome in schizophrenia: Results of a two-year controlled study. *Archives of General Psychiatry, 45,* 797–805.

Hogarty, G. E., McEvoy, J. P., Ulrich, R. F., DiBarry, A. L., Bartone, P., Cooley, S., Hammill, K., Carter, M., Munetz, M. R., & Perel, J. (1995). Pharmacotherapy of impaired affect in recovering schizophrenic patients. *Archives of General Psychiatry, 52,* 29–41.

Hunt, J. J., Singh, H., & Simpson, G. M. (1988). Neuroleptic-induced supersensitivity psychosis: Retrospective studies of schizophrenic inpatients. *Journal of Clinical Psychiatry, 49,* 258–261.

Jablensky, A. (1987). Multi-cultural studies and the nature of schizophrenia: A review. *Journal of the Royal Society of Medicine, 80,* 162–167.

Jeste, D. V., Gilbert, P. L., McAdams, L. A., & Harris, M. J. (1995). Considering neuroleptic maintenance and taper on a continuum: Need for individual rather than dogmatic approach. *Archives of General Psychiatry, 52,* 209–212.

Johns, C. E., Mayerhoff, D. I., Lieberman, J. A., & Kane, J. M. (1990). Schizophrenia: Alternative neuroleptic strategies. In B. Angrist & S. C. Schulz (Eds.), *The neuroleptic-nonresponsive patient: Characterization and treatment* (pp. 51–66). Washington, DC: American Psychiatric Press.

Jones, B. D. (1985). Tardive dysmentia: Further comments. *Schizophrenia Bulletin, 11,* 187–189.

Kahn, R. S., & Davis, K. L. (1995). New developments in dopamine and schizophrenia. In F. E. Bloom & D. J. Kupfer (Eds.), *Psychopharmacology: The fourth generation of progress* (pp. 1193–1203). New York: Raven Press.

Kane, J. M. (1989). The current status of neuroleptic therapy. *Journal of Clinical Psychiatry, 50,* 322–328.

Kane, J. M., & Lieberman, J. A. (Eds.). (1992a). *Adverse effects of psychotropic drugs.* New York: Guilford Press.

Kane, J. M., & Lieberman, J. A. (1992b). Tardive dyskinesia. In J. M. Kane & J. A. Lieberman (Eds.), *Adverse effects of psychotropic drugs* (pp. 235–243). New York: Guilford Press.

Karon, B. (1989). Psychotherapy versus medication for schizophrenia: Empirical comparisons. In S. Fisher & R. P. Greenberg (Eds.), *The limits of biological treatments for psychological distress: Comparisons with psychotherapy and placebo* (pp. 105–150). Hillsdale, NJ: Erlbaum.

Keck, P. E., Jr., Cohen, B. M., Baldessarini, R., & McElroy, S. L. (1989). Time course of antipsychotic effects of neuroleptic drugs. *American Journal of Psychiatry, 146,* 1289–1292.

Kemker, S. S., & Khadivi, A. (1995). Psychiatric education: Learning by assumption. In C. A. Ross & A. Pam (Eds.), *Pseudoscience in biological psychiatry: Blaming the body* (pp. 241–253). New York: Wiley.

Kendler, K. S. (1976). A medical student's experience with akathisia [Letter to the editor]. *American Journal of Psychiatry, 133,* 454–455.

Kennedy, N. J., & Sanborn, J. S. (1992). Disclosure of tardive dyskinesia: Effect of written policy on risk disclosure. *Psychopharmacology Bulletin, 28,* 93–100.

Kerwin, R. W. (1994). The new atypical antipsychotics: A lack of extrapyramidal side-effects and new routes in schizophrenia research. *British Journal of Psychiatry, 164,* 141–148.

Keshavan, M. S., & Kennedy, J. S. (Eds.). (1992). *Drug-induced dysfunction in psychiatry.* New York: Hemisphere.

Kinon, C. J., Kane, J. M., Johns, C., Perovich, R., Ismi, M., Koreen, A., & Weiden, P. (1993). Treatment of neuroleptic-resistant schizophrenic relapse. *Psychopharmacology Bulletin, 29,* 309–314.

Klein, D. F., Gittleman, R., Quitkin, F., & Rifkin, A. (1980). *Diagnosis and drug treatment of psychiatric disorders: Adults and children* (2nd ed., pp. 174–181). Baltimore: Williams & Wilkins.

Kleinman, I., Schacter, D., Jeffries, J., & Goldhamer, P. (1993). Effectiveness of two methods for informing schizophrenic patients about neuroleptic medication. *Hospital and Community Psychiatry, 44,* 1189–1191.

Klitzman, R. (1995, March 4). That way madness lies. *The New York Times,* p. 19.

Kreisman, D., Blumenthal, R., Borenstein, M., Woerner, M., Kane, J., Rifkin, A., & Reardon, G. (1988). Family attitudes and patient social adjustment in a longitudinal study of outpatient schizophrenics receiving low-dose neuroleptics: The family's view. *Psychiatry, 51,* 3–13.

Kuhn, T. (1970). *The structure of scientific revolutions* (2nd ed.). Chicago: University of Chicago Press.

Laborit, H. (1967). Naissance des phénothiazines [Birth of the phenothiazines]. *Le Concours médical, 44,* 7164–7169.

Lader, M., & Lewander, T. (Eds.). (1994). The neuroleptic-induced deficit syndrome [Special issue]. *Acta Psychiatrica Scandinavica, 89*(Suppl. 380), 5–85.

Laporta, M., Archambault, D., Ross-Chouinard, A., & Chouinard, G. (1990). Articulatory impairment associated with tardive dyskinesia. *Journal of Nervous and Mental Disease, 178,* 660–662.

Lauterbach, E., Singh, H., Simpson, G. M., & Morrison, R. (1990). Gait disorders in tardive dyskinesia [letter to the editor]. *Acta Psychiatrica Scandinavica, 82,* 267.

Lavin, M. R., & Rifkin, A. (1991). Psychotic patients' interpretation of neuroleptic side effects [letter to the editor]. *American Journal of Psychiatry, 148,* 1615–1616.

Lavin, M. R., & Rifkin, A. (1992). Neuroleptic-induced parkinsonism. In J. M. Kane & J. A. Lieberman (Eds.), *Adverse effects of psychotropic drugs* (pp. 175–188). New York: Guilford Press.

Lehmann, H. E. (1955). Therapeutic results with chlorpromazine (Largactil) in psychiatric conditions. *Canadian Medical Association Journal, 72,* 91–92.

Lehmann, H. E. (1979). Negative aspects of psychotherapeutic drug treatment. *Progress in Neuro-Psychopharmacology, 3,* 223–229.

Lehmann, H. E. (1989). The introduction of chlorpromazine to North America. *Psychiatric Journal of the University of Ottawa, 14,* 263–265.

Lehmann, H. E. (1993). Before they called it psychopharmacology. *Neuropsychopharmacology, 8,* 291–303.

Lehmann, H. E., & Hanrahan, L. (1954). Chlorpromazine, a new inhibiting agent for psychomotor excitement and manic states. *A.M.A. Archives of Neurology and Psychiatry, 71,* 227–237.

Lemoine, P. (1995). *Le mystère du placebo* [The mystery of the placebo]. Paris: Odile Jacob.

Letailleur, M., Morin, J., & Monnerie, R. (1956). Syndromes transitoires pseudo-parkinsoniens provoqués par la chlorpromazine [Transient pseudo-parkinsonian syndromes provoked by chlorpromazine]. In *Colloque international sur la chlorpromazine et les médicaments neuroleptiques en thérapeutique psychiatrique, Paris, 20, 21, 22 Octobre 1955* (pp. 806–809). Paris: G. Douin et Cie.

Lewander, T. (1994). Neuroleptics and the neuroleptic-induced deficit syndrome. *Acta Psychiatrica Scandinavica, 89*(Suppl. 380), 8–13.

Liberman, R. P., Van Putten, T., Marshall, B. D., Jr., Mintz, J., Bowen, L., Kuehnel, T. G., Aravagiri, M., & Marder, S. R. (1994). Optimal drug and behavior therapy for treatment-refractory schizophrenic patients. *American Journal of Psychiatry, 151,* 756–759.

Lidz, R. W. (1993). The effect of neurotropic drugs on the psychotherapy of schizophrenic patients. In G. Benedetti & P. M. Furlan (Eds.), *The psychotherapy of schizophrenia: Effective clinical approaches—Controversies, critiques & recommendations* (pp. 313–317). Seattle, WA: Hogrefe & Huber.

Manos, N., Gkiouzepas, J., & Logothetis, J. (1981). The need for continuous use of antiparkinsonian medication with chronic schizophrenic patients receiving long-term neuroleptic therapy. *American Journal of Psychiatry, 138,* 184–188.

Matthews, S. M., Roper, M. T., Mosher, L. R., & Menn, A. Z. (1979). A non-neuroleptic treatment for schizophrenia: Analysis of the two-year postdischarge risk for relapse. *Schizophrenia Bulletin, 5,* 322–333.

McEvoy, J. P., Hogarty, G. E., & Steingard, S. (1991). Optimal dose of neuroleptic in acute schizophrenia. *Archives of General Psychiatry, 48,* 739–745.

McIntyre, C., & Simpson, G. M. (1995). How much neuroleptic is enough? *Psychiatric Annals, 25,* 135–139.

McShane, R., Keene, J., Gedling, K., Fairburn, C., Jacoby, R., & Hope, T. (1997). Do neuroleptic drugs hasten cognitive decline in dementia—Prospective study with necropsy follow-up. *British Medical Journal, 314,* 266–270.

Meise, U., Kurz, M., & Fleishacker, W. (1994). Antipsychotic maintenance treatment of schizophrenia patients: Is there a consensus? *Schizophrenia Bulletin, 20,* 215–225.

Melamed, E., Achiron, A., Shapira, A., & Davidovicz, S. (1991). Persistent and progressive Parkinsonism after discontinuation of chronic neuroleptic therapy: An additional tardive syndrome? *Clinical Neuropharmacology, 14,* 273–278.

Meltzer, H. Y. (1992). Treatment of the neuroleptic-nonresponsive patient. *Schizophrenia Bulletin, 18,* 515–542.

Mitchell, P. (1993). Chlorpromazine turns forty. *Psychopharmacology Bulletin, 29,* 341–344.

Montagne, M. (1988). The metaphorical nature of drugs and drug taking. *Social Science and Medicine, 26,* 417–424.

Mosher, L., & Burti, L. (1989). *Community mental health: Principles and practice.* New York: Norton.

Mosher, L., & Menn, A. Z. (1978). Community residential treatment for schizophrenia: Two-year follow-up. *Hospital and Community Psychiatry, 29,* 715–723.

Mukherjee, S. (1984). Tardive dysmentia: A reappraisal. *Schizophrenia Bulletin, 10,* 151–153.

Myslobodsky, M. (1986). Anosognosia in tardive dyskinesia: "Tardive dysmentia" or "tardive dementia"? *Schizophrenia Bulletin, 12,* 1–6.

Myslobodsky, M. (1993). Central determinants of attention and mood disorder in tardive dyskinesia ("tardive dysmentia"). *Brain and Cognition, 23,* 88–101.

Myslobodsky, M. S., Tomer, R., Holden, T., Kempler, S., & Sigal, M. (1985). Cognitive impairment in patients with tardive dyskinesia. *Journal of Nervous and Mental Disease, 173,* 156–160.

Neergard, L. (1996, October 2). FDA OKs schizophrenia drug. *Associated Press.*

Newcomer, J. W., Miller, L. S., Faustman, W. O., Wetzel, M. W., Vogler, J. P., & Csernansky, J. G. (1994). Correlations between akathisia and residual psychopathology: A by-product of neuroleptic-induced dysphoria. *British Journal of Psychiatry, 164,* 834–838.

Oken, R. J., & McGeer, P. L. (1995). Comment on "Schizophrenia: A 100-year retrospective" [letter to the editor]. *American Journal of Psychiatry, 152,* 1693.

Pam, A. (1995). Biological psychiatry: Science or pseudoscience? In C. A. Ross & A. Pam (Eds.), *Pseudoscience in biological psychiatry: Blaming the body* (pp. 7–84). New York: Wiley.

Peralta, V., Cuesta, M. J., Caro, F., & Martinez-Larrea, A. (1994). Neuroleptic dose and schizophrenic symptoms: A survey of prescribing practices. *Acta Psychiatrica Scandinavica, 90,* 354–357.

Pollack, S., Lieberman, J. A., Fleischacker, W. W., Borenstein, M., Safferman, A. Z., Hummer, M., & Kurz, M. (1995). A comparison of European and American dosing regimens of schizophrenic patients on clozapine: Efficacy and side effects. *Psychopharmacology Bulletin, 31*, 315–320.

Ray, W. A., Taylor, J. A., Meador, K. G., Lichenstein, M. J., Griffin, M. R., Fought, R., Adams, M. L., & Blazer, D. G. (1993). Reducing antipsychotic drug use in nursing homes: A controlled trial of provider education. *Archives of Internal Medicine, 153*, 713–721.

Reardon, G. T., Rifkin, A., Schwartz, A., Myerson, A., & Siris, S. G. (1989). Changing patterns of neuroleptic dosage over a decade. *American Journal of Psychiatry, 146*, 726–729.

Rifkin, A., Doddi, S., Karajgi, B., Borenstein, M., & Wachspress, M. (1991). Dosage of haloperidol for schizophrenia. *Archives of General Psychiatry, 48*, 166–170.

Rifkin, A., Quitkin, F., & Klein, D. F. (1975). Akinesia: A poorly recognized drug-induced extrapyramidal behavior disorder. *Archives of General Psychiatry, 32*, 672–674.

Risks and benefits of neuroleptic medication. (n.d.). Toronto: Mount Sinai Hospital.

Ross, C. A. (1995). Errors of logic in biological psychiatry. In C. A. Ross & A. Pam (Eds.), *Pseudoscience in biological psychiatry: Blaming the body* (pp. 85–128). New York: Wiley.

Ross, C. A., & Pam, A. (Eds.). (1995). *Pseudoscience in biological psychiatry: Blaming the body.* New York: Wiley.

Sachdev, P., & Kruk, J. (1994). Clinical characteristics and predisposing factors in acute drug-induced akathisia. *Archives of General Psychiatry, 51*, 963–974.

Sachdev, P., & Loneragan, C. (1991). The present status of akathisia. *Journal of Nervous and Mental Disorders, 179*, 381–391.

Sarbin, T. (1990). Toward the obsolescence of the schizophrenia hypothesis. *Journal of Mind and Behavior, 11*, 259–283.

Schwartz, J. T., & Brotman, A. W. (1992). A clinical guide to antipsychotic drugs. *Drugs, 44*, 981–992.

Segal, S. P., Cohen, D., & Marder, S. R. (1992). Neuroleptic medication and prescription practices with sheltered-care residents: A twelve-year perspective. *American Journal of Public Health, 82*, 846–852.

Semla, T. P., Palla, K., Poddig, B., & Brauner, D. J. (1994). Effect of the Omnibus Reconciliation Act 1987 on antipsychotic prescribing in nursing home residents. *Journal of the American Geriatrics Society, 42*, 648–652.

Simon, R. I. (1992). *Clinical psychiatry and the law.* Washington, DC: American Psychiatric Press.

Simpson, O. M., & Yadalam, K. (1985). Blood levels of neuroleptics: State of the art. *Journal of Clinical Psychiatry, 46*, 22–28.

Singer, S., Richards, C., & Boland, R. J. (1995). Two cases of risperidone-induced neuroleptic malignant syndrome [letter to the editor]. *American Journal of Psychiatry, 152*, 1234.

Singh, H., & Simpson, G. M. (1988). Tardive dyskinesia: Clinical features. In M. E. Wolf & A. Mosnaim (Eds.), *Tardive dyskinesia: Biological mechanisms and clinical aspects* (pp. 67–86). Washington, DC: American Psychiatric Press.

Skelton, J. A., Pepe, M., & Pineo, T. S. (1995). How much better is clozapine? A meta-analytic review and critical appraisal. *Experimental and Clinical Psychopharmacology, 3*, 270–279.

Steck, H. (1954). Le syndrome extra-pyramidal et di-encéphalique au cours des traitements au Largactil et au Serpasil [The extra-pyramidal and di-encephalic syndrome during treatment with Largactil and Serpasil]. *Annales médico-psychologiques, 112*, 737–743.

Steck, H. (1956). Le syndrome extrapyramidal dans les cures de chlorpromazine et serpasil: Sa symptomatologie clinique et son rôle thérapeutique [The extrapyramidal syndrome during chlorpromazine and serpasil treatments: Its clinical symptomatology and therapeutic function]. In *Colloque international sur la chlorpromazine et les médicaments neuroleptiques en thérapeutique psychiatrique, Paris, 20, 21, 22 Octobre 1955* (pp. 783–789). Paris: G. Douin et Cie.

Stone, C. K., & Garver, D. L. (1996). Drs. Stone and Garver reply [letter to the editor]. *American Journal of Psychiatry, 153*, 1109.

Stone, C. K., Garver, D. L., Griffith, J., Hirschowitz, J., & Bennett, J. (1995). Further evidence of a dose-response threshold for haloperidol in psychosis. *American Journal of Psychiatry, 152*, 1210–1212.

Strassman, R. J. (1995). Hallucinogenic drugs in psychiatric research and treatment: Perspectives and prospects. *Journal of Nervous and Mental Disease, 183*, 127–138.

Stuss, D., & Benson, D. (1986). *The frontal lobes.* New York: Raven Press.

Summerfield, A. (1978). Behavioral toxicity: The psychology of pollution. *Journal of Biosocial Science, 10*, 335–345.

Thornton, A., & McKenna, P. J. (1994). Acute dystonic reactions complicated by psychotic phenomena. *British Journal of Psychiatry, 164*, 115–118.

Turnier, L., Desrosiers, P., & Chouinard, G. (1988, December 7). Dyskinésie respiratoire induite par le retrait d'un antidopaminergique [Respiratory dyskinesia induced by withdrawal of an antidopaminergic drug]. *L'Actualité Médicale* (Quebec), pp. 41–42.

Turns, C. N. (1990). Effects of sedatives and neuroleptics [letter to the editor]. *American Journal of Psychiatry, 147*, 1576.

van Kammen, D. P., Kelley, M. E., Gurklis, J. A., Gilberston, M. W., Ya, J. K., & Peters, J. L. (1995). Behavioral vs biochemical prediction of clinical stability following haloperidol withdrawal in schizophrenia. *Archives of General Psychiatry, 52*, 673–678.

Van Putten, T., & Marder, S. R. (1978). "Akinetic depression" in schizophrenia. *Archives of General Psychiatry, 35*, 1101–1107.

Van Putten, T., & Marder, S. R. (1986). Toward more reliable diagnosis of akathisia [letter to the editor]. *Archives of General Psychiatry, 43*, 1015–1016.

Van Putten, T., & Marder, S. R. (1987). Behavioral toxicity of antipsychotic drugs. *Journal of Clinical Psychiatry, 48*(Suppl.), 13–19.

Van Putten, T., Marder, S. R., & Mintz, J. (1990). A controlled dose comparison of haloperidol in newly admitted schizophrenic patients. *Archives of General Psychiatry, 47*, 754–758.

Van Putten, T., & May, P. R. (1978). Subjective response as a predictor of outcome in pharmacotherapy: The consumer has a point. *Archives of General Psychiatry, 35,* 477–480.

Vaughan, S., Oquendo, M., & Horwath, E. (1991). A patient's psychotic interpretation of a drug side effect [Letter to the editor]. *American Journal of Psychiatry, 148,* 393–394.

Volavka, J., Cooper, T. B., Meisner, M., Bitter, I., Czobor, P., & Jager, J. (1990). Haloperidol blood levels and effects in schizophrenia and schizoaffective disorder: A progress report. *Psychopharmacology Bulletin, 26,* 13–17.

Waddington, J. L., Weller, M. P. I., Crow, T. J., & Hirsch, S. R. (1992). Schizophrenia, genetic retrenchment, and epidemiologic renaissance: The Sixth Biennal Winter Workshop on Schizophrenia, Badgastein, Austria, January 26–February 1, 1992. *Archives of General Psychiatry, 49,* 990–994.

Wallace, M. (1994). Schizophrenia—A national emergency: Preliminary observations on SANELINE. *Acta Psychiatrica Scandinavica, 89*(Suppl. 380), 33–35.

Warner, R. (1995). Comment on "Schizophrenia: A 100-year retrospective" [letter to the editor]. *American Journal of Psychiatry, 152,* 1693.

White, K., Kando, J., Park, T., Waternaux, C., & Brown, W. A. (1992). Side effects and the "blindability" of clinical drug trials. *American Journal of Psychiatry, 149,* 1730–1731.

Wiener, M. (1991). Schizophrenia: A defective, deficient, disrupted, disorganized construct. In W. F. Flack, D. R. Miller, & M. Wiener (Eds.), *What is schizophrenia?* (pp. 199–222). New York: Springer-Verlag.

Wilson, I. C., Garbutt, J. C., Lanier, C. F., Moylan, J., Nelson, W., & Prange, A. J. (1983). Is there a tardive dysmentia? *Schizophrenia Bulletin, 9,* 187–192.

Windgassen, K. (1992). Treatment with neuroleptics: The patients' perspective. *Acta Psychiatrica Scandinavica, 86,* 405–410.

Wirshing, W. C., Marder, S. R., Van Putten, T., & Ames, D. (1995). Acute treatment of schizophrenia. In F. E. Bloom & D. J. Kupfer (Eds.), *Psychopharmacology: The fourth generation of progress* (pp. 1259–1266). New York: Raven Press.

Woerner, M., Kane, J. M., Lieberman, J., Alvir, J., Bergmann, K. J., Borenstein M., Schooler, N. R., Mukherjee, S., Rotrosen, J., Rubinstein, M., & Basavaraju, N. (1991). The prevalence of tardive dyskinesia. *Journal of Clinical Psychopharmacology, 11,* 34–42.

Woerner, M., Sheitman, B. B., Lieberman, J. A., & Kane, J. M. (1995). Tardive dyskinesia induced by risperidone? [letter to the editor]. *American Journal of Psychiatry, 153,* 843.

Wolf, M. E., & Brown, P. (1988). Overcoming institutional and community resistance to a tardive dyskinesia management program. In M. E. Wolf & A. Mosnaim (Eds.), *Tardive dysknesia: Biological mechanisms and clinical aspects* (pp. 281–290). Washington, DC: American Psychiatric Press.

Wysosky, D. K., & Baum, C. (1989). Antipsychotic drug use in the United States, 1976–1989. *Archives of General Psychiatry, 46,* 929–932.

Yadalam, K. G., Korn, M. L., & Simpson, G. M. (1990). Tardive dystonia: Four case histories. *Journal of Clinical Psychiatry, 51,* 17–20.

Yassa, R. (1989). Functional impairment in tardive dyskinesia: Medical and psychosocial dimensions. *Acta Psychiatrica Scandinavica, 80,* 64–67.

Yassa, R., & Jeste, D. V. (1992). Gender differences in tardive dyskinesia: A critical review of the literature. *Schizophrenia Bulletin, 18,* 701–715.

Yassa, R., & Lal, S. (1986). Respiratory irregularity and tardive dyskinesia: A prevalence study. *Acta Psychiatrica Scandinavica, 73,* 506–510.

Yassa, R., Nair, V., & Schwartz, G. (1984). Tardive dyskinesia: A two-year follow-up study. *Psychosomatics, 25,* 852–855.

Yassa, R., Nastase, C., Camille, Y., & Belzile, L. (1988). Tardive dyskinesia in a psychogeriatric population. In M. Wolf & A. Mosnaim (Eds.), *Tardive dyskinesia: Biological mechanisms and clinical aspects* (pp. 123–134). Washington, DC: American Psychiatric Press.

Young, C. S., Stewart, J. B., & Fenton, G. W. (1994). Neuroleptic medication for dystonia: Reciprocal relationship between effects on motor function and mood. *British Journal of Psychiatry, 165,* 384–386.

Zito, J. M., & Provenzano, G. (1995). Pharmaceutical decisionmaking: Pharmacoepidemiology or pharmacoeconomics—Who's in the driver's seat? *Psychopharmacology Bulletin, 31,* 735–744.

Zubin, J., Steinhauer, S. R., & Condray, R. (1992). Vulnerability to relapse in schizophrenia. *British Journal of Psychiatry, 161*(Suppl. 18), 13–18.

CHAPTER 6

A Focused Empirical Analysis of Treatments for Panic and Anxiety

WILLIAM G. DANTON and DAVID O. ANTONUCCIO

Anxiety disorders are the most common mental health problem in the United States (Myers et al., 1984; Regier et al., 1988; Regier, Narrow, & Rae, 1990; Robins, Helzer, & Weissmann, 1984). Data from the National Institute of Mental Health Epidemiologic Catchment Area Program (ECA) indicate that in the 6 months preceding the survey, over 6% of the men and 13% of the women in a sample of 18,571 people, had suffered from a *Diagnostic and Statistical Manual of Mental Disorders* (*DSM-III;* American Psychiatric Association [APA], 1987) anxiety disorder. At some point in their lives, over 30 million Americans have suffered from an anxiety disorder (Leon, Portera, & Weissman, 1995).

The overall burden of anxiety disorders on society is large, both in terms of disability and treatment costs. Having a panic disorder doubles the risk for later drug abuse or dependence (Christie et al., 1988). Leon et al. (1995) point out that patients with anxiety disorders are more likely to seek help from emergency rooms and from the specialized mental health system. They also found that men with panic disorder were more likely to be chronically unemployed and to receive disability or welfare. Moreover, treatment costs are not restricted to the anxiety disorders themselves. Overall health care costs are high for patients with these diagnoses as well. Simon, Ormel, VonKorff, and Barlow (1995) found that primary care patients with *DSM-III-R* anxiety disorders incurred roughly twice the health care costs as did patients with subclinical disorders or no anxiety disorders.

229

Although patients with anxiety disorders significantly tax the health care system, it is estimated that only a quarter of those who suffer from these disorders actually receive treatment for their anxiety disorders (Weissman, 1988). The majority of patients who receive treatment are treated in the general health and not the mental health system (Gath & Catalan, 1986; Lyles & Simpson, 1990). A contemporary physician's guide for treatment of anxiety estimates that the typical primary care physician sees at least one patient every day with an anxiety disorder (McGlynn & Metcalf, 1991). Most patients with anxiety disorders who receive treatment are treated by nonpsychiatrist physicians who lack training in psychotherapy, and tend to rely on pharmacological management.

Our review of the literature indicates that pharmacotherapy and psychotherapy—specifically, the behavioral therapies—are the two most researched types of treatment for these disorders. There are conceptual and technical differences between the two approaches, including differences in their active ingredients and in their mechanisms of change (Elkin, Pilkonis, Docherty, & Sotsky, 1988). Is one treatment superior and, if so, in what way? Are medications more cost-effective? Do the treatments complement one another? What are the risks associated with these therapies? The pervasiveness and costs associated with the anxiety disorders make these extremely important questions.

In this chapter we examine research purported to support the use of medications in the treatment of anxiety, particularly panic disorder. We raise concerns about quality and bias in industry-funded efficacy research, and will present findings suggesting that more caution may be warranted in the routine application of these agents. The contemporary comparative literature, including some important meta-analyses, will also be carefully examined.

THE ANXIETY DISORDERS

Anxiety is commonly thought of as a state of uneasiness and distress about future uncertainty. Unlike fear, anxiety is an unrealistic, self-feeding emotion. Fear is adaptive; anxiety is generally not. For psychiatric purposes, anxiety involves more extreme discomfort or avoidance leading to a serious disruption of a person's social or occupational functioning.

The *Diagnostic and Statistical Manual of Mental Disorders* (*DSM-IV*; APA, 1994) specifies 11 diagnoses under the general heading "Anxiety Disorders." It also defines the terms "panic" and "agoraphobia" and while neither of these terms are diagnoses in themselves, they are central to the concept of clinical anxiety. Panic attack is described as a "discrete period of intense fear or discomfort that is accompanied by at least four symptoms of 13 somatic or cognitive symptoms. The attack has a sudden onset and builds to a peak rapidly (usually within 10 minutes or less) . . ." (p. 394). Agoraphobia is defined as "anxiety about being in places or situations from which escape might be difficult (or embarrassing) or in which help might not be available in the event of having a panic attack . . ." (p. 396).

The *DSM-IV* anxiety diagnoses include panic disorder with and without agoraphobia (PD and PD-A), agoraphobia without a history of panic disorder, social phobia, specific phobia, obsessive-compulsive disorder (OCD), posttraumatic stress disorder (PTSD), acute stress disorder, anxiety disorder due to a medical condition or substance use, generalized anxiety disorder (GAD), and anxiety disorder "not otherwise specified." Some authors have suggested that these diagnoses may be roughly divided into two groups depending on whether the anxiety is stimulus dependent or stimulus independent (e.g., Lipman, 1989). Stimulus independent or endogenous anxiety includes diagnoses like GAD and PD. Examples of anxiety disorders associated with an obvious external trigger include simple phobia (e.g., a snake phobia) or social phobia (fear of social embarrassment). This distinction is being challenged today by research suggesting that both types of anxiety are stimulus dependent (e.g., Salkovskis & Clark, 1990). From this perspective, phobic disorders are associated with external triggers, whereas other disorders are associated with internal or proprioceptive triggers. PTSD and OCD are most closely allied with the phobic disorders (Lipman, 1989) and involve special response patterns. PTSD has been called a "traumatic phobia" and consists of a pattern of responses including reexperiencing the traumatic event, avoidance of stimuli associated with the trauma (or numbing of responsiveness) and persistent symptoms of increased arousal. The patient with OCD is compelled to think thoughts or engage in behaviors in order to avoid the anxiety associated with not doing so. Anxiety symptoms differ from anxiety disorders in terms of duration of symptoms and degree of distress.

Anxiety, both phenomenologically and clinically, is complex. It is essential to remember that it is a label for a human experience that occurs against a background of other experiences both personal and social. The state called "anxiety" undoubtedly rests on complex neurobiological events. At the same time, anxiety is phenomenologically connected to conditioned stimuli, troublesome life events and circumstances, and maladaptive styles of information processing (Beck, Emery, & Greenberg, 1985; Clark, 1986).

ANTIANXIETY MEDICATIONS

The purpose of pharmacological treatment of anxiety is to remove the state of anxiety as quickly as possible, treating only what are believed to be the causative mechanisms. The ideal anxiolytic would be selective, allowing patients to live a normal life with no intellectual or psychomotor impairment. Unfortunately, no current anxiolytic meets this criterion (Mosconi, Chiamulera, & Recchia, 1993).

Chloral hydrate and paraldehyde were the first synthetic chemicals to replace alcohol and opiates in the treatment of anxiety. Barbiturates, introduced in the 1930s, showed an exponential growth pattern until the 1950s, when their use leveled off. Problems with dependence, abuse, and danger of overdose led to curtailment of their use. Similar drugs were developed, often accompanied by claims of enhanced safety that later proved to be unfounded. Some examples include ethclorvynol, methaqualone and thalidomide (Lader, 1995).

Benzodiazepines were introduced in 1957. These drugs are advertised as "anxiolytics," and they are the drugs most often prescribed for anxiety disorders. Currently, a good deal of controversy surrounds their use (Lader, 1995; Warneke, 1991). The benzodiazepines are thought to have a prompt onset of action and to provide effective symptom relief with a mild elevation in mood. Although they have been generally regarded as effective (Rosenbaum, 1982), some studies have shown that much of their apparent efficacy is due to placebo response and natural remission (Quality Assurance Project, 1985; A. K. Shapiro, 1978) and their use is associated with side effects and problems of rebound and withdrawal (Pecknold, Swinson, Kuch, & Lewis, 1988; Rickels, Case, Downing, & Winokur, 1983).

All the benzodiazepines are central nervous system (CNS) depressants, similar to alcohol and barbiturates in their clinical effects (Breggin, 1991). The clinical effects of these drugs enable them to be used as anxiolytics, hypnotics, muscle relaxants, and anticonvulsants. Their side effects include sedation, psychomotor and cognitive impairment, amnesiogenic and disinhibitory effects, tolerance and dependence, liability to abuse, and danger of overdose (Essig, 1964). Patients may also have paradoxical psychological effects such as the release of anxiety or hostility while on therapeutic doses of benzodiazepines (C. Wilkinson, 1985). Psychological and physical dependence are serious concerns and may lead patients to become chronic users of these drugs despite the lack of research supporting long-term treatment. As serious as many of these drawbacks appear to be, they have been generally overlooked or ignored, apparently on the assumption that these medications are the most effective treatment alternatives for anxiety disorders. This position warrants an examination of the relevant research literature.

Anxiolytic drugs are intended to treat anxiety by altering the biochemical mechanisms thought to create it (Haefely, 1991). Support for the drug treatment of anxiety has been mostly in the form of uncontrolled clinical trials or comparisons of the active drug with an inert placebo. In general, these studies have found the drug superior to placebo—at least in the short term. Although controlled research is an improvement over clinical trials, many of the controlled studies suffer from methodological problems and problems of inference. A classic example is the Cross-National Collaborative Panic Study, reported by Klerman (1988).

THE CROSS-NATIONAL COLLABORATIVE PANIC STUDY (CNCPS)

The CNCPS was one of the largest controlled clinical trials in the history of psychiatry, involving 1,700 patients at clinical sites in 14 countries. Twenty senior investigators took part in the studies. Klerman (1992) summarized the research by writing that the papers reporting the results of the multicenter trial demonstrated the short-term efficacy of alprazolam compared with placebo. Klerman's conclusion is echoed (and amplified) in much of the prevailing thought about alprazolam today.

In the first study of the series, Ballenger and his colleagues (Ballenger et al., 1988) reported on the efficacy of alprazolam in a placebo-controlled, flexible dose trial in patients who had panic disorder with and without agoraphobia. The study involved 526 patients with 481 completing three weeks of treatment. At Week 1, the drug treatment group showed significant differences in improvement for spontaneous panic attacks, phobic fears, avoidance behavior, anxiety, and secondary disability. At Week 4, 82% of the alprazolam patients were moderately improved or better, whereas only 42% of the placebo group were classified as improved. In the alprazolam group, 50% were panic free, whereas only 28% of the placebo group were free of panic attacks. The authors note that alprazolam decreased the frequency of spontaneous panic attacks, with 59% panic free at Week 8. The drug also reduced phobic avoidance and disability, and it worked more quickly than imipramine or phenalzine.

An examination of the mean frequency of panic attacks across all 8 weeks of the study, shows that at baseline, there were no significant differences between the two groups in terms of panic attacks. At Week 1, the two groups were significantly different on this variable with the alprazolam group reporting significantly fewer panic attacks ($p < .0001$). At Week 4, the groups were still significantly different at the same level. At Week 8, however, the completer analysis showed no significant difference between the two groups. Most of the conclusions about the drug's efficacy were drawn on data comparison at Week 4. The authors of the study also performed an end-point analysis. Although it did show a significant difference between the drug and placebo groups, it is based in part, on how the authors thought the data might look if almost half of the placebo group hadn't dropped out of the study. At Week 8, almost half of the placebo group had dropped out, citing "no treatment effect" as the primary reason. Since there was *no* significant difference between the two remaining groups at Week 8, the authors used subjects' Week 8 data if available, and if not, the last available data carried forward. It is likely this treatment of the data favors the alprazolam group, since the placebo group might have done better had they remained in the study. In fact, a similar study , published by Marks, Swinson, Basoglu, Kuch, et al. (1993) experienced a placebo dropout rate of only 13%. Their placebo group *did* continue to improve on panic measures until Week 8 and study dropouts were less ill than completers (Basoglu, 1992).

Although Klerman pointed out that patients in the placebo group at time of dropout had significantly poorer responses than patients who remained in the study (Klerman, 1992), this ignored the fact that these patients were showing a trend toward improvement. In fact, in the end-point analysis, half of the scores are imputed to have remained unchanged in a sample that was showing continuing improvement. Thus in a short-term comparison, alprazolam was effective at Week 4 and earlier. However, comparing the data on those who completed the study, there was no significant effect at Week 8, suggesting that any real gains were lost by the end of the study. Klerman himself indicated that the completer analysis shows no significant drug effect for "total panic attacks" in either phase of the CNCPS. Some researchers have questioned the FDA's approval of this drug as an "antipanic agent" under the circumstances (Marks, Basoglu, et al., 1993).

Although Klerman repeatedly pointed out that the CNCPS was an examination of the *short-term* efficacy of alprazolam, the study population had *chronic* anxiety disorders of 5 to 9 years' duration. This brings into question the usefulness of the study's conclusions as well as the current practice of prescribing the drug for longer than 4 weeks. Also, the study did not have a psychological treatment component nor a drug-free follow-up in its design. In the Phase II study, which compared the two drugs, alprazolam and imipramine, 22% of the alprazolam versus 8% of the imipramine and 6% of the placebo patients continued taking the medications after the study concluded.

An important question, unanswered in the published report, is why so many subjects in the placebo group dropped out. A partial answer to this question might be that subjects were promised that, should they choose to drop out of the study, they would be provided active treatment. While such a promise might have had less impact if an active placebo had been used, it is suspect with an inert placebo. In fact, after drug taper, one group of Toronto clinicians was asked to guess which patients were in the treatment group and which were in the placebo group. Ninety percent of the time they guessed correctly (Marks et al., 1989). This suggests that neither the clinicians nor the patients in this study were blind to the treatment conditions. Patients who experienced no drug effect and had been given a treatment option at the beginning of the study would certainly be more likely to exercise that option and join the active treatment group.

The cross-national study also concluded that there were few side effects. In fact there were more than a few side effects and these, along with withdrawal symptoms, had significant implications for the patients who suffered from them. Pecknold et al. (1988), published data on panic attacks among patients who completed active treatment and began the drug withdrawal phase of the study. Their data show that most of these patients relapsed. Pecknold defined relapse as a return of panic attacks more severe than baseline. Although all the patients were eventually tapered from the anxiolytic, during the last week of taper the drug treatment patients were worse off than the patients in the placebo group in number of panic attacks—350% worse. In fact, some of these patients were worse off than when they started therapy. At discontinuation of drug therapy, 27% of the patients had rebound anxiety worse than baseline. Thirty percent had mild to moderate withdrawal symptoms. Alprazolam-treated patients also showed significant deterioration on a global assessment scale, relative to the placebo-treated group at both the first and last posttaper weeks.

In summary, alprazolam had a clear though partial effect at Week 4 and some effects at Week 8, but at the price of sedation (48%), ataxia (25%), fatigue (19%), and rebound panic, often worse than the patient's original symptoms. Even though the side effects reported by Pecknold are sobering, there is some suggestion that this study may have underestimated them. The previously mentioned CNCPS follow-up study by Marks, Swinson, Basoglu, Kuch, and colleagues (1993) found significantly more severe sedation, fatigue, irritability, memory problems, impaired mentation, ataxia, slurred speech, appetite decrease, and weight loss in their alprazolam group compared with the placebo group.

In Phase I of the CNCPS, alprazolam was more effective than placebo on most measures according to end-point analysis, but on only 4 of 21 measures in completer analysis. In Phase II, a significant alprazolam effect was found on 5 out of 24 measures in end-point analysis and on only 1 measure in completer analysis (Basoglu, 1992). The effect of alprazolam was impressive only in the end-point analyses in Phase I, but not in Phase II; it was negligible in completer analyses in both studies.

THE MARKS ET AL. CROSS-NATIONAL PANIC STUDY

Marks and his colleagues (1989) were critical of the CNCPS research on several grounds. Their main concerns were that the studies had very high early placebo dropout rates and there were short-term efficacy studies that lacked follow-up, although these patients were suffering from chronic disorders. Additionally, the CNCPS did not compare drug treatment with an effective behavioral therapy.

The Marks et al. (1993) cross-national (Canada-United Kingdom) trial of alprazolam compared exposure therapy (Marks, 1978), alprazolam and placebo for the treatment of chronic panic disorder with agoraphobia. The study improved on the CNCPS in that it employed an exposure therapy comparison group and the authors performed a 6-month drug-free follow-up. The study enjoyed a low placebo dropout rate as well.

One hundred patients were randomly assigned to (a) alprazolam and exposure (combined treatment group), (b) alprazolam and relaxation (psychological placebo), (c) placebo and exposure, or (d) placebo and relaxation (double placebo). Drug taper occurred posttreatment from Weeks 8 to 16. Subjects were followed to Week 43.

Marks, Swinson, Basoglu, Koch, et al. report that the number of major panics decreased for all groups. Panic scores improved as much with placebo as with alprazolam or exposure. The patients who received alprazolam started showing improvement by Week 2, but largely plateaued by Week 4. There was no further improvement in Weeks 4 to 8, with symptoms worsening from then on. On nonpanic variables both exposure and alprazolam were effective by the end of treatment, but exposure had twice the effect size. During Weeks 8 to 16 and on follow-up, gains due to alprazolam were lost, whereas gains due to exposure were maintained. Results showed that the addition of alprazolam to the exposure treatment protocol marginally improved outcome *during* treatment but compromised improvement thereafter. Alprazolam-treated patients compared with controls had stronger beliefs that their improvement was due to medications rather than psychological treatment. Patients who attributed their improvement to medications during treatment did worse at posttaper than those who felt that improvement was due to their own personal efforts.

Unlike the CNCPS, the Marks, Swinson, Basoglu, Koch, et al. study appears to be well designed and well executed. There were no significant differences in main effects between London and Toronto. The outcomes held up across different analytic methods. The study results didn't require endpoint analysis because the study did not suffer the same heavy placebo dropout reported by the CNCPS. Short-term results were similar to previous studies and confirm alprazolam's short-term effects, yet when compared with exposure therapy, the drug was only half as effective. Additionally, there was a high relapse rate when the drug was discontinued. At Week 23, former alprazolam patients were worse off than were the former placebo patients on two phobia and three panic measures. Only in the exposure group did subjects improve and maintain their improvement.

Despite the apparent robustness of Marks et al.'s findings, Spiegel et al. (1993) found fault with the study. These authors criticized Marks on the comparability of his sample (to the CNCPS), the study's methodology, and the analysis and presentation of the data.

Marks, Swinson, Basoglu, Noshirvani, et al. (1993) responded to the concerns cited by Spiegel et al. (1993). In their response, they defend the comparability of the CNCPS and London/Toronto samples both in terms of depression scores and in terms of symptom severity. They point out that the attrition rate during active treatment was lower than that of the CNCPS, despite Spiegel et al.'s assertion to the contrary. Marks successfully addressed a number of other criticisms as well. Perhaps most interesting in this exchange is Marks's concern regarding Spiegel et al.'s motives in attacking the study. Addressing the assertion that their study suffered from methodological flaws, Marks et al. point out that two of the authors of the Spiegel critique helped design, monitor, and analyze the London/Toronto study and the CNCPS. They point out that neither found problems with their study before the results were known. Marks et al. also point out that Upjohn generously supported the design, execution, analysis, and quality assurance of the study. The company was very involved in the study—to a point. Marks et al. (1993) wrote:

> Monitoring and support stopped abruptly when the results became known. Thereafter, Upjohn's response was to invite professionals to critique the study they had nurtured so carefully before. The study is a classic demonstration of the hazards of research funded by industry. (p. 792)

Upjohn funded a number of panic studies to obtain FDA approval for the use of alprazolam in the treatment of panic disorder. They succeeded despite some questionable research methodology and the fact that none of these studies definitively showed alprazolam to be superior to placebo.

OTHER DRUG EFFICACY RESEARCH

Shader and Greenblatt (1983) reviewed the pharmacological, behavioral, and psychotherapeutic treatment approaches available for anxiety disorders. They concluded that nonpharmacological treatments were generally the first treatment of choice in situational and nonincapacitating anxiety. When anxiety was severe and prolonged, they concluded that adjunctive drug treatment was appropriate with the use of antidepressants (ADs) for phobic/panic states and anxiolytics for GAD and mixed anxiety and depression. Benzodiazepines were deemed the anxiolytics of choice at that time.

In a more recent review, Lipman (1989) examined the research on the drug treatment of anxiety and concluded that, despite their popularity, anxiolytic medications were not the most effective drugs for the treatment of anxiety disorders such as simple phobia, social phobia, agoraphobia/panic, OCD, PTSD, and GAD. Lipman noted that the benzodiazepines were the most frequently prescribed medications for the anxiety disorders. Their efficacy, with two exceptions, was not supported by well-controlled studies. The exceptions included the use of benzodiazepines in the short-term treatment of GAD and alprazolam for the treatment of agoraphobia/panic. Lipman also found that ADs demonstrated a moderate level of effectiveness in the treatment of OCD and a relatively greater effectiveness in the treatment of panic/agoraphobia and in long-term treatment of GAD. He concluded that the magnitude of treatment effect for even the ADs left a good deal of room for improvement. Although Lipman's review focused on the pharmacotherapy of anxiety disorders, he felt that psychosocial treatments provide a major source of therapeutic effectiveness. He concluded that the strongest consensus favoring a combination of antidepressant medications and behavioral treatment existed in the panic/agoraphobia area.

Wilkinson, Balestrieri, Ruggeri, and Ballantuone (1991) compared 19 double-blind, placebo-controlled studies of benzodiazepines and ADs. They concluded that drug treatments had a 25% advantage over treatment with placebo. In the short term (less than 14 weeks), the two drug treatments studied were equally effective.

Michelson and Marchione (1991) also evaluated research on pharmacological treatments for panic disorder with agoraphobia. They found that the tricyclic antidepressants (TCAs), especially imipramine, have been the most widely studied medications for this disorder. Indeed, a number of studies have compared imipramine with placebo. Most of these studies have been reviewed by Mavissakalian and Michelson (1986) and Nutt and Glue (1989). Nutt (1990) points out that, apart from a few studies to the contrary (Evans, Kenardy, Schneider & Hoey, 1986; Marks, Gray, Cohen, Hill, Mawson, Ramm & Stern, 1983; Raskin, 1983), all have found imipramine superior to placebo in treating anxiety, especially panic attacks. In controlled trials, imipramine appears to have a selective effect on mood, anxiety, and panic symptoms, but it is less effective against anticipatory anxiety and phobic avoidance. Michelson and Marchione indicate that the selective effects of the drug appear to complement the effects of exposure-based behavioral therapies (BT), which tend to be more effective on anticipatory anxiety and avoidance. Not surprisingly, a fair amount of research has looked at combining TCAs and BT.

Early studies comparing BT and imipramine indicated that imipramine enhanced the effects of both imaginal and in vivo exposure (Zitrin, Klein,

& Woerner, 1978, 1980) but were methodologically flawed (Michelson & Marchione, 1991). Later studies (Agras, Telch, Taylor, Roth, & Brouillard, 1990; Marks et al., 1983; Mavissakalian & Michelson, 1986a, 1986b; Telch, Agras, Taylor, Roth, & Gallen, 1985) have shown that imipramine may improve the outcome of exposure-based treatment in the short run, but that these effects disappear on follow-up. Imipramine appears to exert its primary effect on mood; in combination with BT, it has effects on panic frequency and phobic avoidance. Additionally, the drug is generally effective only in combination with exposure-based treatment and is plagued with side effects that often lead to treatment refusal and dropouts. On follow-up, behaviorally treated patients maintained their treatment gains and showed further improvement, whereas imipramine-treated patients were more likely to relapse.

Patient acceptance is very much a concern with these drugs. They can be unpleasant for many patients because of their side effects. For example, researchers for one study (Uhlenhuth, Matuzas, Glass, & Easton, 1989) experienced a 50% dropout in 8 weeks of patients who were given imipramine. Although the authors concluded that imipramine was effective in treating panic symptoms, the side effects and slow onset of therapeutic action caused a number of patients to drop out. Although some reviews and meta-analyses have suggested that TCAs are the more effective drug treatment for PD (e.g., Clum, Clum, & Surls, 1993; Lipman, 1989), Nutt (1990), in his review of the pharmacological treatment of anxiety, points out that it is now well established that imipramine actually increases anxiety, that it worsens somatic symptoms, and that it precipitates panic attacks. He points out that these effects occur early in treatment and often prompt patients to drop out of therapy (also see Pohl, Yeragani, Balon, & Lycaki, 1988). Nutt notes that the acute effects of imipramine can precipitate full-blown panic attacks and Nutt and Glue (1989) proffer that other tricyclics, including serotonin reuptake blockers, also result in high levels of treatment dropouts due to their side effects. Since the antidepressants tend to be associated with more severe side effects, many of them similar to symptoms of anxiety, one wonders to what extent patient improvement with these agents might be due to attributional effects. That is, patients experience drug side effects similar to their anxiety symptoms but attribute them to the drug. As the variety of side effects associated with the antidepressants increases, it will be interesting to see whether a correlation emerges between the anxiomimetic properties of these drugs and their perceived effectiveness against a given symptom profile.

Research on clomipramine (another TCA), monoamine oxidase inhibitors (MAOIs), and beta-adrenergic blockers was also reviewed by Michelson and Marchione (1991). Clomipramine was found effective in two early studies (Beaumont, 1977; Johnson, Trayer, & Whitsett, 1988); however, the earlier study was an open trial and both studies experienced significant dropouts due to noxious side effects. More recently, McTavish and Benfield (1990) reviewed controlled studies of clomipramine and concluded that the drug is effective in the treatment of panic. Although Michelson and Marchione concluded that clomipramine offered no apparent advantage over imipramine, a more recent study by Modigh, Westperg, and Eriksson (1992) suggested that it may be more efficacious. The MAOIs and beta-blockers have not found strong research support. The MAOIs are associated with greater risks and worse side effect profiles than the TCAs (Raskin, Quitkin, & Harrison, 1984a, 1984b).

In general, controlled research has not supported the use of benzodiazepines in the treatment of PD. Michelson and Marchione (1991) found little research to support the use of low-potency benzodiazepines. In fact, some researchers have found that patients with panic disorder with agoraphobia undergoing exposure therapy experience less improvement when benzodiazepines are added to their treatment protocols (Chambless, Foa, Graves, & Goldstein, 1979; Marks et al., 1993). As was demonstrated in the CNCPS, high-potency benzodiazepines (HBZs) exert some impact on panic symptoms early in treatment but are associated with high relapse, rebound, dependence, and withdrawal problems.

In their review of long-term follow-up studies of medication treatment for PD, Pollack and Otto (1994) suggest that patients do improve with pharmacological treatment but must remain on the medication to sustain benefit. Even on maintenance medication, many patients continue to experience anxiety-related problems. Noyes, Garvey, Cook, and Samuelson (1989) point out, that with an average 2.5 year follow-up, almost two-thirds of the patients treated with medications were still taking them; three-fourths reported at least moderate improvement, but only 14% were free of symptoms. Of patients with at least moderate improvement who attempted to discontinue their medications, over half relapsed within 2 years. Most relapsed within 2 months after discontinuing the drug. Only one-fourth of the patients who discontinued ADs sustained remission two years or longer.

Insofar as drug treatment of PD is concerned, antidepressants appear to be the most effective medications whether used by themselves or in combination with BT (Clum, Clum, & Surls, 1993; Lydiard & Ballenger, 1987; Nutt, 1990). Sedation, dependency, withdrawal, and relapse seriously limit the usefulness of the benzodiazepines. Although they are the preferred drug class, the ADs suffer from limited effectiveness, high relapse rates, and their unpleasant side effect profiles. Obviously, if drugs with more acceptable side effect profiles were available, they would be preferred by clinicians who rely on pharmacotherapy.

NEWER ANXIOLYTICS

Benzodiazepines, due to their faster action and greater consumer acceptability would be even more acceptable if their associated side effects and relapse problems could be controlled. Recent research has focused on developing novel anxiolytics without the traditional problems associated with benzodiazepines such as dependence, sedation, muscle relaxation, and amnesia. One group is the omega (benzodiazepine) receptor ligands alpidem, bretazenil, suriclone, and abecarnil (Sanger, Perrault, Morel, Joly, & Zivkovic, 1991). Although some studies have found drugs in this class no more effective than placebo in the treatment of PD (deJonghe, Swinkels, Tuynman-Qua, & Jonkers, 1989), others have shown them to be roughly comparable to older benzodiazepines, sometimes better tolerated, but still associated with benzodiazepine-like side effects such as sedation and withdrawal (Ballenger et al., 1991; Mavissakalian & Perel, 1995).

One double-blind, placebo-controlled study found alpidem effective compared with placebo in controlling chronic anxiety (Casacchia et al., 1989). Although these authors found that the drug was devoid of significant sedative effects, Morton and Lader (1990), found that alpidem at high doses, like lorazepam, impaired performance on a range of psychomotor tasks. Alpidem appeared to be less disruptive than the benzodiazepine, however.

Early controlled research suggested that alpidem was an effective anxiolytic (Bassi et al., 1989; Morselli, 1990; Murch, Morselli, & Priore, 1988) and safe enough to be recommended for elderly populations (Frattola et al., 1992). However, this drug is unlikely to become a popular replacement for benzodiazepines as several recent studies have suggested that alpidem may be hepatotoxic (Lader, 1995).

Serotonin selective (specific) reuptake inhibitors (SSRIs) such as fluoxetine (Prozac®), sertraline (Zoloft®), paroxetine (Paxil®), and fluvoxamine (Luvox®) are widely considered effective for the treatment of panic disorder although this popularity is based more on clinical practice and uncontrolled clinical trials than on controlled studies (Schneier, Leibowitz, & Davies, 1990). Despite the lack of controlled studies these drugs are now used as first-line treatments for PD when an AD is indicated (Pollack & Otto, 1994). Rickels and Schweizer (1990b) hold that SSRIs do not differ from TCAs in efficacy or onset of action, but feel that they do have a different side effect profile. They appear to provide their effect without sedation, anticholinergic, or cardiotoxic reactions. The most frequent problems associated with these drugs are gastrointestinal upset. While they *appear* to be safer and better tolerated than TCAs, the drug literature is filled with examples of promising new drugs that are discredited by later research.

A limited number of controlled studies have suggested that drugs in this class, especially fluvoxamine, are effective in the treatment of panic disorder (Roy-Byrne, Wagerson, Cowley, & Dager, 1993). An early double-blind, placebo-controlled trial that demonstrated an antipanic effect superior to the heterocylic drug maprotiline was provided by den Boer and Westerberg (1988). Hoehn-Saric, McLeod, and Hipsley (1993) compared fluvoxamine with placebo in a study involving 36 patients with PD. The study used an 8-week, double-blind, parallel groups design. Both groups improved on all measures; however, the fluvoxamine group showed significantly fewer panic attacks beginning at Week 3 and significantly lower anxiety, depression, and disability from Week 6 on. There were no differences in mean ratings of severity of major attacks and of severity and frequency of minor attacks. At 8 weeks, significantly more patients on fluvoxamine were free of major and minor panic attacks. The study is vulnerable to many of the criticisms applied to drug efficacy research: There was no behavioral treatment condition in the design, the researchers used an inert placebo, and they assessed patients at posttreatment while they were still taking the drug.

Black, Wesner, Bowers, and Gabel (1993) compared the effectiveness of fluvoxamine with cognitive therapy and found that 81% of the medication-treated patients were panic-free at 8 weeks compared with 53% of the cognitive therapy patients. The authors did not provide data on avoidance, and it is not known whether this treatment impacted patients' avoidant behavior. Additionally, since the patients were still taking the medication at final assessment, the findings do not take into account relapse rates on discontinuation of medications that typically range from 20% to 90% (Rickels, Schweizer, Weiss, & Zavodnick, 1993).

A study by deBeurs, vanBalkom, Lange, Koele, and vanDyck (1995) examined the use of fluvoxamine in combination with in vivo exposure in the treatment of PD with agoraphobia. deBeurs and colleagues compared the double-blind, placebo administered SSRI fluvoxamine with the behavioral techniques of repeated hyperventilation and respiratory training. These interventions were followed by in vivo exposure and compared with in vivo exposure alone. Outcome was assessed by self-report measures, a multitask behavioral avoidance task and continuous monitoring of panic attacks. All treatments were deemed effective and resulted in significant decrease in agoraphobic avoidance. The combination of fluvoxamine and exposure was the most effective treatment. It had twice the effect on self-reported agoraphobic avoidance as did psychological panic management with exposure. Psychological panic management combined with exposure was not superior to exposure alone.

The deBeurs et al. (1995) study is flawed in its methodology and over-general in its conclusions. Patients were allowed to continue their use of benzodiazepines if they had been taking them for over 3 months. The apparent rationale for this decision was that (a) many patients, if asked to stop taking tranquilizers, will surreptitiously take them anyway, and (b) treatment gains would be artificially inflated by increasing pretest psychopathology resulting from drug withdrawal. This decision does not take into account the possibility of drug interaction: Although the authors state that benzodiazepine users were evenly distributed across conditions, drug interaction would occur only in the fluvoxamine condition.

The dependent variables included self-reported agoraphobia, depression, and somatic anxiety (comprising composite scores derived from various self-report instruments), behavioral task avoidance and associated anxiety, panic attacks, and goal attainment outcomes. The authors do not characterize the types of goals patients set in goal attainment scaling and it is not clear whether these goals included intended improvement in avoidance behaviors, cognitions, or both. Scores on all three self-report measures significantly decreased over time; however, self-reported agoraphobia responded best to fluvoxamine plus exposure as did mean goal attainment scores.

There was no fluvoxamine alone condition, which would allow appraisal of the drug effects in isolation. All treatments resulted in a significant improvement in task avoidance, and there were no differences between conditions. This is a curious finding since there was a differential treatment effect on patients' reports of reduced agoraphobia on the self-report composite but no concomitant effect on behavioral avoidance. Psychological panic management plus exposure produced the fewest panic-free patients by the end of the study. The authors admit that their sample was atypical in reporting 60% fewer panic attacks than is average for this population. The distributions of PAs were quite skewed as well. Additionally, the panic management intervention was crude by contemporary standards. Finally, and perhaps most importantly, patients were still taking medication when assessed at the end of the study. Conclusions regarding symptom suppression might be more appropriate than assertions of anxiety treatment that imply recovery.

The older monoamine oxidase inhibitors (MAOIs) have many adverse side effects that limit their usefulness, but they may soon be replaced by RIMAs (reversible inhibitors of monoamine oxidase-A). Controlled studies on these new drugs are not yet available.

The selective serotonin-1A receptor partial agonist anxiolytics were reviewed by Feighner and Boyer (1989). The authors suggest that drugs such as buspirone, gepirone, and ipsapirone have several new and unique features. They appear to evidence no cross-tolerance with alcohol or benzodiazepines, are less likely to be abused, and less likely to result in withdrawal symptoms or rebound anxiety on cessation of therapy (Murphy, Owen, & Tyerer, 1989). Proponents suggest that these drugs have no muscle relaxant, sedative, or anticonvulsant properties, do not cause euphoria (Perry, 1985), and do not seem to impair psychomotor functioning. They do have slower onset than benzodiazepines and the side effect profile is quite different. Side effects include gastrointestinal symptoms such as nausea and diarrhea, headache, dizziness, restlessness, and giddiness (Olajide & Lader, 1987).

Buspirone is an azapirone derivative that is structurally different from the benzodiazepines and has very different biochemical and pharmacological actions. Its effects are believed due to its ability to decrease serotonergic function (Nutt, 1990). The absence of sedation as a clinical marker and the gradual onset of effect appear to decrease patient satisfaction, however. Another problem associated with buspirone is that patients who have had previous exposure to benzodiazepine therapy do poorly on this drug and tend to report unwanted side effects such as restlessness. The most common side effects associated with this drug are dizziness, nausea, and headache (which lead to discontinuation in 10% to 20% of the patients).

Buspirone, like other new drugs received great press when it was first introduced (Cohn, Bowden, Fisher, & Rodos, 1986; Feighner, Merideth, & Hendrickson, 1982; Goldberg & Finnerty, 1979; Rickels et al., 1982). Later reviews have been less enthusiastic. Sanger (1994) notes that efforts to develop partial agonist anxiolytics with lesser effects on memory have failed, as these newer drugs also disrupt learning processes. Reports in the animal literature also show that buspirone disrupts acquisition avoidance learning and retention (e.g., Venault et al., 1986). At least two studies have shown buspirone ineffective in the treatment of PD (Pohl, Balon, Yeragani, & Gershon, 1989; Sheehan, Davidson, Manschreck, et al., 1983). Sanger was led to conclude that there may be an unavoidable link between anxiety, memory, and learning. He points out that the same limbic structures are implicated in both anxiety and memory and that it is overly optimistic to expect the development of anxiolytics devoid of negative effects on cognition in humans.

Overall, drug studies suggest that medications are generally more effective than placebo in the treatment of anxiety disorders. The quality of the research, the limited effect sizes, and the documented side effects must be kept in mind, however. Benzodiazepines may be useful for their immediate anxiolytic effect but there is a countertherapeutic offset of dependence, adverse side effects, and relapse. Some ADs and the newer SSRIs may be more useful than the benzodiazepines in long-term management of anxiety; however, the ADs are associated with unpleasant and sometimes dangerous side effects. The newer agents, despite their current popularity, have very few controlled studies supporting their use. Finally, with all drug treatment, there is the problem of outcome attribution. Patients do not attribute their improvement to their own efforts and may be more vulnerable to future problems.

CURRENT BEHAVIORAL TREATMENT

Psychological treatments and specifically behavioral treatments are generally effective in the treatment of anxiety (Lipsey & Wilson, 1993; Zinbarg, Barlow, Brown, & Hertz, 1992). Dropout rates are very low (mean of 8%) compared with other forms of therapy (Hunt & Andrews, 1992). Recent meta-analyses have consistently shown strong treatment effects for behavior therapy (Berman, Miller, & Massman, 1985; Clum, 1989; Clum et al., 1993; Gould, Otto, & Pollack, 1995; Michelson & Marchione, 1991). One meta-analysis (Trull, Nietzel, & Main, 1988) examined 19 behavioral therapy studies of subjects who had PDA. Behavior therapy involved programmed practice, imaginal exposure, gradual in vivo exposure, flooding, and relaxation. There was a clinically significant response to exposure 60% to 75% of the time (50% if attrition and nonresponders are considered). The benefits of treatment were well maintained.

Chambless and Gillis (1993) reviewed and contrasted 14 studies of cognitive-behavioral therapy (CBT) for GAD, PD with and without agoraphobia, and social phobia. The studies in their sample used cognitive, exposure-based, and relaxation interventions. They calculated effect sizes for pretest and posttest improvements (within subject comparison) as well as gains relative to a control group. Their results indicate that CBT is consistently more effective than waiting list and placebo control groups. They also concluded that in general, CBT is more beneficial than supportive therapy. Comparisons between behavior treatments showed variability. The authors suggest that cognitive change is a strong predictor of treatment outcome but that such change can be produced by a number of therapeutic approaches.

Different behavioral treatments may appear to be equally effective in the short run. However, long-term outcome may tell a different story. Durham and Turvey (1987) looked at BT and CBT in the treatment of GAD and found no difference at treatment's end, but a tendency for the CBT group to maintain or improve while the BT group tended to revert toward pretreatment scores. Butler (1984) found that subjects who received anxiety management training did better than exposure-only subjects and that they continued to improve after treatment. Generally speaking, the skills learned in CBT may enable patients to continue to improve, whereas exposure may be a more symptomatic intervention. More research is needed to address the issue, however.

Other types of psychotherapy do not appear to be as effective as the behavioral treatments for these disorders. A controlled study by Beck, Sokal, Clark, Berchick, and Wright (1992), compared the relative efficacy of focused cognitive therapy (FCT) and Rogerian supportive therapy on patients with PD and PDA. The FCT was aimed at breaking the cycle of panic resulting from catastrophic misattributions of somatic symptoms. Although this study has been criticized for possibly confounding the cognitive therapy with exposure (Arcierno, Hersen, & Van Hasselt, 1993), the results were nonetheless impressive. Subjects in the FCT condition showed reductions in panic frequency of 84% at posttest. Clinician's ratings showed reductions of 93%. Supportive therapy showed reductions of 36% and 30% respectively. FCT subjects showed significant reductions on Beck Depression (Beck, Ward, Mendelson, Mock, & Erbaugh, 1961) and Anxiety (Beck, Epstein, Brown, & Steer, 1988) Inventories. After one year, 85% of the FCT subjects remained panic-free. Similar results were obtained by Craske, Maidenberg, and Bystritsky (1995) who compared CBT and nondirective, supportive therapy. Other researchers have looked at psychodynamic therapy and found it to be less effective as well (Durham et al., 1994).

Alternative forms of treatment, some of which lend themselves to being added to behavioral protocols, are being evaluated. Some researchers have found support for the use of paradoxical intention (Michelson & Ascher, 1984) and for paradoxical intention with reframing in treating these disorders. Raglin and Morgan (1985) found that vigorous exercise was associated with reductions in state anxiety. Going one step further, Petruzzello, Landers, Hatfield, Kubitz, and Salazar (1991) performed a meta-analysis of studies that examined the relationship between exercise and anxiety and found that aerobic exercise of at least 21 minutes' duration achieved significant reductions in anxiety. These authors see exercise as a clear treatment alternative.

Other, less therapist-intensive behavioral approaches have been examined in controlled studies as well. A number of therapists have treated patients with anxiety disorders in group settings using CBT with good results (Cadbury, Childs-Clark, & Sandhu, 1990; Long & Bluteau, 1988; Michelson et al., 1990; Shapiro, Sank, Shaffer, & Donovan, 1982). Jannoun, Munby, Catalan, and Gelder (1980) tested a successful home-based program for agoraphobia that featured relaxation procedures. One group of researchers (Sorby, Reavley, & Huber, 1991) followed PD patients who were given anxiety management booklets by medical general practitioners. Many of the patients showed significant improvement. Welkowitz et al. (1991) trained practitioners at a traditional pharmacological center to use breathing control, cognitive restructuring, and exposure to successfully treat their patients. Milne, Jones, and Walters (1989) used former anxiety patients as therapists for 14 new patients and found this approach successful.

THE SEARCH FOR PSYCHOSOCIAL TREATMENT RECIPES

A current trend in the behavioral therapy field is the identification of the "active ingredients" of therapy and the packaging of these techniques into theoretically coherent treatment protocols (Barlow, Craske, Cerny, & Klosko, 1989). Barlow et al. found strong support for the effectiveness of component treatments that focus on several potential etiologic pathways. Interventions such as relaxation, breathing retraining, exposure to interoceptive stimuli, and cognitive reappraisal of somatic cues provide an effective, lasting treatment for panic symptoms.

Barlow (1990) reviewed the literature on long-term outcome of patients with PD who were treated with CBT. Barlow concluded that exposure-based treatment of agoraphobia was "reasonably effective" but felt that few patients were cured. He proposed a new cognitive-behavioral treatment based on a psychobiological model of PD. He suggests that some people are predisposed to panic, especially under stress. Some of these patients develop anxiety about the possibility of another panic attack and become sensitive to the panic cues. This "biocognitive" model is similar to that proposed by Clum (1989) and supported by others (Margraf, Ehlers, & Roth, 1986; Reiss, Peterson, Gursky, & McNally, 1986). Barlow's group uses systematic exposure to somatic events associated with panic, breathing retraining, and corrective information about attacks and catastrophic cognitions associated with panic to treat their patients.

Interventions for specific anxiety disorders will continue to be fine-tuned as research defines patient response patterns. The most effective psychotherapies for situational anxieties appear to be exposure and cognitive behavioral treatments. The three principal approaches to nonsituational panic attacks are applied relaxation, anxiety management, and cognition modification (Gelder, 1990). Ost, Jerremalm, and Jansson (1982) found that, in treating claustrophobia, the treatment (exposure vs. applied relaxation) worked best when it matched the response type (behavioral vs. physiological reactors). Similar conclusions were drawn by Lustman and Sowa (1983). Matching the appropriate anxiety disorder with the right treatment combination can be complicated, however. For example, the relationship between treatment and response type may vary by diagnosis. Ost et al. (1982) found that the two types of treatment were not differentially effective with the two responder types in the treatment of agoraphobia. On the other hand, exposure, while very effective for the treatment of some anxiety disorders, is not necessarily effective for them all (e.g., Foa & Rothbaum, 1989).

Combined Medication and Behavioral Treatments

The impact of adding medication to behavioral therapy treatment has been examined in controlled studies. Telch, Agras, Taylor, Roth, and Gallen (1985) compared three treatment conditions: imipramine without exposure, imipramine with exposure, and placebo with exposure. They found that the imipramine without exposure and placebo with exposure conditions resulted in no decrease in panic attacks whereas the drug plus exposure condition resulted in a significant reduction in panic attacks. They concluded that both medication and exposure are necessary to reduce panic attacks. This conclusion should be viewed cautiously however, since Clum et al. (1993) have shown that this finding may hold only when outcome is unidimensionally appraised by frequency of panic attacks.

Ballenger (1986) asserts that both TCAs and MAOIs produce moderate to marked improvement in 60% to 75% of patients with PDA, but the addition of exposure boosts the rate to 90%. As Ballenger points out, the problem is that some patients don't tolerate the side effects of these drugs very well. The benzodiazepines, on the other hand, may actually diminish the effectiveness of exposure. Marks and associates (1993) found no increased benefit from adding alprazolam to exposure therapy. The withdrawal of alprazolam actually diminished gains patients had made from exposure therapy. Concern is often expressed that medications may interfere with exposure either by interrupting the biological mechanism that facilitates habituation or by interfering with a full cognitive reappraisal of the safety of interoceptive cues by substituting the medication as a perceived safety cue (Barlow, 1988; Otto, Gould, & Pollack, 1994). Otto et al. (1994) argue that interoceptive exposure and cognitive restructuring might have helped Marks's patients deal with medication withdrawal; however, this seems a bit inefficient. Why add drug treatment to effective behavioral treatment if yet more behavioral treatment has to be used to ameliorate the iatrogenic effect of the drug? Current meta-analyses suggest that there is no specific advantage in adding drug therapy to effective behavioral therapy (e.g., see Clum et al., 1993; Gould et al., 1995; Mattick, Andrews, Hadzi-Pavlovic, & Christensen, 1990).

COMPARATIVE STUDIES

A number of meta-analyses have sought to compare the relative efficacy of various anxiety treatments. Michelson and Marchione (1991) estimated successful treatment outcomes based on their review of the literature, meta-analyses, and recent clinical research. Starting with a hypothetical cohort of 100 patients, they calculated the number of "survivors" after attrition and relapse who improved in each treatment category. Their data provide strong support for the notion that exposure is a relatively beneficial treatment for PDA. It also points out that rapid, focused relaxation training is relatively useful. Cognitive-behavioral treatment had an effect size of .83 compared with untreated controls. Overall cognitive therapy (CT) and graduated exposure (GE) were the most effective treatments they evaluated. Their empirically based, hypothetical illustration shows cognitive therapy with exposure and cognitive therapy to be the optimal treatments for PD both in terms of short- and long-term outcomes.

Four of the six studies they reviewed showed benzodiazepines to be superior to the alternative treatments studied. However, no controlled studies show them to be better than placebo. Low-potency benzodiazepines did decrease anxiety but resulted in dependency, tolerance, and side effects. Because these factors are considered in Michelson and Marchione's index, their results show a low efficiency index for these agents. Although the authors were unimpressed by the quantity of supportive research, they recommended the use of imipramine and other TCAs over benzodiazepines. Early studies on the MAOIs showed small effect sizes, but increased dosage and longer treatment led to greater successes. However, potential toxicity and multiple side effects make these agents less attractive. MAOIs are not first-line antidepressants and they lack FDA approval for use in the treatment of anxiety disorders.

Several papers have reported meta-analytic comparisons of psychotherapy and pharmacotherapy. The first of these (Clum, 1989) compared two decades of CBT and pharmacotherapy panic research. Clum estimated the relative merits of psychological and pharmacological interventions using an imaginary cohort composed of PDA patients and those with PD alone. He looked at termination (attrition), treatment success or failure, and relapse. Clum went beyond looking at treatment outcome alone, arguing that this approach ignores dropout and relapse rates. He argued that if treatment dropouts are due to the side effects of treatment, than the claimed effectiveness of the treatment should be adjusted accordingly. For example, if a drug with a 70% success rate carries a 30% dropout rate, it is in fact successful with only 70% of the remaining 70% or 49% of the original sample. Similarly he argues, relapse rates should be included in calculating treatment effectiveness. If suppression of symptoms is the goal of treatment then that should be made explicit by researchers. If treatment is to imply elimination of symptoms then relapse should be considered a part of the outcome. Clum's analysis of the available literature included relapse, dropout, and effectiveness data.

Clum's composite Efficacy Index showed cognitive behavioral therapy (CBT) to be superior to beta-blockers, low-potency benzodiazepines, and antidepressant medications. CBT had a 74% success rate. Clum notes that combining treatments reduced success rates compared with either treatment alone. This was especially true for behavior therapy, high-potency benzodiazepines (HBZs), and ADs. Overall, psychological treatment and HBZs had the best outcomes. Psychological treatments had a much lower relapse rate than did pharmacological treatment. If ADs were combined with behavior therapy, the relapse rate was lower than for antidepressant therapy alone, but higher than for behavior therapy alone. Clum's analysis suggests behavior therapies that target panic attacks had the highest success rate and lowest relapse rate.

Mattick, Andrews, Hadzi-Pavlovic, and Christensen (1990) examined 54 studies to determine relative pre-post treatment effect sizes for in vivo exposure, alternative psychological treatment, and medication in the treatment of patients with agoraphobia and panic disorder. The authors also looked at follow-up data, when available.

Their analysis of 40 studies that employed in vivo exposure demonstrated a mean effect size of 1.7 on measures of phobia and .96 on measures of panic. Effect sizes on measures of anxiety and depression were 0.68 and 0.69. Improvements were stable at follow-up after an average of 16 months.

Nine studies employed various BT techniques such as imaginal exposure, relaxation, assertion therapy, and cognitive therapy without the use of in vivo exposure. Collectively, these therapies demonstrated a significant effect on phobia (0.96) and a modest effect on panic (0.47).

Mattick et al. examined 16 studies employing CBT combined with exposure. The combined treatment appeared to have a wider impact on symptoms. While studies employing these techniques evidenced less impact on measures of phobia (1.43), they showed larger effect sizes on panic (1.29), anxiety (1.04), and depression (0.84). As the authors point out, the reduced effect on phobia may have been due to less emphasis having been placed on exposure in the combined intervention studies.

Analysis of the drug studies provided some interesting data. Alprazolam evidenced the largest treatment effects on measures of panic (1.04). Imipramine demonstrated a similar effect size on panic (1.01), but was most effective (compared with other treatments) against depression (0.89 compared with 0.41 for alprazolam). Diazepam yielded an effect size of only 0.56.

Studies that examined combined psychological treatment with imipramine showed that the addition of psychological treatments enhanced drug therapy, but the combination was no more effective than exposure alone. There were a total of 12 studies in this group.

Cox, Endler, Lee, and Swinson (1992) reviewed studies performed between 1980 and 1990 on patients with and without agoraphobia who were treated with imipramine, alprazolam, or exposure. Thirty-four studies meeting their inclusion criteria were analyzed. Combination treatments and studies of agoraphobia without panic were excluded. The dependent measures were global pre-post ratings by clinicians. The largest effect sizes were found for exposure (3.42) followed by alprazolam (2.1) and imipramine (1.16).

In a later report, Clum et al. (1993) acknowledged problems with their earlier study (Clum, 1989). First, the original analysis used panic attacks as the only dependent variable. Second, all the studies were equally weighted in the analysis, regardless of their rigor (i.e., some studies lacked a control group or included only completers in the final analysis). Some bias was introduced because studies that used no-treatment controls had better outcomes than those that used placebo controls (the former were more likely to have been used with BT studies). Finally, the double-blind method, most often associated with drug studies, may have produced less impressive outcomes.

Addressing these concerns in the later analysis, Clum and his colleagues (1993) examined 47 studies published between January 1964 and January 1990. This more robust analysis used only 29 of the 47 studies (only those with control groups). Clum's efficacy data on mean effect sizes of treatments compared with placebo indicated that psychological coping skills, flooding, combination treatments, and ADs exerted therapeutic effects across the spectrum of dependent variables. When the data were collapsed across dependent variables, psychological coping emerged with a larger treatment effect than flooding or antidepressants, which in turn, showed a larger effect than HBZs.

Psychological coping strategies were significantly more effective than HBZs and other drugs (primarily minor tranquilizers and beta-blockers; $p < .05$). A combination of BT and AD medication was significantly more effective than HBZs and other drugs ($p < .05$). Although it is commonly held that HBZs and ADs were the treatments of choice, only the ADs had large treatment effects and that group still suffered a high number of dropouts. Clum interprets these results as indicating that ADs were the drug treatment of choice when drugs were combined with behavior therapy. Of the psychological techniques, psychological coping (relaxation training, cognitive restructuring, and exposure) showed the greatest treatment effect. Flooding or exposure alone were also successful.

The results in this study differed from previous studies because in this analysis, the authors computed effect sizes using a range of dependent variables. If one looks only at frequency of panic attacks, then ADs and combined AD/BT show the greatest effect size while HBZs and psychological coping have a lesser and about equal effect size. Clum and his colleagues concluded that psychological coping strategies and flooding or exposure are the treatment of choice for PDA.

This study also examined the outcome effects of comorbid agoraphobia, the duration of the primary disorder, and the type of control group used in the study. Drug placebos were used most often as a control, followed by exposure, waiting list control, and progressive relaxation. The type of control group proved to be very important since statistically significant differences depended on the type of control used. Whether PD presented with or without agoraphobia was not related to effect size. If the experimenter was not blind to the treatment, there was a modest but nonsignificant influence toward increasing the effect size. Behavioral assessment was significantly less likely to show a treatment effect than were other types of assessment.

Van Balkom, Nauta, and Bakker (1995) criticized earlier meta-analyses on the grounds that they have methodological problems, especially the inclusion of between-study contrasts which they believe risk confusing confounding variables with true between-treatment effects. Van Balkom et al. selected 25 within-study contrasts published between 1964 and 1993. Nine studies contrasted imipramine and high-potency benzodiazepines. Eleven studies compared exposure combined with panic control therapies versus exposure alone or versus panic control alone. Two studies compared exposure combined with imipramine versus imipramine alone, while single studies compared CBT with alprazolam, CBT with fluvoxamine, and alprazolam with exposure against each treatment by itself.

The single trial comparisons (which often involved small sample sizes) suggest that CBT was more effective than alprazolam. Although difficult to interpret due to sampling bias, comparison between fluvoxamine and CBT suggested that there was no difference between the two treatments on measures of panic. Fluvoxamine was more effective if measures of anxiety and depression were considered. Alprazolam with exposure was more effective than exposure alone and exposure alone was more effective than alprazolam alone. Two studies showed imipramine and exposure to be more effective than imipramine alone.

In the 11 studies that compared panic management techniques with in vivo exposure, in vivo exposure emerged as the more effective treatment. The addition of panic control techniques did not improve outcome.

Nine studies compared imipramine and high-potency benzodiazepines. There was no significant between-treatment effect for either completer or intent-to-treat samples. The dropout rate for imipramine was much larger than that for alprazolam (27% vs. 13%).

Gould et al. (1995), expanded on the studies by Clum et al. (1993) by examining 43 controlled studies (published or presented between 1974 and March 1994 with data on 76 separate treatment interventions). This analysis also examined short and longer term outcome as well as looked at more specific treatment components than were analyzed by Clum and his colleagues (1993). Finally, the study included a cost analysis for CBT and phar-macological treatments.

Gould and his colleagues calculated two effect sizes for each study. An overall effect size was calculated by averaging the effect sizes of all the de-pendent measures within each study. A second effect size statistic was calculated for panic frequency. Studies were broken down by type of in-tervention: pharmacotherapy, CBT, or combination of the two approaches. Pharmacotherapy studies were further classified by type of drug adminis-tered: AD, BZ, and "others," as well as by type of control group used. Cognitive-behavioral studies were broken down by type: cognitive alone, cognitive restructuring plus exposure, cognitive-restructuring plus intero-ceptive exposure, and "other" interventions. Building on recommenda-tions presented by Clum et al. (1993), this study also considered the type of comparison or control group because this variable has been shown to af-fect treatment effect size.

Interoceptive exposure and cognitive restructuring yielded an effect size of 0.88, ADs yielded an effect size of 0.55, and benzodiazepines yielded an effect size of 0.40. Gould and his colleagues concluded that for short-term outcome, CBT, pharmacotherapy, and combined treatments were more effective than control conditions. Contrary to Clum et al.'s (1993) findings, ADs and BZs were equally effective in short-term treat-ment of PDA, but the ADs were not as well tolerated. They found that CBT was associated with relatively large overall effect sizes, low attrition, lower panic frequency, and a high panic-free outcome. However, the effect sizes associated with these studies enjoy a slight advantage because of using wait-list rather than pill placebo control. These authors also found that the most effective CBT interventions included a combination of cog-nitive restructuring and exposure. Studies that combined the relatively older CBT techniques with pharmacotherapy showed this combination to not be as effective as CBT alone. The newer CBT protocols in combination with the older drugs and the newer antidepressants (SSRIs), either alone or in combination with the newer cognitive treatments, were not included in the analysis because efficacy research was not available.

The Gould et al. (1995) analysis also looked at outcome 6 months or more posttreatment. They found that pharmacological interventions were least likely to maintain gains realized through treatment although most of the studies analyzed had discontinued treatment medications at follow-up. Results for CBT suggested that, on the average, treatment effects were maintained at about the same level enjoyed by subjects at the conclusion of the acute treatment phase.

Well-designed studies that show strong treatment effects for CBT are not likely to result in changes in market emphasis so long as those outcomes are offset by assumptions of prohibitive costs. Gould et al. addressed this

issue by comparing average costs for CBT and drug treatment. Their estimates will surprise many people. Imipramine and group CBT were the
lowest cost interventions. Individual CBT was less costly than higher dose
alprazolam and fluoxetine treatments at the end of one year and less costly
than lower dose alprazolam by the end of the second year. The authors note
that CBT has a lower dropout rate and approximately the same efficacy rating as imipramine.

The NIH Consensus Conference on PD concluded that the available
evidence supports the short-term efficacy of pharmacological and CBT
treatments for PD (National Institutes of Health, 1991). Otto et al. (1994)
conclude that there is good evidence for the short-term efficacy of CBT for
PD. They also note that well-controlled studies show treatment using cognitive restructuring and interoceptive exposure have been associated with
panic-free rates of 71% to 80% for short-term treatment in individual and
group formats. These rates are better than the 50% to 70% range reported
for benzodiazepine and AD treatment. In the short term, treatment differences are often not statistically significant but when long-term outcome is
considered, they are. Many patients who are treated with drugs require
ongoing medication treatment and remain symptomatic despite that treatment. Longitudinal studies show that 40% of these patients continue
to have panic attacks and 50% to 80% continue to remain symptomatic in
follow-ups from 1.5 to 6 years. Additionally, discontinuation of pharmacotherapy is often associated with relapse and withdrawal. In contrast, patients treated with cognitive therapy show panic-free rates in excess of 80%
in 1 to 2-year follow-ups.

Drug treatments alone are not as effective as psychological interventions
in the treatment of panic disorder with and without agoraphobia, even if
severe. Behavioral therapies involving exposure demonstrate considerable
effectiveness on avoidance behaviors and are effective in reducing panic.
Cognitive interventions are effective against panic with agoraphobia, when
combined with exposure techniques.

Research does not support drug therapies as being more effective than
psychological interventions in the long-term treatment of anxiety. Despite
popular belief, drugs appear to be neither a more robust form of treatment,
nor more effective in the long run. It may be that, all things considered,
they are more expensive as well.

DRUG SIDE EFFECTS

Although relative efficacy and cost are important considerations in the
selection of an appropriate treatment, they are certainly not the only factors to be considered. Consumer safety should be considered as well.

Medical treatments are often seen as alternatives to psychological interventions, and their more dangerous attributes are ignored. Problems with dependency, treatment attribution, learning, and physical and reproductive risk have been documented in the research literature.

DRUG DEPENDENCE

Anxiety disorders are often the result of the patient's herculean efforts to avoid feeling anxious. Treatment with antianxiety medication may inadvertently conspire in this avoidance, ultimately making matters worse. Patients get into a "robbing Peter to pay Paul" situation, trading drug dependence for short-term anxiety control. The problem is not one of whether anxiolytic drugs work; the problem is that they do work, in the short term. Patients must then face the unpleasant task of giving them up. Even if physical dependence were not a problem, psychological dependence might be a concern. After all, contingent removal of an unpleasant feeling reinforces the instrumental behavior. As patients use medication to reduce anxiety, their dependence on the medication is strengthened.

Physical dependence is marked by the need to continue using a drug to avoid withdrawal symptoms. Benzodiazepine withdrawal syndrome occurs when the drug dose is diminished or withdrawn. Sussman (1993) notes that while it is more likely to result from high-dose, long-term therapy, withdrawal symptoms can occur after short-term, normal dose therapy. Studies have shown that physical dependence can occur within 2 to 3 weeks following high-dose therapy and after 6 to 8 months with normal dosing (Lader & File, 1987; Winokur, Rickels, Greenblatt, Snyder, & Schatz, 1980). The most frequent symptoms of withdrawal are almost impossible to distinguish from the typical symptoms of anxiety.

Balter, Manheimer, Mellinger, and Uhlenhuth (1984) found that in a given year approximately 11% of the general population uses a benzodiazepine (other than as a hypnotic); most use them for less than 4 months. However, Barnas et al. (1991) found a mean use time of 4.5 years in a pharmacy population. The subpopulation abuse data presented by Sussman (1993) suggests that some individuals may not take benzodiazepines for their intrinsic reinforcement qualities, but rather for their ability to control negative symptoms associated with discontinuing the anxiolytic or coming down from other drugs (including alcohol).

Rickels and Schweizer (1990a) examined the withdrawal syndrome resulting from the abrupt discontinuation of therapeutic doses of short and long half-life benzodiazepines in patients who had daily use for over one year. Interestingly, despite a mean daily dose of 14.1 mg diazepam equivalents, they noted residual symptoms of anxiety and depression in their sample. From 58% to 100% of their patients experienced a withdrawal reaction. Return to benzodiazepine use occurred in 27% of the patients taking long half-life and 57% of the patients taking short half-life benzodiazepines. Schweizer, Rickels, Case, and Greenblatt (1990) compared short and long half-life benzodiazepines on gradual (25% per week) taper. They found that 90% of the patients experienced a mild to moderate withdrawal reaction. Nonetheless, 32% of the long half-life and 42% of the short half-life patients were unable to achieve a drug-free state.

Not all patients become dependent on benzodiazepines. Indeed, a patient's willingness to take these drugs, let alone become dependent on them, depends on the patient's subjective response to the drug (DeWit, Uhlenhuth, & Johanson, 1986; McCracken, deWit, Uhlenhuth, & Johanson, 1990). For example, patients who chose diazepam in blind choice experiments report negligible drug effects, while nonchoosers report significant subjective effects, predominately sedative. Again, not all patients treated with benzodiazepines become dependent, but for those who do, discontinuing drugs can be a formidable challenge.

Long-term outcome is most important to patients with chronic disorders (Marks, Swinson, Basoglu, et al., 1993). Although studies establish the short-term efficacy of anxiolytics, many of these same studies show that patients encounter problems discontinuing them. Most patients, when slowly tapered after short-term therapy, are able to discontinue benzodiazepines without a great deal of difficulty (Balter, Ban, Uhlenhuth, & Eberhard, 1993). Patients treated in long-term therapy at higher doses however, may experience greater difficulty. A return of the original condition (relapse) during discontinuation can greatly complicate clinical management.

Problems associated with discontinuing these medications at higher doses suggest that it may be even more difficult to discontinue newer HBZs. Cole and Kando (1993) reviewed published case reports and discovered some interesting differences between alprazolam, a high-potency benzodiazepine, and the older benzodiazepines. The older benzodiazepines were more likely to be associated with adverse events than was alprazolam (with the exception of mania or hypomania). Alprazolam was more likely to be associated with worsening in PTSD and increased impulsivity with borderline personality disorder. They point out however, that the latter conditions are less likely to have been treated with low-potency benzodiazepines and more likely to have been treated with alprazolam. Although alprazolam is approved for use with PD, panic disorder patients have a more difficult time discontinuing the medication than do patients with GAD (Klein, Colin, Stolk, & Lenox, 1994).

Rickels, Schweizer, Weiss, and Zavodnick (1993) studied 48 patients who completed eight months of maintenance treatment with alprazolam, imipramine, or placebo. Rickels and colleagues gave a gradual 4-week taper. A withdrawal syndrome was observed in almost all alprazolam-treated but in only a few of the imipramine- or placebo-treated patients. A total of 33% of the alprazolam-treated patients were unable to discontinue their medication. Severity of panic attacks at baseline, but not daily alprazolam dose was a significant predictor of taper difficulty.

Nagy, Krystal, Charney, Merikangas, and Woods (1993) interviewed 28 patients who had received a 4-month program of behavior therapy combined with imipramine, 1 to 5 years postdischarge. Half the patients were medication free, 8 were using a reduced dose, 2 were using the same dose they had been using at discharge, and 4 were receiving other antipanic medications. The patients all seemed to have benefited from the treatment. Long-term outcome was independent of additional therapy during follow-up.

Finally, Tesar (1990) notes that discontinuation of alprazolam is particularly difficult and is sometimes associated with serious rebound and withdrawal symptoms. Uhlenhuth, DeWit, Balter, Johanson, and Mellinger (1988) reported that despite a sharp decline in benzodiazepine prescriptions over the previous 10 years, reservations about their use continued to escalate. These authors believe risk is low but feel that benzodiazepine addiction can occur when a clinical dose is taken for about 6 months. Ladar (1995) asserts that about one-third of long-term users have clinically significant withdrawal, even after tapering the dose. After high doses, almost all patients show withdrawal phenomena, which can be severe. Abstinence rates vary according to Ladar, but only about half the patients achieve long-term success and some of those patients become chronically depressed. Although there may be disagreement about the degree of abuse and dependency liability associated with anxiolytics, few would deny such liability exists.

OUTCOME ATTRIBUTION AND THE THERAPEUTIC RELATIONSHIP

Another concern is that drug treatment, when used by itself, may impoverish the clinician-patient relationship. Treatment with anxiolytics may mask other problems, such as a developing illness, a deteriorating marriage, or alcohol abuse. A continuing dysphoria may serve as a signal to the psychotherapist that unresolved problems remain to be addressed; drug therapy may mute that signal. Routine prescription of these medications may distract the clinician (and the patient) from the need for concern, support, and time.

One component of psychotherapy for patients with anxiety disorders is helping them take an active role in solving their problems. Although anxiety may be unpleasant, it can also be adaptive. It can motivate individuals to make life changes and facilitate psychological development. Patients who have participated in successful treatment leave with a sense of self-efficacy that is likely to transfer to other situations. Prescription of anxiolytics may encourage passivity and acceptance in patients instead of mastery or active problem-solving. Instead of self-attribution, the patient may attribute improvement to the proximal cause, the medication. Marks, Swinson, Basoglu, et al. (1993) found that patients who attributed their therapeutic gains to the medication they received during treatment did significantly worse at posttaper than those who believed their improvement was a result of their own efforts during psychological treatment. From a slightly different perspective, Otto, Pollack, Meltzer-Brody, and Rosenbaum (1992), note that when anxiety symptoms emerge during or after medication taper, patients' untreated fears of anxiety sensations retrigger catastrophic misinterpretation and can start the problem all over again.

An unfortunate extension of the biological model of anxiety treatment may be a somewhat mechanistic, "fix it" mentality (Butz,1994). Anxiety is not seen as a reaction to something gone wrong, but rather it becomes the focus of treatment. The attempt to establish a kind of biochemical homeostasis through drug treatment ignores the possibility that the resolution of tension systems and chaos may lead to the emergence of a new, more adaptive order.

Learning Problems

It is important to be aware of research suggesting that some anxiolytics may impair learning (Basoglu, 1992; Gray, 1987; Lucki, Rickels, Giesecke, & Geller, 1987; Marks et al., 1993; Rickels, Case, Warren, & Schweizer, 1988; Romney & Angus, 1984). The benzodiazepines appear to disrupt the consolidation process in semantic memory (Curran, 1991). Gorenstein, Bernik, and Pompeia (1994) and Lader (1995) found that in long-term users of benzodiazepines, tolerance to these learning effects may never develop. Patients may complain of poor subjective memory and experience difficulty recalling information presented during treatment. Some research has suggested that the use of diazepam as an adjunct to therapies emphasizing learning may be contraindicated (Angus & Romney, 1984; Durham & Allan, 1993; Marks, Swinson, Basoglu, Kuch, et al., 1993). Amnestic episodes may occur as well and this is a particular problem in the elderly where chronic use may lead to pseudo-dementia (Ancill, Embury, Mac-Ewan, & Kennedy, 1987; Klerman, 1988). Although attempts have been made to develop anxiolytics that do not cause this side effect, the effect itself may be biochemically linked to anxiolysis (Sanger, 1994).

PHYSICAL RISKS

Researchers have expressed concerns about increased physical risk to patients, both from bodily injury and from drug interactions. Use of benzodiazepine tranquilizers increases the risk of accidental injury requiring medical attention (Oster, Huse, Adams, Imbimbo, & Russell, 1990). Additionally, anxiolytics are the third most commonly mentioned drugs involving emergency room visits (Sussman 1993). Benzodiazepines (diazepam and lorazepam) as well as benzodiazepine-like anxiolytics (alpidem, suriclone) can produce marked and pervasive driving impairment, which can persist throughout treatment. (O'Hanlon, Vermeeren, Uiterwijk, van Veggel, & Swijgman, 1995; also see Linnoila & Hakkinen, 1974; O'Hanlon, Haak, Blaauw, & Riemersma, 1982).

While benzodiazepines remain the most popular drug class for treating anxiety disorders, they can have serious side effects such as sedation, muscular disorders, abuse liability, and synergistic effects with alcohol and central nervous system depressant drugs (Mosconi, Chiamulera, & Ricchia, 1993). Interactions with other drugs such as beta-blockers, antihistamines, and alcohol are also a concern, especially since the use of nonprescription medications can be difficult to control. Older patients are particularly at risk with these drugs because of enhanced sensitivity due to pharmacokinetic and pharmacodynamic factors (Lader, 1995).

Patients with anxiety disorders are not always treated with anxiolytics. Some are prescribed antidepressants (ADs). However, these drugs are associated with problems of their own. Underlying medical illness and drug interactions may make the use of many AD agents problematic (Stoudemire, Moran, & Fogel, 1991). This is especially true for patients with cardiovascular problems. Thus the prescription of ADs for those with PD may be of special concern since patients with PD may be at increased risk for cardiovascular morbidity and mortality (Taylor & Hayward, 1990).

REPRODUCTIVE CONCERNS

Iatrogenic sexual dysfunction may be yet another worry. One study (Balon, Yeragani, Pohl, & Ramesh, 1993) found a 43% incidence of sexual dysfunction among men and women receiving ADs for anxiety and mood disorders. More women than men suffer from anxiety disorders (Sheehan, Sheehan, & Minichiello, 1981), and women of childbearing age should be spared exposure to drug therapies whenever possible. The chronic use of benzodiazepines during any phase of pregnancy or breast feeding is contraindicated (Mortola, 1989).

CONTEMPORARY PRACTICE

There is a logical premise for prescribing anxiolytic drugs for the treatment of anxiety disorders. If an individual is complaining of unpleasant feelings, drugs are available to remove the symptom or at least the degree of unpleasantness the person is experiencing. In the short term, drugs, such as benzodiazepines are effective in reducing dysphoria and the patient's response to them is, for all practical purposes, immediate. Patients are often pleased with their new-found ability to control unpleasant sensations, and clinicians feel they have been of help to the patient. Today, the prevailing opinion is that anxiolytic therapy is quick, effective, and less expensive than psychotherapy. As a result, this approach is very popular. In 1989, more than 36.4 million new prescriptions for minor tranquilizers were written in the continental United States. The majority (81%) were written for benzodiazepines; the rest were for hydroxyzine, meprobamate, and buspirone. The primary diagnosis associated with these prescriptions was "anxiety state" 25% of the time. Psychiatrists accounted for 20% of the new prescriptions, just behind internists at 21% (Anti-anxiety drug usage, 1989).

Benzodiazepines, introduced into clinical practice in 1960, are among the most widely prescribed psychotherapeutic drugs in the United States today (Martin, 1987; Swartz et al., 1991). Swartz et al., (1991) also report that these drugs tend to be used more by the elderly, whites, women, less educated individuals, and the separated or divorced. Given their side effect profiles and potential interactions with other medications, there is concern about their overuse with elderly patients. Nolan and O'Malley (1987) found that the mean number of drugs per prescription increased linearly from 1.5 in children 0 to 9 years of age to 2.8 in those 80 and older. The rate of prescribing benzodiazepines increased markedly with advancing age. Psychotropic drugs were among the most frequently prescribed for those over 65.

Psychiatric experts seem unconcerned about the abundant use of benzodiazepines in clinical practice. Balter et al. (1993) polled a select international panel of psychiatric experts (assembled through a multistage peer nomination process) about the treatment of anxiety and depressive disorders. Although sometimes divided, agreement was generally high that the benzodiazepines have a good benefit-to-risk ratio. The panel also agreed that qualitative differences in abuse liability are minimal, physical dependence at therapeutic dose is not a major clinical problem and when physical dependence occurs, it can be handled by the treating physician.

Uhlenhuth, Balter, Ban, and Yang (1995), reporting on clinical features that affect experts' recommendations, note that when there was a high level of functional impairment the experts more often recommended psychosocial procedures for adjustment disorder. Medications were recommended for agoraphobia, social phobia, OCD, and adjustment disorder. Polypharmacy was most often recommended for agoraphobia.

Undoubtedly, there is a biological bias in the types of treatment patients are likely to receive in outpatient medical settings. Medical clinicians are likely to rely on treatments that are most comfortable and familiar to them. But new pressures being brought to bear on these practitioners make it even more likely they will rely on pharmacological management of mental health problems. This added pressure has some physicians concerned. A recent featured article in *The Wall Street Journal* (Pollock, 1995) expressed concern with managed care's reliance on the use of psychiatric drugs and noted that many doctors were alarmed by this trend. In the article, managed care officials extol the cost savings of drug treatments for mental health disorders. They argue that their approach reflects the "best of modern medicine" by providing effective treatment to patients who wouldn't have responded as well to psychotherapy. Their stated goal is to get "as many patients better as fast as possible" (p. 1). They are concerned that the financial and emotional incentives (of psychotherapists) prolong treatment with psychotherapy. Most treatment of anxiety disorders takes place in the primary care sector and is provided by medically trained clinicians who are encouraged to use drugs by both managed care firms and pharmaceutical manufacturers. It is unlikely many patients will encounter psychological treatments early in the course of their disorders.

Taylor et al. (1989) surveyed 794 subjects who had volunteered for PD studies. Fewer than 15% had undergone in vivo exposure, although a majority had received some form of counseling and had used benzodiazepines. Goisman et al. (1993) analyzed treatment data as part of a multicenter longitudinal anxiety study in New England (231 patients in 9 sites). Behavioral therapy was used less frequently than supportive therapy, medication, or psychodynamic therapy. Although there is strong evidence supporting the effectiveness of behavioral techniques in treating anxiety symptoms and disorders, treatment of anxiety in the medical setting has tended to be almost exclusively pharmacological (Alexander, Selby, & Calhoun, 1987; Drummond, 1993). Not only are patients initially treated with anxiolytics, the tendency is to try a different drug if the first one doesn't work, rather than refer the patient for psychotherapy.

Baldessarini (1978) in *The Harvard Guide to Psychiatry* called for anxiolytics to be used minimally, for the shortest practical duration. In recent years, however, the trend has grown toward viewing anxiety as a chronic biological disorder. Analogies are drawn to diabetes and other chronic medical conditions and a rationale is thus created to keep patients on maintenance medications (Lyles & Simpson, 1990; Talley, 1990). Since these drugs do little to *cure* anxiety disorders, many patients who try to stop using medications and who have not been provided psychotherapy must face their original disorder as well as the discomfort of discontinuing their medication. This is a significant problem as most of these patients will be treated by general practitioners who lack training in psychotherapy.

The prevailing perspective is that these "lifelong illnesses" are best treated with medication. If anxiety returns when medications are discontinued, it is simply taken as evidence of the chronic nature of the disorder and not of failed treatment. The often frustrating, impenetrable logic used to justify the chronic use of medications seems more akin to religious dogma than to science.

Many practicing clinicians from a variety of mental health disciplines believe that anxiolytic medication is an appropriate, if not necessary adjunct to psychotherapy, particularly in cases of severe anxiety. We strongly question this belief since the global efficacy of anxiolytic drugs has been strongly challenged in the comparative and meta-analytic research literature presented in this chapter. Most of these same studies support the notion that psychotherapy alone can be as effective or more effective than medications. The fact is, psychotherapy may be preferred by patients (Gath & Catalan, 1986; Halberstam, 1978; Sanua, 1995) and, when side effects, relapse rates, and long-term improvements are considered, therapy may be less costly as well (Fisher & Greenberg, 1989, p. 328; Gould, Otto, & Pollack, 1995).

CONCLUSION

There is a vast amount of literature on the drug treatment of anxiety. The use of a new antianxiety agent often begins with clinical trials, basically anecdotal reports, that comment on the drug's believed efficacy in treating certain disorders. In clinical settings, a good deal of excitement may be generated about the use of the new agent, based solely on clinical folklore. Additional interest in the agent is generated when it is promoted at conferences or through research grants. Almost without fail, new medications are believed to have fewer or more benign side effects than their predecessors. It may take a number of years for good research to indicate otherwise.

Less than 15 years ago, Murray (1984) reviewed available research on the effects of the benzodiazepines (Valium® and Librium®) on human psychomotor and cognitive functions. He concluded that the benzodiazepines were "remarkable drugs" and that they "have no gravely harmful side effects, little addictive potential (and) danger from overdosage is minimal" (p. 169). He also concluded that these drugs, ". . . have little, if any, adverse effect on well established, higher mental functions . . ." (p. 169). Murray's paper was followed by reports over the next 5 years, suggesting abuse potential (Funderburk et al., 1988), impoverished performance on visual analog scales and computer tests (von Frenckell, Ansseau, & Bonnet, 1986), increased aggression (Gantner & Taylor, 1988), decrements in psychomotor performance and failure to improve performance (McLeod, Hoehn-Saric, Labib, & Greenblatt, 1988), seizures on withdrawal from high-dose therapy (Zaccara, Innocenti, Bartelli, Casini, et al., 1986), decrements in anterograde episodic memory and attention (Welkowitz, Weingartner, Thompson, & Pickar, 1987), long-lasting alterations in neural substrates of rats (Kellogg, Simmons, Miller, & Ison, 1985), sedation (Rickels et al., 1985), delusional depression on withdrawal from long-term use (Keshavan, Moodley, Eales, Joyce, & Yeragani, 1988), and withdrawal reactions, even with short-term, moderate doses, when combined with ADs (Feet, Larsen, Lillevold, & Roebuck, 1988). Despite early optimism, the benzodiazepines have proven to be a undeservedly popular treatment for anxiety disorders with serious drawbacks for the patients who use them.

Leonard (1994) notes that the dependence potential of the classical benzodiazepines became apparent only after their widespread clinical use, some years after their introduction. It can be anticipated that the dependence potential of the new benzodiazepines will similarly become evident in the future. Zopiclone, one of the newer medications, has been in widespread use as a hypnotic the longest, and there is already evidence it produces physical dependence, though less so than diazepam (Thakore & Dinan, 1992). It is ironic that often the best source of information on the adverse side effects of older medications is to be found in literature promoting a new medication as a "significant advance" over previous therapies.

Despite concerns about the safety and logic of anxiolytic therapy, articles continue to be published in psychiatric journals touting the effectiveness of psychopharmacology and downplaying the usefulness of behavioral approaches. Gorman and Papp (1990) write, "Anxiety disorders are chronic illnesses requiring long-term treatment. Relapse is typical and should not be considered treatment failure. . . . The efficacy of nonpharmacological treatments alone is, with very few exceptions, unsubstantiated at present" (p. 11). In our view, this position is no longer defensible.

The enthusiastic promotion of antianxiety drugs as a first-line treatment for anxiety disorders should not come as a surprise. These products are developed by businesses that profit from their sale. Strategies that bring drugs to market and promote their use are likely to be preferred over those that do not. The application of rigorous scientific methodology may not be in the best interest of business. As a result, marketing needs dictate research outcomes rather than the reverse.

Controlled drug research is often contaminated with concomitant exposure and psychosocial contact between experimenter and patient. The continued use of inert placebos in drug research seriously challenges the assertion that these studies are double-blind (Fisher & Greenberg, 1993). Experimenter bias is then a concern. Negative outcome research may not be published. When research is published, it may be presented in such a way as to suggest that the studied drug is more useful than the research would indicate. Although these problems do not discredit all drug efficacy research, they greatly complicate the interpretation of this literature.

Biological interventions have a great deal of appeal. They provide a "no-fault" explanation for troublesome behaviors and a simple solution for their amelioration. Medications are easy to prescribe, easy to take, and thought to be effective by both laypeople and clinicians. Medications are the most often used treatments for anxiety in the United States. Most people who suffer from anxiety are treated in the general medical sector by nonpsychiatric physicians who tend to rely on these therapies. Although psychiatrists have traditionally been more conservative than primary practice physicians in the use of anxiolytics, there is an ever-increasing biological emphasis in psychiatry, and today psychiatrists are writing nearly as many prescriptions for anxiolytics as are generalists. Psychologists, longtime advocates of psychotherapeutic treatment, are showing increased interest in drug therapies as well.

Research on the behavioral treatment of anxiety disorders has demonstrated robust, long-lasting treatment outcomes. The comparative literature strongly suggests the superiority of behavioral therapy over pharmacotherapy. When the weaker treatment outcomes of medications are combined with the documented problems of relapse and dangerous side effects, behavior therapy appears to be the treatment of choice for panic disorder and agoraphobia.

REFERENCES

Agras, W. S., Telch, M. J., Taylor, C. B., Roth, W. T., & Brouillard, M. E. (1990, June). *Imipramine and exposure therapy for agoraphobia.* Paper presented at the meeting of the International Conference on Panic Disorders, Gothenberg, Sweden.

Alexander, M., Selby, J., & Calhoun, L. (1987). Physician attitudes toward office based non-pharmacological treatment of anxiety. *Family Medicine, 19*(5), 376–377.

American Psychiatric Association. (1987). *Diagnostic and statistical manual of mental disorders* (3rd ed., rev.). Washington, DC: Author.

American Psychiatric Association. (1994). *Diagnostic and statistical manual of mental disorders* (4th ed.). Washington, DC: Author.

Ancill, R., Embury, G. D., MacEwan, G. W., & Kennedy, J. S. (1987). Lorazepam in the elderly: A retrospective study of the side effects in 20 patients. *Journal of Psychopharmacology, 2,* 126–127.

Angus, W. R., & Romney, D. M. (1984). The effect of diazepam on patients' memory. *Journal of Clinical Pharmacy, 4*(4), 203–206.

Anti-anxiety drug usage in the United States, 1989. (1991). *Statistical Bulletin—Metropolitan Insurance Companies, 72*(1), 18–27.

Arcierno, R., Hersen, M., & Van Hasselt, V. B. (1993). Interventions for panic disorder: A critical review of the literature. *Clinical Psychology Review, 13,* 561–578.

Arntz, A., Hildebrand, M., & van den Hout, M. (1994). Overprediction of anxiety, and disconfirmatory processes in anxiety disorders. *Behavior Research & Therapy, 32*(7), 709–722.

Baldessarini, R. J. (1978). Chemotherapy. In A. M. Nicholi (Ed.), *The Harvard guide to modern clinical psychiatry* (pp. 387–433). Belknap Press.

Ballenger, J. (1986). Pharmacotherapy of the panic disorders. *Journal of Clinical Psychiatry, 47,* 27–32.

Ballenger, J., Burrows, G. D., DuPont, R. L., Lesser, I. M., Noyes, R., Pecknold, J. C., Rifkin, A., & Swinson, R. P. (1988, May). Alprazolam in panic disorder and agoraphobia: Results from a multi-center trial. *Archives of General Psychiatry, 45,* 413–421.

Ballenger, J., McDonald, S., Noyes, R., Rickels, K., Sussman, N., Woods, S., Patin, J., & Singer, J. (1991). The first double-blind, placebo-controlled trial of a partial benzodiazepine agonist abecarnil (ZK 112-119) in generalized anxiety disorder. *Psychopharmacology Bulletin, 27*(2), 171–179.

Balon R., Yeragani, K., Pohl, R., & Ramesh, C. (1993). Sexual dysfunction during antidepressant treatment. *Journal of Clinical Psychiatry, 54*(6), 209–212.

Balter, M., Ban, T. A., Uhlenhuth, E.H., & Eberhard, H. (1993). International study of expert judgment on therapeutic use of benzodiazepines and other psychotherapeutic medications: 1. Current concerns. *Human Psychopharmacology, 8*(4), 253–261.

Balter, M., Manheimer, D. I., Mellinger, G. D., & Uhlenhuth, E. H. (1984). A cross-national comparison of anti-anxiety/sedative drug use. *Current Medical Research and Opinion, 85,* 5–20.

Barlow, D. (1988). *Anxiety and its disorders: The nature and treatment of anxiety and panic.* New York: Guilford Press.

Barlow, D. (1990). Long-term outcome for patients with panic disorder treated with cognitive-behavioral therapy. *Journal of Clinical Psychiatry, 51*(Suppl. A), 17–23.

Barlow, D., Craske, M. G., Cerny, J. A., & Klosko, J. S. (1989). Behavioral treatment of panic disorder. *Behavior Therapy, 20,* 261–282.

Barnas, C., Fleischhaker, W. W., Whitworth, A. B., Schett, P., Stuppack, C., & Hinterhuber, H. (1991). Characteristics of benzodiazepine long-term users: Investigation of benzodiazepine consumers among pharmacy customers. *Psychopharmacology, 103,* 233–239.

Basoglu, M. (1992). Pharmacological and behavioral treatment of panic disorder. *Psychotherapy and Psychosomatics, 58*(2), 57–59.

Bass, C., Chambers, J. B., Kiff, P., Cooper, D., & Gardner, W. N. (1988). Panic anxiety and hyperventilation in patients with chest pain: A controlled study. *Quarterly Journal of Medicine, 69*(260), 949–959.

Bassi, S., Albizzati, M. G., Ferrarese, C., Frattola, L., Cesona, B., Piolti, R., & Farolfi, A. (1989). Alpedem, a novel anxiolytic drug. A double-blind, placebo-controlled study in anxious outpatients. *Clinical Neuropharmacology, 12*(1), 67–74.

Bates, G. W., Cambell, I. M., & Burgess, P. M. (1990). Assessment of articulated thoughts in social anxiety: Modification of the ATSS procedure. *British Journal of Clinical Psychology, 29*(1), 91–98.

Beaumont, G. (1977). A large open multi-centered trial of clomipramine (anafranil) in the management of phobic disorders. *Journal of International Medical Research, 5,* 116–123.

Beck, A. T., Emery, G., & Greenberg, R. L. (1985). *Anxiety disorders and phobias: A cognitive perspective.* New York: Basic Books.

Beck, A. T., Epstein, N., Brown, G., & Steer, A. (1988). An inventory for measuring clinical anxiety: Psychometric properties. *Journal of Consulting and Clinical Psychology, 56*(6), 893–897.

Beck, A. T., Laude, R., & Bognert, M. (1974). Ideational components of anxiety neurosis. *Archives of General Psychiatry, 31,* 319–325.

Beck, A. T., Sokal, L., Clark, D. A., Berchick, R., & Wright, F. (1992). A crossover study of focused cognitive therapy for panic disorder. *American Journal of Psychiatry, 149,* 778–783.

Beck, A. T., Ward, C. H., Mendelson, M., Mock, J., & Erbaugh, J. (1961). An inventory for measuring depression. *Archives of General Psychology, 4,* 561–571.

Berman, J., Miller, R. C., & Massman, P. J. (1985). Cognitive therapy verses systematic desensitization: Is one treatment superior? *Psychological Bulletin, 97,* 451–461.

Black, D., Wesner, R., Bowers, W., & Gabel, J. (1993). A comparison of fluvoxamine, cognitive therapy and placebo in the treatment of panic disorder. *Archives of General Psychiatry, 50,* 44–50.

Borkovec, T. D., & Costello, E. (1993). Efficacy of applied relaxation and cognitive-behavioral therapy in the treatment of generalized anxiety disorder. *Journal of Consulting and Clinical Psychology, 61*(4), 611–619.

Borkovec, T. D., & Inz, J. (1990). The nature of worry in generalized anxiety disorder: A predominance of thought activity. *Behavioral Research and Therapy, 28*(2), 153–158.

Breggin, P. (1991). *Toxic psychiatry* (pp. 240–265). New York: St. Martin's Press.

Butler, G. (1984). Exposure and anxiety management in the treatment of social phobia. *Journal of Consulting and Clinical Psychology, 52*(4), 642–650.

Butler, G. (1993). Predicting outcome after treatment for generalized anxiety disorder. *Behavior Research and Therapy, 31*(2), 211–213.

Butz, M. (1994). Psychopharmacology: Psychology's Jurassic Park? *Psychotherapy, 31*(4), 692–699.

Cadbury, S., Childs-Clark, A., & Sandhu, S., (1990). Group anxiety management: Effectiveness, perceived helpfulness and follow-up. *British Journal of Clinical Psychology, 29*(2), 245–247.

Casacchia, M., Farolfi, A., Priore, P., Magni, G., Stratta, P., Cesana, B., & Rossi, A. (1989). A double blind, placebo-controlled study of alpidem, a novel anxiolytic of imidazopyridine structure, in chronically anxious patients. *Acta Psychiatrica Scandinavica, 80*(2), 137–141.

Chambless, D. L., Foa, E. B., Graves, G., & Goldstein, A. J. (1979). Flooding with methohexitone in the treatment of agoraphobia. *Behavioral Research and Therapy, 17*, 243–251.

Chambless, D. L., & Gillis, M. M. (1993). Cognitive therapy of anxiety disorders. *Journal of Consulting and Clinical Psychology, 61*(2), 248–260.

Christie, K., Burke, J. D., Regier, D. A., Rae, D. S., Boyd, J. H., & Locke, B. Z. (1988). Epidemiologic evidence for early onset of mental disorders and higher risk of drug abuse in young adults. *American Journal of Psychiatry, 145*(8), 971–975.

Clark, D. (1986). A cognitive approach to panic. *Behavior Research and Therapy, 24*, 461–470.

Clark, D., Taylor, C., Roth, W. T., Hayward, C., Ehlers, A., Margraf, J., & Agras, W. S. (1990). Surreptitious drug use by patients in a panic disorder study. *American Journal of Psychiatry, 147*(4), 507–509.

Clum, G. A. (1989). Psychological interventions vs. drugs in the treatment of panic. *Behavior Therapy, 20*, 429–457.

Clum, G. A., & Borden, J. W. (1989). Etiology and treatments of panic disorders. *Progress in Behavior Modification, 24*, 192–222.

Clum, G. A., Clum, G. A., & Surls, R. (1993). A meta-analysis of treatments for panic disorder. *Journal of Consulting and Clinical Psychology, 61*(2), 317–326.

Cohn, J. B., Bowden, C. L., Fisher, J. G., & Rodos, J. J. (1986). Double-blind comparison of buspirone and clorazepate in anxious outpatients. *American Journal of Medicine, 80*(3B), 10–16.

Cole, J. O., & Kando, J. C. (1993). Adverse behavioral events reported in patients taking alprazolam and other benzodiazepines. *Journal of Clinical Psychiatry, 54*(10), 49–61.

Cooke, D. (1979). Hyperventilation: Its treatment and relation to anxiety. *Behavior Therapist, 2*(5), 32–33.

Cox, B. J., Endler, N. S., Lee, P. S., & Swinson, R. P. (1992). A meta-analysis of treatments for panic disorder with agoraphobia: Imipramine, alprazolam and *in vivo* exposure. *Journal of Behavior Therapy & Experimental Psychiatry, 23*(3), 175–182.

Craske, M. G., Maidenberg, E., & Bystritsky, A. (1995). Brief cognitive-behavioral verses nondirective therapy for panic disorder. *Journal of Behavior Therapy and Experimental Psychiatry, 26*(2), 113–120.

Curran, H. (1991). Benzodiazepines, memory and mood: A review. *Psychopharmacology, 105,* 1–8.

deBeurs, E., vanBalkom, A., Lange, A., Koele, P., & vanDyck, R. (1995). Treatment of panic disorder with agoraphobia: Comparison of fluvoxamine, placebo, and psychological panic management combined with exposure and of exposure *in vivo* alone. *American Journal of Psychiatry, 152*(5), 683–691.

deJonghe, F., Swinkels, J., Tuynman-Qua, H., & Jonkers, F. (1989). A comparative study of suriclone, lorazepam and placebo in anxiety disorder. *Pharmacopsychiatry, 22*(6), 266–271.

den Boer, J. A., & Westerberg, G. M. (1988). Effect of serotonin and noradrenaline uptake inhibitor in panic disorder: A double-blind comparative study with fluvoxamine maprotiline. *Informational Clinical Psychopharmacology, 3,* 59–74.

de Ruiter, C., Garssen, B., Rijken, H., & Kraaimaat, F. (1989). The hyperventilation syndrome in panic disorder, agoraphobia and generalized anxiety disorder. *Behaviour Research and Therapy, 27*(4), 447–452.

DeWit, H., Uhlenhuth, E. H., & Johanson, C. E. (1986). Individual differences in the reinforcing and subjective effects of amphetamine and diazepam. *Drug and Alcohol Dependence, 16*(4), 341–360.

Downing, R., & Rickels, K. (1983). Physician prognosis in relationship to drug and placebo response in anxious and depressed psychiatric outpatients. *Journal of Nervous and Mental Disease, 171*(3), 182–185.

Downing, R., Rickels, K., Wittenborn, E., & Mattson, N. B. (1971). Interpretation of data from investigations assessing the effectiveness of psychotropic agents. In J. Levine, B. C. Schiele, & C. Bouthilet (Eds.), *Principles and problems in establishing the efficacy of psychotropic agents* (pp. 321–369). Washington, DC: U.S. Government Printing Office.

Drummond, L. (1993). Behavioral approaches to anxiety disorders. *Postgraduate Medical Journal, 69*(809), 222–226.

Durham, R., & Allan, T. (1993). Psychological treatment of generalised anxiety disorder. A review of the clinical significance of results in outcome studies since 1980. *British Journal of Psychiatry, 163,* 19–26.

Durham, R., Murphy, T., Allan, T., Richard, K., Treliving, L. R., & Fenton, G. W. (1994). Cognitive therapy, analytic psychotherapy and anxiety management training for generalized anxiety disorder. *British Journal of Psychiatry, 165*(3), 315–323.

Durham, R., & Turvey, A. (1987). Cognitive therapy vs. behaviour therapy in the treatment of chronic general anxiety. *Behaviour Therapy and Research, 25*(3), 229–234.

Elkin, I., Pilkonis, P. A., Docherty, J. P., & Sotsky, M. D. (1988). Conceptual and methodological issues in comparative studies of psychotherapy and pharmacotherapy: 1. Active ingredients and mechanisms of change. *American Journal of Psychiatry, 145*(8), 909–1076.

Essig, C. (1964). Addiction to nonbarbiturate sedative and tranquilizing drugs. *Clinical Pharmacology and Therapeutics, 5,* 334–343.

Evans, I. (1972). A conditioning model of a common neurotic pattern—fear of fear. *Psychotherapy: Theory, Research and Practice, 9,* 238–241.

Evans, L., Kenardy, J., Schneider, P., & Hoey, H. (1986). Effects of a selective serotonin uptake inhibitor in agoraphobia with panic attacks: A double-blind comparison of zimelidine. *Acta Psychiatrica Scandinavica, 73,* 49–53.

Fava, G., Zielezny, M., Savron, G., & Grandi, S. (1995). Long-term effects of behavioral treatment for panic disorder with agoraphobia. *British Journal of Psychiatry, 166,* 87–92.

Feet, P., Larsen, S., Lillevold, P. E., & Roebuck, O. H. (1988). Withdrawal reactions to diazepam in combined imipramine/diazepam treatment of primary nonagitated depressed outpatients. *Acta Psychiatrica Scandinavica, 78*(3), 341–347.

Feighner, J., & Boyer, W. (1989). Serotonin-1A anxiolytics. *Psychopathology, 22*(1), 21–26.

Feighner, J., Merideth, C., & Hendrickson, G. (1982). A double-blind comparison of buspirone and diazepam in outpatients with generalized anxiety disorder. *Journal of Clinical Psychiatry, 43,* 103–107.

Fisher, S., & Greenberg, R. P. (Eds.). (1989). *The limits of biological treatments for psychological distress: Comparisons with psychotherapy and placebo* (p. 328). Hillsdale, NJ: Erlbaum.

Fisher, S., & Greenberg, R. P. (1993). How sound is the double-blind design for evaluating psychotropic drugs? *Journal of Nervous and Mental Disease, 181,* 345–350.

Foa, E., & Rothbaum, B. O. (1989). Behavioral psychotherapy for post-traumatic stress disorder: Behavioral psychotherapy into the 1990's [Special Issue]. *International Review of Psychiatry, 1*(3), 219–226.

Frattola, L., Piolti, R., Bassi, S., Albizzati, M. G., Cesona, B. M., Botloni, M. S., Priore, P., Borglic, C., & Morselli, P. C. (1992). Effects of alpedem in anxious elderly outpatients: A double-blind, placebo-controlled trial. *Clinical Neuropharmacology, 15*(6), 477–487.

Funderburk, F., Griffiths, R. R., McLeod, D. R., Bigelow, G. E., Mackinzie, A., Liebson, I. A., & Nemeth-Coslett, R. (1988). Relative abuse liability of lorazepam and diazepam: An evaluation in "recreational" drug users. *Drug and Alcohol Dependence, 22*(3), 215–222.

Gantner, A. B., & Taylor, S. P. (1988). Human physical aggression as a function of diazepam. *Personality and Social Psychology Bulletin, 14*(3), 479–484.

Gath, D., & Catalan, J. (1986). The treatment of emotional disorders in general practice: Psychological methods versus medication. *Journal of Psychosomatic Research, 30,* 381–386.

Gelder, M. G. (1990). Psychological treatment of panic anxiety. *Psychiatric Annals, 20*(9), 529–532.

Glaudin, V., Smith, W. T., Ferguson, J. M., DuBoff, E. A., Rosenthal, M. H., & Mee-Lee, D. (1994). Discriminating placebo and drug in generalized anxiety disorder (GAD) trials: Single vs. multiple clinical raters. *Psychopharmacology Bulletin, 30*(2), 175–178.

Goisman, R., Rogers, M., Steketee, G., Warshaw, M. G., Cuneo, P., & Keller, M. B. (1993). Utilization of behavioral methods in a multicenter anxiety disorders study. *Journal of Clinical Psychiatry, 54*(6), 213–218.

Goldberg, H. L., & Finnerty, R. J. (1979). The comparative efficacy of buspirone and diazepam in the treatment of anxiety. *American Journal of Psychiatry, 136,* 1184–1187.

Goldstein, A. J., & Chambliss, D. L. (1978). A reanalysis of agoraphobia. *Behavior Therapy, 9,* 47–59.

Gorenstein, C., Bernik, M. A., & Pompeia, S. (1994). Differential acute psychomotor and cognitive effects of diazepam on long-term benzodiazepine users. *International Clinical Psychopharmacology, 9*(3), 145–153.

Gorman, J. M., & Papp, L. A. (1990). Chronic anxiety: Deciding the length of treatment. *Journal of Clinical Psychiatry, 51*(Suppl.), 11–15.

Gould, R., Otto, M. W., & Pollack, M. H. (1995). A meta-analysis of treatment outcome for panic disorder. *Clinical Psychology Review, 15*(8), 819–844.

Gray, J. (1987). Interactions between drugs and behavior therapy. In H. Eysenck & M. Martin (Eds.), *Theoretical foundations of behavior therapy* (pp. 433–447). New York: Plenum Press.

Haefely, W. (1991). Psychpharmacology of anxiety. *European Neuropsychopharmacology, 1,* 89–95.

Halberstam, M. (1978). An office study of patient attitudes toward tranquilizing medication. *Southern Medical Journal, 71*(2), 15–17.

Hecker, J., Fink, C. M., & Fritzler, B. K. (1993). Acceptability of panic disorder treatments: A survey of family practice physicians. *Journal of Anxiety Disorders, 7,* 373–384.

Hoehn-Saric, R., McLeod, D. R., & Hipsley, P. A. (1993). Effect of fluroxamine on panic disorder. *Journal of Clinical Psychopharmacology, 13*(5), 321–326.

Hunt, C., & Andrews, G. (1992). Drop-out rate as a performance indicator in psychotherapy. *Acta Psychiatrica Scandinavica, 85*(4), 275–278.

Jannoun, L., Munby, M., Catalan, J., & Gelder, M. (1980). A home-based treatment program for agoraphobia: Replication and controlled evaluation. *Behavior Therapy, 11*(3), 294–305.

Johnson, D. G., Trayer, I. E., & Whitsett, S. E. (1988). Clomipramine treatment of agoraphobia in females: An eight week controlled trial. *Archives of General Psychiatry, 45,* 453–459.

Keane, T. (1995). The role of exposure therapy in the psychological treatment of PTSD. *Clinical Quarterly: National Center for Post Traumatic Stress Disorder, 5*(4), 1–6.

Kellogg, C., Simmons, R. D., Miller, R. K., & Ison, J. R. (1985). Prenatal diazepam exposure in rats: Long-lasting functional changes in the offspring. *Neurobehavioral Toxicology & Teratology, 7*(5), 483–488.

Kenardy, J., Evans L., & Oei, T. P. (1992). The latent structure of anxiety symptoms in anxiety disorders. *American Journal of Psychiatry, 149*(8), 1058–1061.

Keshavan, M. S., Moodley, P., Eales, M., Joyce, E., & Yeragani, V. K. (1988). Delusional depression following benzodiazepine withdrawal. *Canadian Journal of Psychiatry, 33*(7), 626–627.

Klein, D. (1964). Delineation of two drug responsive anxiety syndromes. *Psychopharmacologica Berlina, 5,* 397–408.

Klein, E., Colin, V., Stolk, J., & Lenox, R. H. (1994). Alprazolam withdrawal in patients with panic disorder and generalized anxiety disorder: Vulnerability and effect of carbamazepine. *American Journal of Psychiatry, 151*(12), 1760–1766.

Klerman, G. L. (1988, May). Overview of the cross-national collaborative panic study. *Archives of General Psychiatry, 45,* 407–412.

Klerman, G. L. (1992). Drug treatment of panic disorder. Reply to comment by Marks and associates. *British Journal of Psychiatry, 161,* 465–471.

Klosko, J. S., Barlow, D. H., Tassinari, R., & Cerny, J. A. (1990). A comparison of alprazolam and behavior therapy in treatment of panic disorder. *Journal of Consulting & Clinical Psychology, 58*(1), 77–84.

Lader, M. (1995). Clinical pharmacology of anxiolytic drugs: Past, present and future. *Advances in Biochemical Psychopharmacology, 48,* 135–152.

Lader, M., & File, S. (1987). The biological basis of benzodiazepine dependence. *Psychological Medicine, 17,* 539–547.

Leon, A., Portera, L., & Weissman, M. M. (1995). The social costs of anxiety disorders. *British Journal of Psychiatry, 166*(Suppl.), 19–22.

Leonard, B. (1993). Commentary on the mode of action of benzodiazepines. Conference on panic and anxiety: A decade of progress. *Journal of Psychiatric Research, 27*(1), 193–207.

Leonard, B. (1994). Sleep disorders and anxiety: Biochemical antecedents and pharmacological consequences. *Journal of Psychosomatic Research, 38*(1), 69–87.

Linnoila, M., & Hakkinen, S. (1974). Effects of diazepam and codeine, alone and in combination with alcohol, on simulated driving. *Clinical Pharmacology and Therapeutics, 15,* 368–373.

Lipman, R. S. (1989). Pharmacotherapy of the anxiety disorders. In S. Fisher & R. P. Greenberg (Eds.), *The limits of biological treatments for psychological distress: Comparisons with psychotherapy and placebo* (pp. 69–103). Hillsdale, NJ: Erlbaum.

Lipman, R. S., Park, L. C., & Rickels, K. (1966). Paradoxical influence of a side-effect interpretation. *Archives of General Psychiatry, 15,* 462–474.

Lipsey, M., & Wilson, D. B. (1993). The efficacy of psychological, educational and behavioral treatment: Confirmation from meta-analysis. *American Psychologist, 48*(12), 1181–1209.

Loebel, A., Hyde, T. S., & Dunner, D. L. (1986). Early placebo response in anxious and depressed patients. *Journal of Clinical Psychiatry, 47*(5), 230–233.

Long, C., & Bluteau, P. (1988). Group coping skills training for anxiety and depression: Its application with chronic patients. *Journal of Advanced Nursing, 13*(3), 358–364.

Lucki, I., Rickels, K., Giesecke, M. A., & Geller, A. (1987). Differential effects of the anxiolytic drugs, diazepam and buspirone, on memory function. *British Journal of Clinical Pharmacology, 23*(2), 207–211.

Lustman, P., & Sowa, C. J. (1983). Comparative efficacy of biofeedback and stress inoculation for stress reduction. *Journal of Clinical Psychology, 39*(2), 191–197.

Lydiard, R. B., & Ballenger, J. C. (1987). Antidepressants in panic disorder and agoraphobia. *Journal of Affective Disorders, 13,* 153–168.

Lyles, W. B., & Simpson, B. (1990). Advances in the treatment of anxiety and depressive disorders. *Journal of the Florida Medical Association, 77*(8), 731–734.

Margraf, J., Ehlers, A., & Roth, W. T. (1986). Biological models of panic disorder and agoraphobia: A review. *Behaviour Research and Therapy, 24,* 553–567.

Margraf, J., Ehlers, A., Roth, W., Clark, D., Sheik, J., Agras, W., & Taylor, C. (1991). How "blind" are double blind studies? *Journal of Consulting and Clinical Psychology, 59*(1), 184–187.

Margraf, J., Tayler, C., Ehlers, A., Roth, W. T., & Agras, W. S. (1987). Panic attacks in the natural environment. *Journal of Nervous and Mental Disease, 175*(9), 558–565.

Marks, I. (1978). *Living with fear.* New York: McGraw-Hill.

Marks, I. (1981). *Cure and care of neuroses: Theory and practice of behavioral psychotherapy.* New York: Wiley.

Marks, I. (1983). The benzodiazepines: For good and evil. *Neuropsychobiology, 10,* 115–126.

Marks, I., Basoglu, M., Noshirvani, H., Greist, J., Swinson, R. P., & O'Sullivan, G. (1993). Drug treatment of panic disorder: Further comment. *British Journal of Psychiatry, 162,* 795–796.

Marks, I., de Albuquerque, A., Cottraux, J., & Gentil, V. (1989, July). The "efficacy" of alprazolam in panic disorder and agoraphobia:A critique of recent reports. *Archives of General Psychiatry, 46,* 668–669.

Marks, I., Gray, S., Cohen, D., Hill, R., Mawson, D., Ramm, E., & Stern, R. S. (1983). Imipramine and brief therapy aides exposure in agoraphobics having self-exposure homework. *Archives of General Psychiatry, 40,* 153–162.

Marks, I., Swinson, R. P., Basoglu, M., Kuch, K., Noshirvani, H., O'Sullivan, G., Lelliot, P. T., Kirby, M., McNamee, G., Sengun, S., & Wickwire, K. (1993). Alprazolam and exposure alone and combined in panic disorder with agoraphobia. *British Journal of Psychiatry, 162,* 776–787.

Marks, I., Swinson, R. P., Basoglu, M., Noshirvani, H., Kuch, K., O'Sullivan, G., & Lelliott, P. T. (1993). Reply to comment on the London/Toronto Study. *British Journal of Psychiatry, 162,* 790–794.

Martin, I. (1987). The benzodiazepines and their receptors: 25 years of progress [Review]. *Neuropharmacology, 26*(7B), 957–970.

Mattick, R. P., Andrews, G., Hadzi-Pavlovic, D., & Christensen, H. (1990). Treatment of panic and agoraphobia: An integrative review. *Journal of Nervous and Mental Disease, 178*(9), 567–576.

Mavissakalian, M. R., & Michelson, L. (1986a). Agoraphobia: Relative and combined effectiveness of therapy assisted in *in vivo* exposure and imipramine. *Journal of Clinical Psychiatry, 47,* 117–122.

Mavissakalian, M. R., & Michelson, L. (1986b). Two-year follow-up of exposure and imipramine treatment of agoraphobia. *American Journal of Psychiatry, 143*(9), 1106–1112.

Mavissakalian, M. R., & Perel, J. M. (1995). Imipramine treatment of panic disorder with agoraphobia: Dose ranging and plasma level-response relationships. *American Journal of Psychiatry, 152*(5) 673–682.

McCracken, S., deWit, H., Uhlenhuth, E. H., & Johanson, C. E. (1990). Preference for diazepam in anxious adults. *Journal of Clinical Psychopharmacology, 10*(3), 190–196.

McGlynn, T. J., & Metcalf, H L. (1991). *Diagnosis and treatment of anxiety disorders: A Physician's Handbook* (2nd ed.). Washington, DC: American Psychiatric Press.

McLeod D. R., Hoehn-Saric, R., Labib, A. S., & Greenblatt D. J. (1988). Six weeks of diazepam treatment in normal women: Effects on psychomotor performance and psychophysiology. *Journal of Clinical Psychopharmacology, 8*(2), 83–99.

McNair, D., & Kahn, R. J. (1981). Imipramine and chlordiazepoxide for agoraphobia. In D. F. Klein & J. G. Rabkin (Eds.), *Anxiety: New research and changing concepts.* (pp. 169–180). New York: Raven Press.

McTavish, D., & Benfield, P. (1990). Clomipramine: An overview of its pharmacological properties and a review of its therapeutic use in obsessive-compulsive disorder and panic disorder. *Drugs, 39,* 136–153.

Michelson, L., &. Ascher, L. M. (1984). Paradoxical intention in the treatment of agoraphobia and other anxiety disorders. *Journal of Behavior Therapy and Experimental Psychiatry, 15*(3), 215–220.

Michelson, L., & Marchione, K. (1991). Behavioral, cognitive and pharmacological treatments of panic disorder with agoraphobia: Critique and synthesis. *Journal of Consulting and Clinical Psychology, 59*(1), 100–114.

Michelson L., Marchione, K., Greenwald M., Glanz, L., Testa, S., & Marchione, N. (1990). Panic disorder: Cognitive-behavioral treatment. *Behavior Research and Therapy, 28*(2), 141–151.

Milne, D., Jones, R., & Walters, P. (1989). Anxiety management in the community: A social support model and preliminary evaluation. *Behavioral Psychotherapy, 17*(3), 221–236.

Modigh, K., Westperg, P., & Eriksson, E. (1992). Superiority of clomipramine over imipramine in the treatment of panic disorder: A placebo-controlled trial. *Journal of Clinical Psychopharmacology, 12,* 251–261.

Morselli, P. L. (1990). On the therapeutic action of alpidem in anxiety disorders: An overview of the European data. *Pharmacopsychiatry, 23*(3), 129–134.

Mortola, J. (1989). The use of psychotropic agents in pregnancy and lactation. *Psychiatric Clinics of North America, 12*(1), 69–87.

Morton, S., & Lader, M. (1990). Studies with alpidem in normal volunteers and anxious patients. *Pharmacopsychiatry, 23*(3, Suppl.), 120–123.

Mosconi, M., Chiamulera, C., & Recchia, G. (1993). New anxiolytics in development. *International Journal of Clinical Pharmacology Research, 13*(6), 331–344.

Murch, B., Morselli, P. L., & Priore, P. (1988). Clinical studies with the new anxiolytic alpidem in anxious patients: An overview of the European experiences. *Pharmacology, Biochemistry and Behavior, 29*(4), 803–806.

Murphy, S., Owen, R., & Tyerer, P. (1989). Comparative assessment of efficacy and withdrawal symptoms after 6 and 12 weeks' treatment with diazepam or buspirone. *British Journal of Psychiatry, 154,* 529–534.

Murray, J. (1984). The effects of the benzodiazepines Valium (diazepam) and Librium (chlordiazepoxide) on human psychomotor and cognitive functions. *General Psychology Monographs, 109*(2), 167–197.

Myers, J. K., Weissman, M. M.,Tischer, G. L., Holzer, C. E., Leaf, P. J., Orvaschel, H., Anthony, J. C., Boyd, J. H., Burke, J. D., Kramer, M., & Stoltzman, R. (1984). Six-month prevalence of psychiatric disorders in three communities: 1980 to 1982. *Archives of General Psychiatry, 41,* 959–967.

Nagy, L., Krystal, J. H., Charney, D. S., Merikangas, K. R., & Woods, S. W. (1993). Long-term outcome of panic disorder after short-term imipramine and behavioral group treatment: 2.9-year naturalistic follow-up study. *Journal of Clinical Psychopharmacology, 13*(1), 16–24.

National Institutes of Health. (1991). Treatment of panic disorder. *NIH Bulletin, 9*(2), 25–27.

Newman, M., Hofmann, S., Trabert, W., Roth, W., & Taylor, C. (1994). Does behavioral treatment of social phobia lead to cognitive changes? *Behavior Therapy, 25*(3), 503–517.

Nolan, L., & O'Malley, K. (1987). Age-related prescribing patterns in general practice. *Comprehensive Gerontology. Section A, Clinical and Laboratory Sciences, 1*(3), 97–101.

Noyes, R., Garvey, M. J., Cook, B. L., & Samuelson, L. (1989). Problems with tricyclic antidepressant use in patients with panic disorder or agoraphobia: Results of a naturalistic follow-up study. *Journal of Clinical Psychiatry, 50*(5), 163–169.

Nutt, D. (1990). The pharmacology of human anxiety. *Pharmacology and Therapeutics, 47*(2), 233–266.

Nutt, D., & Glue, P. (1989). Clinical pharmacology of anxiolytics and antidepressants: A pharmacological perspective. *Pharmacology and Therapeutics, 44,* 309–334.

O'Hanlon, J., Haak, T. W., Blaauw, G. J., & Riemersma, J. B. (1982). Diazepam impairs lateral position control in highway driving. *Science, 217,* 79–81.

O'Hanlon J., Vermeeren, A., Uiterwijk, M. M., van Veggel, L. M., & Swijgman, H. F. (1995). Anxiolytics' effects on the actual driving performance of patients and healthy volunteers in a standardized test. An integration of three studies. *Neuropsychobiology, 31*(2), 81–88.

Olajide, D., & Lader, M. (1987). A comparison of buspirone, diazepam, and placebo in patients with chronic anxiety states. *Journal of Clinical Psychopharmacology, 7*(3), 148–152.

Ost, L., Jerremalm, A., & Jansson, J. (1982). Individual response patterns and the effects of different behavioral methods in the treatment of claustrophobia. *Behavior Research and Therapy, 20*(5), 445–460.

Ost, L., Jerremalm, A., & Jansson, J. (1984). Individual response patterns and the effects of different behavioral methods in the treatment of agoraphobia. *Behavior Research and Therapy, 22*(6), 697–707.

Oster, G., Huse, D. M., Adams, S., Imbimbo, J., & Russell, M. W. (1990). Benzodiazepines tranquilizers and the risk of accidental injury. *American Journal of Public Health, 801*(2), 1467–1470.

Otto, M., Gould, R. A., & Pollack, M. H. (1994). Cognitive-behavioral treatment of panic disorder: Considerations for the treatment of patients over the long term. *Psychiatric Annals, 24*(6), 307–315.

Otto, M., Pollack, M., Meltzer-Brody, S., & Rosenbaum, J. (1992). Cognitive-behavioral therapy for benzodiazepine discontinuation in panic disorder patients. *Psychopharmacology Bulletin, 28*(2), 123–130.

Pecknold, J. C., Swinson, R. P., Kuch, K., & Lewis, C. P. (1988, May). Alprazolam in panic disorder and agoraphobia: Results from a multicenter trial: 3. Discontinuation effects. *Archives of General Psychiatry, 45*, 429–436.

Perry, P. (1985). Assessment of addiction liability of benzodiazepines and buspirone. *Drug Intelligence and Clinical Pharmacology, 19*, 657–659.

Petruzzello, S., Landers, D. M., Hatfield, B. D., Kubitz, K. A., & Salazar, W. (1991). A meta-analysis on the anxiety-reducing effects of acute and chronic exercise. Outcomes and mechanisms. *Sports Medicine, 11*(3), 143–182.

Pigott, T., L'Heureux, F., Hill, J., Bihari, K., Bernstein, S., & Murphy, D. (1992). A double-blind study of adjuvant buspirone hydrochloride in clomipramine-treated patients with obsessive-compulsive disorder. *Journal of Clinical Psychopharmacology, 12*(1), 11–18.

Pitman, R., Altman, B., Greenwald, E., Longpre, R. E., Macklin, M. L., Poire, R. E., & Steketee, G. S. (1991). Psychiatric complications during flooding therapy for posttraumatic stress disorder. *Journal of Clinical Psychiatry, 52*(1), 17–20.

Pohl, R., Balon, R., Yeragani, V. K., & Gershon, S. (1989). Serotonergic anxiolytics in the treatment of panic disorder: A controlled study with buspirone. *Psychopathology, 22*(Suppl.), 60–67.

Pohl, R., Yeragani, V. K., Balon, R., & Lycaki, H. (1988). The jitteriness syndrome in panic disorder patients treated with antidepressants. *Journal of Clinical Psychiatry, 49*, 100–104.

Pollack, M. H., & Otto, M. W. (1994). Long-term pharmacologic treatment of panic disorder. *Psychiatric Annals, 24*(6), 291–298.

Pollock, E. (1995, December 1). Managed care's focus on psychiatric drugs alarms many doctors. *Wall Street Journal*, p. 1.

Popper, C. (1993). Psychopharmacologic treatment of anxiety disorders in adolescents and children. *Journal of Clinical Psychology, 54*(5, Suppl.), 52–62.

Quality Assurance Project. (1985). Treatment outlines for the management of anxiety states. *Australian and New Zealand Journal of Psychiatry, 19*, 138–151.

Raglin, J., & Morgan, W. P. (1985). Influence of vigorous exercise on mood state. *Behavior Therapist, 8*(9), 179–183.

Raskin, A. (1983, November. The influence of depression on the antipanic effects of antidepressant drugs [Abstract]. *Psychiatric Clinics in North America, 4–6*.

Raskin, J., Quitkin, F., & Harrison, W. (1984a). Adverse reactions to monoamine oxidase inhibitors: A comparative study. *Journal of Clinical Psychopharmacology, 4*, 270–278.

Raskin, J., Quitkin, F., & Harrison, W. (1984b). Adverse reactions to monoamine oxidase inhibitors: Treatment correlates and clinical management. *Journal of Clinical Psychopharmacology, 5*, 2–9.

Regier, D., Boyd, J. H., Burk, J. D., Jr., Rae, D. S., Myers, J. K., Kramer, M., Robins, L. N., George, L. K., Karno, M., & Locke, B. Z. (1988). One-month prevalence of mental disorders in the United States: Based on five epidemiologic catchment area sites. *Archives of General Psychiatry, 45*, 977–986.

Regier, D., Narrow, W. E., & Rae, D. S. (1990). The epidemiology of anxiety disorders: The epidemiologic catchment area (ECA) experience. *Journal of Psychiatric Research, 24*(2), 3–14.

Reiss, S., &. McNally, R. J. (1985). Expectancy model of fear. In S. Reiss & R. R. Bootzin (Eds.), *Theoretical issues in behavior therapy* (pp. 107–121). New York: Academic Press.

Reiss, S., Peterson, R. A., Gursky, D. M., & McNally, R. J. (1986). Anxiety, sensitivity, anxiety frequency and the predictors of fearfulness. *Behaviour Research and Therapy, 24*, 1–8.

Rickels, K., Downing, R., Case, G., Csanalosi, I., Chung, H., Winokur, A., & Gingrich, R. (1985). Six week trial with diazepam: Some clinical observations. *Journal of Clinical Psychiatry, 46*(11), 479–474.

Rickels, K., Case., G., Downing, R. W., & Winokur, A. (1983). Long-term diazepam therapy and clinical outcome. *Journal of the American Medical Association, 250*, 767–771.

Rickels, K., Case, W., Warren, G., & Schweizer, E. (1988). The drug treatment of anxiety and panic disorder. Inaugural Conference of the International Society for the Investigation of Stress Symposium: Drugs and stress (1988, Munich, Federal Republic of Germany). *Stress Medicine, 4*(4), 231–239.

Rickels, K., & Schweizer, E. (1990a). The clinical course and long-term management of generalized anxiety disorder. *Journal of Clinical Psychopharmacology, 10*(3, Suppl.), 101S–110S.

Rickels, K., &. Schweizer, E. (1990b). Clinical overview of serotonin reuptake inhibitors. *Journal of Clinical Psychiatry, 51*(Suppl. B), 9–12.

Rickels, K., Schweizer, E., Weiss, S., & Zavodnick, S. (1993). Maintenance drug treatment for panic disorder: 2. Short-term and long-term outcome after drug taper. *Archives of General Psychiatry, 50*, 61–68.

Rickels, K., Weisman, K., Norstad, N., Singer, M., Stoltz, D., Brown, A., & Danton, J. (1982). Buspirone and diazepam in the treatment of anxiety: A controlled study. *Journal of Clinical Psychiatry, 43*, 81–86.

Robins, L. N., Helzer, J. E., & Weissman, M. M. (1984). Lifetime prevalence of specific psychiatric disorders in three sites. *Archives of General Psychiatry, 41*, 949–958.

Romney, D. M., & Angus, W. R. (1984). A brief review of the effects of diazepam on memory. *Psychopharmacology Bulletin, 20*(2), 313–316.

Rosenbaum, J. F. (1982). The drug treatment of anxiety. *New England Journal of Medicine, 306*, 401–404.

Rosenberg, R., Bech, P., Mellergard, M., & Ottosson, J. O. (1991). Alprazolam imipramine and placebo treatment of panic disorder: Predicting therapeutic response. *Acta Psychiatrica Scandinavica-Supplementum, 365,* 46–52.

Roy-Byrne, P., Wagerson, D., Cowley, D., & Dager, S. (1993). Psychopharmacologic treatment of panic, general anxiety disorders and social phobia. *Psychopharmacology II, 16*(4), 719–735.

Salkovskis, P. (1991). The importance of behavior in the maintenance of anxiety and panic: A cognitive account: The changing face of behavioural psychotherapy [Special issue]. *Behavioural Psychotherapy, 19*(1), 6–19.

Salkovskis, P., & Clark, D. (1990). Affective responses to hyperventilation: A test of the cognitive model of panic. *Behaviour Research and Therapy, 28*(1), 51–61.

Sanger, D. (1994). Neuropharmacology of anxiety: Prospectives and prospects. *TiPS, 15,* 36–39.

Sanger, D., Perrault, G., Morel, E., Joly, D., & Zivkovic, B. (1991). Animal models of anxiety and the development of novel anxiolytic drugs. *Progress in Neuropsychopharmacology and Biological Psychiatry, 15*(2), 205–212.

Sanua, V. (1995). "Prescription privileges" vs. psychologists' authority: Psychologists do better without drugs. *The Humanistic Psychologist, 23,* 187–212.

Sargant, W., & Dally, P. (1962). Treatment of anxiety states by antidepressant drugs. *British Medical Journal, 1,* 6–9.

Schneier, F., Leibowitz, M. R., & Davies, S. O. (1990). Fluoxetine in panic disorder. *Journal of Clinical Psychopharmacology, 10,* 119–121.

Schweizer, E., Rickels, K., Case, W. G., & Greenblatt, D. J. (1990). Long-term therapeutic use of benzodiazepines: 2. Effects of gradual taper. *Archives of General Psychiatry, 47*(10), 908–915.

Schweizer, E., Rickels, K., Weiss, S., & Zavodnick, S. (1993). Maintenance drug treatment of panic disorder: 1. Results of a prospective, placebo-controlled comparison of alprazolam and imipramine. *Archives of General Psychiatry, 50*(1), 51–60.

Shader, R., & Greenblatt, D. J. (1982). Management of anxiety in the elderly: The balance between therapeutic and adverse effects. *Journal of Clinical Psychiatry, 43*(9), 8–18.

Shader, R., & Greenblatt, D. J. (1983). Some current treatment options for symptoms of anxiety. *Journal of Clinical Psychiatry, 44*(11-2), 21–29.

Shapiro, A. K.(1978). Placebo effects in medical and psychological therapies. In S. L. Garfield & A. E. Bergen (Eds.), *Handbook of psychotherapy and behavior change* (2nd ed., pp. 369–410). New York: Wiley.

Shapiro, F. (1995). *Eye movement desensitization and reprocessing.* New York: Guilford Press.

Shapiro, J., Sank, L., Shaffer, E., & Donovan, D. (1982). Cost effectiveness of individual vs. group cognitive behavior therapy for problems of depression and anxiety in an HMO population. *Journal of Clinical Psychology, 38*(3), 674–677.

Sheehan, D., Davidson, J., Manschreck, T., & VanWyck Fleet, T. (1983). Lack of efficacy of a new antidepressant (bupropion) in the treatment of panic disorder with phobias. *Journal of Clinical Psychopharmacology, 3,* 28–31.

Sheehan, D., Sheehan, K., & Minichiello, W. (1981). Age of onset of phobic disorders: A reevaluation. *Comprehensive Psychiatry, 22*(6), 544–553.

Simon, G., Ormel, J., VonKorff, M., & Barlow, D. (1995). Health care costs associated with depressive and anxiety disorders in primary care. *American Journal of Psychiatry, 152*(3), 352–357.

Sorby, N. G., Reavley, W., & Huber, J. W. (1991). Self help programme for anxiety in general practice: Controlled trial of an anxiety management booklet. *British Journal of General Practice, 41*(351), 417–420.

Spiegel, D., Roth, M., Weissman, M., Lavori, P., Gorman, J., Rush, J., & Ballenger, J. (1993). Comment on the London/Toronto study of alprazolam and exposure in panic disorder with agoraphobia. *British Journal of Psychiatry, 162,* 788–789.

Stoudemire, A., Moran, M. G., & Fogel, B. S. (1991). Psychotropic drug use in the medically ill: Part 2. *Psychosomatics, 32*(1), 34–46.

Sussman, N. (1993). Treating anxiety while minimizing abuse and dependence. *Journal of Clinical Psychiatry, 54*(5, Suppl.), 44–51.

Sutton-Simon, K., &. Goldfried, M. R. (1979). Faulty thinking patterns in two types of anxiety. *Cognitive Therapy and Research, 3*(2), 193–203.

Swartz, M., Landerman, R., George, L. K., Melville, M. L., Blazer, D., & Smith, K. (1991). Benzodiazepine anti-anxiety agents: Prevalence and correlates of use in a southern community. *American Journal of Public Health, 81*(5), 592–596.

Talley, J. (1990). But what if a patient gets hooked? Fallacies about long-term use of benzodiazepines. *Post Graduate Medicine, 87*(1), 187–203.

Taylor, C., & Hayward, R., (1990). Cardiovascular considerations in selection of anti-panic pharmacotherapy. *Journal of Psychosomatic Research, 24*(2), 43–49.

Taylor, C., King, R., Margraf, J., Ehlers, A., Telch, M., Roth, W. T., & Agras, W. S. (1989). Use of medication and *in vivo* exposure in volunteers for panic disorder research. *American Journal of Psychiatry, 146*(11), 1423–1426.

Taylor, C., Sheikh, J., Agras, W. S., Roth, W. T., Margraf, J., Ehlers, A., Maddock, R. J., & Gossard, D. (1986). Ambulatory heart rate changes in patients with panic attacks. *American Journal of Psychiatry, 143*(4), 478–482.

Telch, M. J., Agras, W. S., Taylor, C. B., Roth, W. T., & Gallen, C. (1985). Combined pharmacological and behavioral treatment for agoraphobia. *Behavioral Research and Therapy, 23,* 325–335.

Tesar, G. E. (1990). High-potency benzodiazepines for short-term management of panic disorder: The U.S. experience. *Journal of Clinical Psychiatry, 51*(Suppl.), 4–10.

Thakore, J., & Dinan, T. G. (1992). Physical dependence following zopiclone usage: A case report. *Human Psychopharmacology, 7,* 142–146.

Trull, T., Nietzel, M. T., & Main, A. (1988). The use of meta-analysis to assess the clinical significance of behavior therapy for agoraphobia. *Behavior Therapy, 19,* 527–538.

Uhlenhuth, E., Balter, M. B., Ban, T. A., & Yang, K. (1995). International study of expert judgment on therapeutic use of benzodiazepines and other psychotherapeutic medications: 3. Clinical features affecting experts' therapeutic recommendations. *Psychopharmacology Bulletin, 31*(2), 289–296.

Uhlenhuth, E., Balter, M. B., Mellinger, G. D., Cisin, I. H., & Clinthorne, J. (1983). Symptom checklist syndromes in the general population: Correlations with psychotherapeutic drug use. *Archives of General Psychiatry, 40,* 1167–1173.

Uhlenhuth, E., DeWit, H., Balter, M. B., Johanson, C. E., & Mellinger, G. D. (1988). Risks and benefits of long-term benzodiazepine use. *Journal of Clinical Psychopharmacology, 8*(3), 161–167.

Uhlenhuth, E., Matuzas, W., Glass, R. M., & Easton, C. (1989). Response of panic disorder to fixed doses of alprazolam or imipramine. *Journal of Affective Disorders, 17*(3), 261–270.

Van Balkom, A. J., Nauta, M. C., & Bakker, A. (1995). Meta-analysis on the treatment of panic disorder with agoraphobia: Review and examination. *Clinical Psychology and Psychotherapy, 2,* 1–14.

Venault, P., Chapouthier, G., deCavallo, L., Simiand, J., Morre, M., Dodd, R., & Rossier, J. (1986). Benzodiazepine impairs and b-carboline enhances performance in learning and memory tasks. *Nature, 321,* 864–866.

von Frenckell, R., Ansseau, M., & Bonnet, D. (1986). Evaluation of the sedative properties of PK 8165 (pipequaline), a benzodiazepine partial agonist, in normal subjects. *International Clinical Psychopharmacology, 1*(1), 24–35.

Warneke, L. (1991). Benzodiazepines: Abuse and new use. *Canadian Journal of Psychiatry, 36,* 194–205.

Weissman, M. (1985). The epidemiology of anxiety disorders: Rates, risks and familial patterns. In A. H. Tumard & J. D. Maser (Eds.), *Anxiety and the anxiety disorders* (pp. 275–296). Hillsdale, NJ: Erlbaum.

Weissman, M. (1988). The epidemiology of anxiety disorders: Rates, risks and familial patterns. *Journal of Psychiatric Research, 22*(Suppl. 1), 99–114.

Welkowitz, L., Papp, L., Cloitre, M., Liebowitz, M., Martin, L. Y., & Gorman, J. M. (1991). Cognitive-behavior therapy for panic disorder delivered by psychopharmacologically oriented clinicians. *Journal of Nervous and Mental Disease, 179*(8), 473–477.

Wilkinson, C. (1985). Effects of diazepam (Valium) and trait anxiety on human physical aggression and emotional state. *Journal of Behavior Medicine, 8,* 101–113.

Wilkinson, G., Balestrieri, M., Ruggeri, M., & Bellantuone, C. (1991). Meta-analysis of double-blind placebo-controlled trials of antidepressants and benzodiazepines for patients with panic disorders. *Psychological Medicine, 21*(4), 991–998.

Wilson, S. A., Becker, L. A., & Tinker, R. H. (1995). Eye movement desensitization and reprocessing (EMDR) treatment for psychologically traumatized individuals. *Journal of Consulting and Clinical Psychology, 63*(6), 928–937.

Winokur, A., Rickels, K., Greenblatt, D. J., Snyder, P. J., & Schatz, N. J. (1980). Withdrawal reaction from long-term, low dosage administration of diazepam: A double-blind, placebo-controlled case study. *Archives of General Psychiatry, 37,* 101–105.

Wolkowitz, O. M., Weingartner, H., Thompson, K., & Pickar, D. (1987). Diazepam-induced amnesia: A neuropharmacological model of an "organic amnesia." *American Journal of Psychiatry, 144*(1), 25–29.

Wolpe, J. (1993). Commentary: The cognitivist oversell and comments on symposium contributions. *Journal of Behavior Therapy and Experimental Psychiatry, 24*(2), 141–147.

Zaccara, G., Innocenti, P., Bartelli, M., Casini, R., Tozzi, F., Rossi, L., & Zappoli, R. (1986). Status epilepticus due to abrupt diazepam withdrawal: A case report. *Journal of Neurology, Neurosurgery and Psychiatry, 49*(8), 959–960.

Zinbarg, R., Barlow, D., Brown, T., & Hertz, R. (1992). Cognitive-behavioral approaches to the nature and treatment of anxiety disorders. *Annual Review of Psychology, 43*, 235–267.

Zitrin, C. M., Klein, D. F., & Woerner, M. G. (1978). Behavior therapy, supportive psychotherapy, imipramine, and phobias. *Archives of General Psychiatry, 35*, 307–316.

Zitrin, C. M., Klein, D. F., & Woerner, M. G. (1980). Treatment of agoraphobia with group exposure *in vivo* and imipramine. *Archives of General Psychiatry, 37*, 63–72.

CHAPTER 7

Pharmacological Treatments for Borderline Personality Disorder: A Critical Review of the Empirical Literature

ROBERT F. BORNSTEIN

FEW WORDS STRIKE fear into the heart of the practicing clinician as easily as the word *borderline,* and with good reason. Borderline patients are notoriously difficult to treat. Clinicians describe them as manipulative, labile, self-centered, self-destructive, demanding, disheartening, and just plain frustrating (Egan, 1986; Millon, 1981, 1996; Perry, 1989; Stein, 1996). Their transference reactions are intense and unpredictable, and the countertransference strain they elicit can test the commitment of even the most devoted practitioner (Coen, 1992; Kernberg, 1975). The terrible reputation of the borderline patient is such that the mere appearance of a borderline personality disorder (BPD) diagnosis in a patient's treatment record is sufficient to ensure that many clinicians will avoid taking the case if at all possible.

Clinicians' negative impressions of borderline patients are in many ways quite understandable. Studies confirm that work with borderline patients is extremely difficult and often stressful (Gunderson, 1989; Leibovich, 1983; Perry, 1989), a finding that has been echoed in informal, anecdotal accounts of treatment experiences with borderlines (Kernberg, 1984; Paris, 1994). The following vignette describes an episode in the life of a 22-year-old female patient with BPD:

The patient . . . had been admitted to the hospital following a serious over-dose, which had been her third suicide attempt. . . . When she lost her job as a secretary, she felt her life was out of control and took a bottle of antide-pressant medication that had been prescribed by her outpatient thera-pist. . . . Shortly before her suicide attempt, she cut her wrists superficially when her therapist announced that he was going on vacation. This was the 30th time she had engaged in wrist-scratching since adolescence. . . . Upon admission to the inpatient unit, this patient reported hearing babies crying out and, on one occasion, seeing bugs crawling on her legs. . . . She was highly manipulative, deceptive and repeatedly threatened to elope and kill herself during dysphoric periods, when she felt her needs were not being met. [She] reinforced the seriousness of her threats by turning in pieces of glass and other objects with which she could harm herself [and] continued to complain of suicidal impulses that were out of control. (Hull, Clarkin, & Alexopoulos, 1993)

Given such eccentric and bizarre behavior, it is not surprising that re-searchers have devoted a great deal of time and energy trying to discern the etiology and dynamics of borderline symptoms, and attempting to ex-plain the "stable instability" characteristic of borderlines. More than a century ago, Hughes (1884, p. 297) noted that "the borderland of insanity is occupied by many persons who pass their whole life near that line, sometimes on one side, sometimes on the other." Several decades later, Kraepelin (1915) and Kretschmer (1925) echoed Hughes's (1884) observa-tions, describing the precursor of what would later become BPD in the of-ficial psychiatric nomenclature. Both Kraepelin and Kretschmer linked the borderline syndrome to severe long-standing disturbances in affect and thought processes.

The first modern use of the borderline concept is found in the work of Stern (1938), who—like Hughes (1884)—contended that persons with bor-derline symptoms were on the "border" between neurosis and psychosis. Following this line of thinking, several theorists suggested that the term *borderline* was best used as a descriptor pertaining to a primitive level of personality organization (Kernberg, 1970), or a particularly severe form of personality pathology (Millon, 1969), rather than a diagnostic category per se. Throughout the 1970s, clinicians debated whether BPD reflected an underlying affective disturbance, thought disorder, or both (Akiskal, Djenderedjian, Rosenthal, & Khani, 1977; Klein, 1977; Perry & Klerman, 1978). Although this controversy lost much of its strength after 1980, when the *Diagnostic and Statistical Manual of Mental Disorders* (DSM-III; American Psychiatric Association [APA], 1980) officially classified BPD as an Axis II personality disorder, the issue is not resolved completely: It still resur-faces periodically in the diagnostic and treatment literature (Blatt, 1991; Brinkley, 1993; Egan, 1986; Tuinier & Verhoeven, 1995; Westen, 1991).

The most comprehensive and heuristic conceptualization of borderline pathology ultimately came from psychodynamic theory. Integrating clinical data with findings from cognitive and developmental psychology, Kernberg (1970, 1975), Kohut (1971, 1977), Blatt (1990, 1991) and others have argued that the core difficulties characterizing BPD lie in three areas. First, the borderline patient has an extremely tenuous sense of self, which may decompensate—quite literally fragment and disappear—under stress (Kernberg, 1984). Second, the borderline patient is incapable of maintaining stable mental representations of significant figures when these figures are not physically present (what Blatt [1991] refers to as a deficit in "evocative constancy"). Finally, the borderline patient has a rigid, maladaptive defensive style, overrelying on the defense mechanism of splitting (as well as other primitive defenses like projection and denial) to cope with anxiety (Blatt & Auerbach, 1988; Greene, Rosenkrantz, & Muth, 1985; Kohut, 1971, 1977).

Given the high degree of dysfunction and self-destructiveness associated with BPD, coupled with the heterogeneity of behavioral deficits associated with this disorder, it is not surprising that clinicians and clinical researchers have had great difficulty determining which treatment modalities—if any—are useful in treating borderline pathology. Numerous treatment approaches have been implemented during the past several decades, including psychodynamic psychotherapy (Kernberg, 1984), behavior therapy (Lazarus, 1982), cognitive therapy (Freeman & Leaf, 1989), and humanistic therapy (Langley, 1994). Many biologically oriented clinicians also advocate pharmacotherapy for BPD, either alone or in conjunction with more traditional psychotherapeutic approaches.

Pharmacotherapy for BPD has typically involved one of two goals. Some clinicians and researchers argue that pharmacotherapy alone is the treatment of choice for this disorder (see, e.g., Silk, 1994). Others contend that pharmacological treatments for BPD are best conceptualized as an adjunct to more traditional psychotherapeutic approaches (e.g., Paris, 1994). In contrast to those who regard pharmacotherapy for BPD as an end in itself, these researchers view pharmacotherapy as a means to an end—a procedure for managing the more flagrant BPD symptoms so that psychotherapy may be used to promote adaptive long-term functioning.

Regardless of whether pharmacotherapy is used as the sole treatment for BPD or as an adjunct to other forms of treatment, studies assessing the efficacy of drug treatments for BPD have invariably focused on the same issue: the extent to which different pharmacological agents ameliorate one or more BPD, or BPD-related, symptoms. Thus, the key outcome measures in these investigations are always the same: reductions in symptom levels and enhanced functioning in one or more domains (e.g., mood, sociability, impulse control). Within this general framework about a dozen controlled clinical trials assessing the efficacy of BPD drug treatments have been conducted within the past 15 years. A variety of different medications have been used in these investigations, and both inpatients and outpatients have taken part in these trials, which generally last from several weeks to several months.

The purpose of this chapter is to review the empirical literature on pharmacological treatment of BPD, with the aim of determining which (if any) pharmacological agents have demonstrated efficacy in the treatment of this puzzling and debilitating disorder. I first describe the *DSM-IV* symptoms of BPD (APA, 1994) and discuss how these symptoms relate to findings regarding the psychodynamics of borderline pathology. Next, I discuss special treatment issues in work with BPD patients, to place the ensuing discussion into the proper context. Third, I assess the BPD drug treatment literature, describing the best and most recent studies of each of the major pharmacological agents used to treat this disorder. Finally, I discuss the implications of this treatment literature, exploring the methodological limitations of extant studies in this area, and the relationship of drug treatment to other forms of treatment for BPD patients.

BPD: SYMPTOMS AND PSYCHODYNAMICS

According to the *DSM-IV* (APA, 1994, p. 654), the essential feature of BPD is "a pervasive pattern of instability in interpersonal relationships, self-image, and affects, and marked impulsivity beginning by early adulthood and present in a variety of contexts." The *DSM-IV* goes on to describe nine separate symptoms of BPD; the patient must have five or more of these symptoms to receive the BPD diagnosis. These symptoms are:

1. Frantic efforts to avoid real or imagined abandonment.
2. A pattern of unstable, intense interpersonal relationships.
3. Identity disturbance and a markedly unstable sense of self.
4. Impulsivity that is potentially self-damaging (e.g., binge eating, promiscuous sex).
5. Suicidal behavior, gestures, or threats.
6. Affective instability.
7. Chronic feelings of emptiness.
8. Inappropriate, intense anger, or difficulties controlling anger.
9. Transient stress-related paranoid ideation or dissociative symptoms.

Two things are noteworthy regarding these symptom criteria. First, they are generally consistent with clinical and empirical findings regarding the psychodynamics of BPD. The tenuous self-concept and unstable interpersonal relationships that psychodynamic researchers have found to be central to borderline pathology are both captured in the essential feature of BPD as described in the *DSM-IV* (see Blatt, 1991; Blatt & Auerbach, 1988).

Second, the *DSM-IV* BPD symptom criteria include three separate domains of personality dysfunction. Symptoms 1, 2, 4, and 5 are primarily behavioral, whereas symptoms 2, 3, and 9 reflect cognitive difficulties, and symptoms 6, 7, and 8 describe disturbances in affect or emotional responding. Paralleling clinical observations that BPD is a disorder which manifests itself in many ways (Millon, 1981, 1996), the *DSM-IV* BPD symptom criteria require the diagnostician to focus on several different aspects of the patient's functioning to assign the BPD diagnosis.

SPECIAL TREATMENT ISSUES IN WORK WITH BPD PATIENTS

All Axis II personality disorders present special challenges for the clinician, but the treatment difficulties associated with BPD are unique. Some of the more problematic treatment issues in clinical work with borderline patients include the following.

SYMPTOM HETEROGENEITY

Borderline patients present an unusually varied and confusing array of symptoms (Gunderson & Phillips, 1991). There is no doubt that BPD meets the essential criteria for an Axis II disorder (see APA, 1994, p. 633). However, BPD also shares a number of features with Axis I symptom disorders (e.g., substance abuse, binge eating, suicidal behavior). Researchers have even speculated that BPD might have an organic basis: BPD patients show a number of physiological abnormalities, including biochemical imbalances, cortical dysfunctions, and aberrant electroencephalograph (EEG), magnetic resonance imaging (MRI), and positron emission tomography (PET) scan readings (Kutcher, Blackwood, & St. Clair, 1987; Kutcher, Papatheodorou, Reiter, & Gardner, 1995).

DIAGNOSTIC UNRELIABILITY

Diagnostic reliability for Axis II disorders is marginal at best, and diagnostic reliability for BPD tends to be even lower than that of other personality disorders (McCann, 1991). In part this is because BPD symptoms show considerable overlap with symptoms of certain other Axis II disorders (e.g., schizotypal, narcissistic, paranoid). In part, the low reliability estimates often reported for BPD reflect that it has become something of a catchall category for personality dysfunction that cannot be classified elsewhere (Weissman, 1993). Whatever the cause, the diagnostic unreliability of BPD makes treatment planning more difficult, and has made research on BPD treatment difficult to interpret.

COMORBIDITY

Compounding BPD's diagnostic unreliability, BPD shows high rates of comorbidity with Axis I diagnoses, including mood disorders, eating disorders, and posttraumatic stress disorder (Gunderson & Zanarini, 1987; Shea, Widiger, & Klein, 1992). On Axis II, BPD shows high rates of comorbidity with histrionic, schizotypal, paranoid, narcissistic, antisocial, and dependent personality disorders (Bornstein, 1995). As several researchers have noted, these comorbidity data might well reflect the co-occurrence of BPD with other disorders. However, an equally plausible interpretation of these data is that the symptom criteria for BPD lack discriminant validity.

LABILITY

From the perspective of the clinician, the unpredictability of borderline behavior is a central obstacle to successful treatment for several reasons (Stein, 1996). First, the lability of the borderline patient often results in countertransference strain severe enough to hinder the clinician's judgment (Goldstein, 1995). Second, the BPD patient's unpredictability interferes with implementation of a cohesive long-term treatment plan. Third, when frightened or frustrated, the borderline patient has the potential to act out in verbally or physically aggressive ways (Greene et al., 1985).

SELF-DESTRUCTIVENESS

The borderline patient's propensity to self-medicate, coupled with the tendency to make suicidal gestures when frightened or threatened, makes pharmacological treatment of these patients especially risky (see Linehan, Tutek, Heard, & Armstrong, 1994; Russ, Roth, Kakuma, Harrison, & Hull, 1994). The possibility that the patient will accidentally or deliberately overdose on prescription drugs is significant. Moreover, the possibility that prescribed medications will interact with one or more recreational drugs being used by the borderline patient must always be considered: Studies suggest that more than 50% of all BPD patients use some form of recreational drug during outpatient treatment (Kernberg, 1984; Nace, 1992).

PHARMACOLOGICAL TREATMI
A CRITICAL REVIEW OF
EMPIRICAL LITERATU

Two forces converged in the mid-1960s to stimula logical treatment of borderline conditions. First, lief among clinicians that borderline patients us unpleasant symptoms. Dyrud (1972, p. 163) sugge "are self-medicating, not in the sense of recreatic̲̲̲ ̲̲̲̲ ̲̲ ̲̲ ̲̲̲̲̲ ̲̲̲̲ necessarily, but [as a way of] adjusting an intolerable feeling state." If borderline patients were already self-medicating and were likely to continue to do so (the thinking was), then it would be best if their drug use was controlled and monitored by physicians (see Brinkley, Beitman, & Friedel, 1979, for a detailed discussion of this issue).

Second, there was a growing sense of desperation among clinicians who had found no reliable treatment for borderline patients. A hope arose that pharmacological agents might facilitate more traditional forms of psychotherapy (Grinker, Werble, & Drye, 1968; Havens, 1968; Kernberg, 1968, 1975).

Between 1968 and 1979 there were very few controlled clinical trials involving pharmacological treatment of borderline symptoms (Brinkley, 1993; Brinkley et al., 1979). The situation changed somewhat in 1980, when the *DSM-III* criteria for BPD were published (allowing researchers to use a consistent set of criteria to select patients for inclusion in studies), and a wider variety of pharmacological agents became available (allowing researchers to test more systematically the relative effects of different drugs on BPD symptoms).

In the following sections, I limit my review to those studies published after 1980. These studies have been divided into five categories, reflecting the different types of pharmacological agents used: antidepressants, anxiolytics, antipsychotics, anticonvulsants, and lithium.

ANTIDEPRESSANTS

Interest in the use of antidepressant medications in the treatment of BPD is rooted in the long-standing (but still controversial) notion that affective disturbances play a key role in the etiology and dynamics of borderline symptoms (Klein, 1975, 1977). Ironically, most antidepressant BPD studies have assessed the efficacy of monoamine oxidase inhibitors (MAOIs) rather than tricyclic antidepressants, although in recent years tricyclic medications have been the overwhelming treatment of choice for a wide range of mood disorders (Brinkley, 1993).

..., there have been more than 20 open (i.e., nonblind) trials ex-
...the effects of antidepressant medications on BPD symptoms (e.g.,
...ro, Astill, & Herbert, 1990; Cornelius, Soloff, & Perel, 1990, 1991;
...wdry & Gardner, 1988; Hull et al., 1993; Markowitz, Calabrese, &
Schulz, 1991; Norden, 1989). However, there have been only six double-
blind placebo-controlled studies assessing the efficacy of antidepressants
in the treatment of BPD. Four of these studies involved phenelzine, one
study assessed amitriptyline, and one investigation focused on fluoxetine.

In the first published study in this area, Liebowitz and Klein (1981)
compared the effects of phenelzine and placebo in a sample of 11 female
BPD patients who were undergoing traditional insight-oriented psychotherapy throughout the 3-month period during which the study took
place. Dosage levels ranged from 15 to 75 milligrams (mg) per day; blood
plasma levels were not assessed in this investigation. Although a large
number of patient- and therapist-rated dimensions of functioning were
assessed in this study (increasing substantially the possibility of a Type I
error), no differences were found between the drug and placebo groups
on any outcome measure.

A decade later, Soloff, Cornelius, and George (1991) obtained only
slightly more encouraging results in a similar study comparing the efficacy
of phenelzine versus placebo in a mixed-sex sample of 68 BPD patients followed over 5 weeks: Numerous outcome measures were taken, with differences emerging only in the areas of anger and hostility (phenelzine-treated
patients showed greater improvement than placebo-treated patients on
both dimensions). This investigation was subsequently criticized by Brinkley (1993, p. 864), who noted that a "defect of this study is a potentially inadequate phenelzine dosage ceiling (60 mg/day) and a required MAO
inhibition level of 70%."

Similar results were also obtained by Cornelius, Soloff, Perel, and Ulrich
(1993), who compared phenelzine and placebo effects in a mixed-sex sample of 36 BPD-diagnosed outpatients followed over 16 weeks. A variety of
therapist-rated outcome measures were used (13 in all), although no data
regarding interrater reliability were reported in this study. In line with
the findings reported by Soloff et al. (1991), Cornelius et al. (1993) found
statistically significant drug-placebo differences in only 2 of 13 areas:
Phenelzine-treated patients showed less depression and less irritability
than controls.

The strongest results obtained to date regarding the efficacy of
phenelzine in the treatment of BPD came from Parsons et al. (1989), who
followed a large, heterogeneous sample of BPD patients concurrently
diagnosed with major depression. Relative to control (i.e., placebo-
treated) patients, phenelzine-treated patients in Parsons et al.'s study

showed marked improvement in a number of areas, including a significant reduction in the number and severity of BPD symptoms.

This was one of the few investigations to include a placebo "washout period" prior to the start of data collection: Before the study began, all potential subjects went through a 10-day placebo trial, and only nonresponders were included in the study proper. Although extant findings indicate that inclusion of a placebo washout period does not influence the magnitude of therapeutic effects obtained in an antidepressant study (Greenberg, Fisher, & Riter, 1995; Reinherr, Ward, & Byerly, 1989; Trivedi & Rush, 1994), this methodological variation may limit the generalizability of the results obtained by Parsons et al. (1989).

In the only double-blind, placebo-controlled study of amitriptyline in the treatment of BPD, Soloff, George, Nathan, Schulz, and Perel (1986) found a significant decrease in depressive symptoms in 45 amitriptyline-treated outpatients relative to 45 outpatient controls. One unexpected finding emerged from this investigation, however: A substantial portion of amitriptyline-treated patients became significantly worse during the investigation showing increases in impulsive, assaultive, and/or suicidal behavior (Soloff, George, & Nathan, 1987).

Finally, Salzman et al. (1995) obtained mixed results when they compared fluoxetine and placebo effects in a mixed-sex sample of 21 BPD outpatients followed over a 13-week period. Two-thirds of the patient sample met criteria for BPD diagnosis; the remaining patients "exhibited [borderline] traits" (Salzman et al., 1995, p. 24). Positive results were obtained in one area: Over time, fluoxetine-treated patients showed significant decreases in therapist-rated anger relative to control patients. Negative results were obtained in three areas: No fluoxetine-placebo differences were found for therapist ratings of patient mood, depression, and global level of functioning.

Taken together, studies of the effects of antidepressant medications on BPD and BPD-related symptoms have produced weak and unconvincing results. Many investigations have reported minimal advantages of antidepressants over placebos, and even those studies which obtain positive results in some areas almost invariably obtain nonsignificant results on the majority of dimensions assessed. Moreover, virtually every investigation in this area has suffered from at least one methodological flaw significant enough to call into question the results obtained in the study.

ANXIOLYTICS

In many ways, anxiolytic medications would appear to be the drugs of choice for BPD. Although borderline patients show a wide range of symptoms, it seems that anxiety (or more precisely, the BPD patient's inability to modulate anxiety) plays a critical role in the dynamics of borderline pathology (Freeman & Leaf, 1989; Millon, 1981). Moreover, clinical and empirical findings confirm that increases in anxiety levels exacerbate longstanding BPD symptoms, including rage, impulsivity, and self-destructive behavior (Blatt, 1990; Greene et al., 1985; Kernberg, 1984).

In light of the key role that anxiety appears to play in the etiology and dynamics of BPD, it is surprising that there have been no double-blind, placebo-controlled studies examining the effects of anxiolytic medications on BPD symptoms. In fact, the only two studies examining the effects of anxiolytic medications on BPD symptoms used an open (nonblind) design and involved extremely small sample sizes ($n = 3$ in each study). The conclusions that can be drawn from these trials are very limited. In any case, Faltus (1984) reported that administration of alprozalam resulted in widespread symptom reduction in BPD patients (i.e., decreases in rage, anxiety, psychotic thinking, and depression). Similar results were obtained by Freinhar and Alvarez (1985), who also noted decreases in impulsivity in clonazepam-treated borderline patients. The absence of a placebo control makes these studies susceptible to rater bias and unreliability effects, both of which undermine the conclusions drawn in these studies (see Greenberg, Bornstein, Greenberg, & Fisher, 1992a, 1992b, for detailed discussions of this issue).

ANTIPSYCHOTICS

Although early speculation that BPD is linked to the schizophrenic spectrum (see Hoch & Polatin, 1949) has now been disproven (Brinkley, 1993; Kendler, Gruenberg, & Strauss, 1981), researchers continue to examine the effects of antipsychotic drugs on borderline symptoms. In part, these studies are based on the observation that BPD patients show substantial cognitive slippage and thought disorder, and may even experience micropsychotic or dissociative episodes when under stress (Millon, 1981). Some of the better-designed pharmacological treatment studies of BPD have involved neuroleptics.

Two studies compared the effects of different antipsychotic medications on BPD symptoms, but both studies lacked a placebo control group. Because of this limitation, the only conclusions that can be drawn from these investigations concern the relative efficacy of different antipsychotics. As it happens, both studies found no differences in the effects of the different drugs. Leone (1982) reported that both loxapine and chlorpromazine enhanced mood and decreased anger in a sample of 80 BPD patients followed over a 6-week period. Serban and Siegel (1984) obtained more wide-ranging effects, noting that both haloperidol and thiothixene reduced anxiety, depression, paranoia, and self-image problems in a sample of 52 borderline patients followed for 12 weeks.

Since 1980, there have been four double-blind, placebo-controlled studies assessing the efficacy of antipsychotic medications on BPD symptoms. Three of these investigations assessed the efficacy of haloperidol; the fourth study assessed the effects of thiothixene.

Investigations of haloperidol have produced mixed results. Whereas Soloff, George, Nathan, Schulz, Ulrich, and Perel (1986) found a significant increase in global ratings of functioning in a mixed-sex sample of 40 haloperidol-treated BPD patients followed over a 5-week period, Soloff and Millward (1983), using a similar design and a larger ($n = 70$) patient sample, found no advantage of haloperidol over placebo in BPD patients. Unfortunately, the 1983 study had a substantial dropout rate (55% in the haloperidol group and 43% in the placebo group), a problem common to many drug treatment studies (see Dewan & Koss, 1989). The 1986 study also suffered from a limitation common to many psychotropic drug investigations: wide variations in haloperidol dosage levels (2 to 12 mg/day), and a similarly wide variation in blood plasma levels (see Greenberg & Fisher, 1989, for a detailed discussion of this issue).

Cornelius, Soloff, George, Ulrich, and Perel (1993) obtained results diametrically opposed to those of Soloff et al. (Soloff & Millward, 1983; Soloff, George, Nathan, Schulz, Ulrich, et al., 1986), finding a significant increase in both depression and hypersomnia in a sample of 36 BPD-diagnosed outpatients treated with haloperidol for 16 weeks. These unexpected results led the researchers to question whether whatever positive short-term effects may result from this medication (e.g., those obtained by Soloff & Millward, 1983; Soloff, George, Nathan, Schulz, Ulrich, et al., 1986) are effective in the long term. Cornelius, Soloff, George, et al. (1993, p. 336) noted that their "findings demonstrate a lack of efficacy in the continuation therapy of BPD patients."

Consistent with the findings obtained in studies of haloperidol effects, the only placebo-controlled study assessing the efficacy of thiothixene produced very modest results. Relative to many other investigations in this area, the study conducted by Goldberg et al. (1986) was well-designed, with well-validated measures administered to a large ($n = 50$) patient sample by raters blind to treatment condition on eight separate occasions during the study. In addition, this was the only pharmacological treatment study of BPD wherein an active (i.e., side-effect-producing) placebo was used, maximizing the likelihood that patients and raters would provide symptom reports uncontaminated by knowledge of treatment condition (see Fisher & Greenberg, 1989b; Greenberg et al., 1992a, 1992b).

Goldberg et al. (1986) found significant decreases in ideas of reference, psychotic thinking, and obsessive-compulsive behavior in their thiothixine-treated patients (but not the placebo-treated patients) during the 12-week course of the study. On the negative side, however, Goldberg et al. found no significant change on the majority of symptom dimensions assessed in this investigation.

As was the case with antidepressant studies, the majority of studies assessing the effects of antipsychotic medications on BPD symptoms have been methodologically flawed. The best designed study in this area (Goldberg et al., 1986) produced mixed results, but this investigation raises the possibility that thiothixine might have some utility in reducing psychotic thinking and obsessive-compulsive behavior in BPD patients. The modest effects obtained in this investigation more than 10 years ago, as well as the ongoing need for replication in the psychopharmacology treatment literature, suggest that a replication and extension of this promising study is clearly in order.

ANTICONVULSANTS

Initial interest in the use of anticonvulsants in BPD treatment can be traced to the numerous studies demonstrating brain and central nervous system abnormalities in BPD patients (see Cowdry, Pickar, & Davies, 1986; Paris, 1994; Russ et al., 1994). Although the causal links between neurological dysfunction and BPD remain open to question, use of anticonvulsant drugs in the treatment of borderline symptoms has become increasingly popular in recent years.

Four published studies have assessed the effects of anticonvulsant medications on BPD symptoms, but two of these investigations (Stein, Simeon, Frenkel, Islam, & Hollander, 1995; Wilcox, 1994) used open designs. The two double-blind, placebo-controlled studies in this area both examined the effects of carbamazepine on BPD (and BPD-related) symptoms.

Cowdry and Gardner (1988) assessed the efficacy of carbamazepine versus placebo in 16 female BPD patients over an 8-week period, and obtained mixed results. On the positive side, therapist ratings of mood and behavioral dyscontrol showed significant improvements in the carbamazepine group but not in the placebo group. On the negative side, patients' self-ratings of mood did not differ in the drug and placebo groups. In addition, this study had a high dropout rate (45%), suggesting that the results obtained may be an overestimate of the actual therapeutic effect of this drug on BPD symptoms. The finding of stronger effects for therapist than patient ratings is not unusual in these studies, especially for those investigations that do not employ an active placebo (Greenberg, Bornstein, Zborowski, Fisher, & Greenberg, 1994).

Negative results in this area were also obtained by De la Fuente and Lotstra (1994), who compared carbamazepine and placebo in 20 borderline inpatients over a 4-week period. Although 13 different outcome measures were used in this study, with each measure administered to each patient at two different dates, no differences were found between the drug and placebo groups on any outcome measure.

Anticonvulsant drugs do not look promising in the treatment of borderline symptoms. Of the two studies conducted to date, one produced mixed results, and the other found no advantage whatsoever of anticonvulsant over placebo. Future investigations involving other anticonvulsants—or higher carbamazepine levels—might well produce more positive findings.

LITHIUM

The rationale underlying use of lithium in BPD treatment is unclear. Some researchers have argued that lithium may be useful in treatment of borderline symptoms because of its aggression-reducing effects (Sheard, Marini, & Bridges, 1976). Others contend that the primary reason to explore lithium treatment of BPD is that lithium has proven to have mood-stabilizing properties in many bipolar patients (LaWall & Wesselius, 1982). At any rate, lithium treatment of BPD symptoms remains in the exploratory stage.

Links, Steiner, Boiago, and Irwin (1990) conducted the only double-blind, placebo-controlled study of lithium in the treatment of BPD patients, following 19 patients over 22 weeks. Only two patients (11% of the initial sample) completed the entire 22-week treatment course; the others dropped out of the study due to side effect problems or lack of therapeutic effect. In any case, no statistically significant findings emerged in this study, even for measures taken earlier in the trial period, when a higher percentage of patients were still participating in the investigation. No lithium-placebo differences were found for level of depression, anger, or suicidal ideation. As is typical in pharmacological treatment studies, therapist ratings of change showed somewhat greater trends toward significance than did patient ratings of change (Greenberg et al., 1994). More (and better) data are needed before the therapeutic effects of lithium on BPD symptoms can be evaluated meaningfully.

DISCUSSION

A review of the available data on pharmacological treatment of BPD indicates that while some positive results have been obtained in isolated studies, no medication has proved consistently effective in reducing BPD symptoms. The effects of the antipsychotic drug thiothixine may be somewhat more powerful than those of other drugs assessed thus far, but even this conclusion must be considered tentative insofar as it is based on the results of a single clinical trial involving 60 subjects and a 12-week assessment period (Goldberg et al., 1986). Additional research examining pharmacological treatment of BPD is warranted, and as new psychotropic medications are developed and refined, it is possible that stronger and more consistent results will be obtained. At present, however, the most reasonable and conservative conclusion to be drawn is that no single pharmacological agent has demonstrated efficacy in the treatment of borderline symptoms.

The question remains: Why have studies in this area produced such inconsistent and inconclusive results? Two reasons come to mind. First, many studies of pharmacological treatments of BPD proceed in "scatter-shot" fashion and lack a sound theoretical base (see Brinkley, 1993, for a detailed discussion of this issue). In part, the absence of a single over-arching theoretical framework reflects disagreement about the etiology of BPD, and about the physiological causes—if any—that underlie this disorder (Egan, 1986; Silk, 1994). Unless the physiological basis of BPD is more firmly established, it will be difficult for drug treatment studies to advance in a cohesive, integrative manner.

Second, almost every study published in this area during the past 15 years suffers from one or more significant methodological flaws. These include the absence of an active placebo control group, small sample sizes in many investigations, high subject dropout rates, and the use of questionable outcome measures of psychological functioning and symptom levels (see Fisher & Greenberg, 1989a, for a review of these and other methodological flaws in contemporary drug treatment studies).

To be sure, many psychotherapy outcome studies suffer from similar methodological flaws (most importantly, the absence of an "active placebo" control group). Moreover, psychotherapy outcome studies involving BPD-diagnosed patients, like pharmacological treatment studies, have generally produced only modest results (see Linehan et al., 1994; Links, Mitton, & Steiner, 1990; Stevenson & Meares, 1992; Tucker, Bauer, Wagner, Harlam, & Sher, 1987). Still, it is remarkable that despite their methodological limitations, which for the most part tend to exaggerate the observed efficacy of pharmacological agents used in BPD treatment, no published studies in this area have produced unambiguously positive results (see also Jacobson & Hollon, 1996; Sommers-Flanagan & Sommers-Flanagan, 1996, for related discussions of the antidepressant treatment literature).

To some extent, the methodological problems characterizing BPD treatment studies are understandable and unavoidable: Ethical constraints limit the kinds of experimental manipulations that may be employed in these investigations, and the welfare of patients participating in these studies must always take precedence over the collection of methodologically "pure" clinical data. Nonetheless, pharmacological treatment studies are extremely expensive to implement and carry out, and given the ever-diminishing pool of research funds available for these and other treatment investigations, greater precautions must be taken to ensure that those studies actually performed are of the highest possible quality (see Klein, 1996). One or two well-designed studies in this area would be preferable to a plethora of flawed clinical trials.

Two methodological problems common to virtually every study in this area warrant brief discussion in this context. First, reliability data for BPD diagnoses are almost never reported in these investigations. In fact, every double-blind study reviewed in this chapter used existing diagnoses, often derived from chart records, to select subjects for inclusion in the investigation. As noted earlier, interdiagnostician reliability for psychiatric diagnoses is modest at best, and quite poor for most Axis II disorders (see Bornstein, 1995). Future studies in this area must take greater precautions to ensure that treatment groups are homogeneous with respect to diagnostic profile and symptom severity.

In addition, the absence of any long-term follow-up data prevent us from knowing the degree to which short-term treatment effects produced by these pharmacological agents persist over an extended period. Long-term efficacy studies will be particularly important in this domain because of the high recidivism rates for borderline patients (Kernberg, Selzer, Koenigsberg, Carr, & Appelbaum, 1989), and the high risk of drug-induced side effects in many pharmacological treatment regimens (Dewan & Koss, 1989). This latter issue is, unfortunately, likely to be even more problematic for BPD patients than for patients with other Axis II disorders (Silk, 1994; Smith, Koenigsberg, Yeomans, & Clarkin, 1995).

Given the practical and ethical constraints involved in designing methodologically sound pharmacological treatment studies for BPD, coupled with the well-recognized difficulties associated with all forms of BPD treatment, it may be time to shift the focus of research in this area. To date, drug studies of BPD have invariably assessed the effects of one or more psychotropic medications on BPD-related symptoms. The goal of these studies is maximal symptom reduction. Given the modest results produced thus far, in these and other areas of pharmacological treatment research, perhaps symptom reduction per se should no longer be the primary outcome measure in these investigations.

I propose that future BPD drug treatment studies assess the effects of different pharmacological agents on the patient's capacity to benefit from psychotherapy, rather than on psychological symptoms themselves. In other words, BPD drug treatment studies should always be conducted with patients currently undergoing some well-established mode of psychotherapy, and the outcome measures used in these studies should focus on psychotherapeutic efficacy (or the patient's ability to engage in productive therapeutic work) rather than on psychological symptom reduction.

To be sure, there is no empirical evidence indicating that pharmacological treatments are likely to produce stronger results in facilitating therapy than in reducing psychological symptom. Nonetheless, such an approach—while speculative—has three significant advantages over the current research strategy.

First, it allows researchers to include in their investigations patient- and therapist-rated outcome measures of psychotherapy process and outcome that have well-established construct validity. Several such measures are currently available (see Luborsky & Crits-Christoph, 1990; Weiss & Sampson, 1986). Others are now being developed and will be available in the near future (Bornstein & Bowen, 1995). Although not without their limitations, these therapy-based outcome measures typically produce stronger reliability and validity data than most of the symptom-oriented outcome measures used in pharmacological treatment studies (Murray, 1989).

Second, examining the effects of pharmacological agents on psychotherapy progress is likely to produce better results than traditional drug treatment studies, in part because these investigations can actually capitalize on the modest effects produced by many psychotropic drugs. When the efficacy of a pharmacological agent is assessed in terms of psychotherapeutic efficacy, it may actually be the case that modest drug effects are more useful than powerful drug effects. As clinical research has long indicated, traditional forms of psychotherapy tend to be most effective when a patient is experiencing a moderate degree of psychological discomfort (Clarke, 1995; Weisz, Weiss, Han, & Granger, 1995). Too little discomfort results in a lack of motivation to engage in productive therapeutic work; too much discomfort can be inhibiting and counterproductive (Cashdan, 1973, 1988; Clementer, Malan, & Trauer, 1990). Thus, whereas the "ideal" outcome in a traditional drug treatment study is wholesale symptom reduction (which few pharmacological agents are able to provide), the ideal outcome in a therapy-based drug treatment study is modest symptom reduction (which may be a more realistic aim for most of the pharmacological agents currently available).[1]

---

[1] It is important to distinguish capacity to benefit from psychotherapy from the degree of improvement resulting from therapy. Although a plethora of findings confirm that patients who show the highest "cure rates" in therapy are those who have the least severe and least debilitating symptoms to start with (e.g., Parloff, 1984; Smith, Glass, & Miller,

Finally, a modified approach to pharmacological treatment of BPD allows the clinician to use every tool available to work with the BPD patient, employing a multimodal approach rather than a unidimensional one. As Goldstein (1995) noted, diagnosis and treatment of BPD will be enhanced if and when clinicians focus on understanding the borderline patient's strengths and coping skills rather than focusing more or less completely on the BPD patient's symptoms and deficits. Combined psychological and pharmacological treatment of BPD may be an important step in that direction.

CONCLUSION

By shifting the emphasis of BPD drug treatment studies from symptom reduction to psychotherapy enhancement, researchers will in many respects have come full circle. Several decades ago, interest in pharmacological treatment of BPD was stimulated in part by clinicians' and clinical researchers' frustration regarding the ostensible failure of traditional insight-oriented psychotherapy to ameliorate BPD symptoms (see Brinkley et al., 1979). During the 1980s and 1990s, BPD treatment studies have focused more and more on pharmacological rather than psychological interventions (Kernberg et al., 1989; Linehan et al., 1994; Paris, 1994). By "joining forces," psychotherapy and pharmacotherapy researchers have an opportunity to produce stronger results in BPD treatment than either camp has been able to produce alone.

An integrated psychotherapeutic-pharmacological approach to BPD treatment is also consistent with the viewpoint that BPD, like many other Axis I and Axis II disorders, cannot be classified neatly as being "psychological" or "physiological" in nature. It is both. BPD symptoms reflect the interplay of biological factors and psychological processes, although additional research is needed to disentangle the causal relationships between these variables (Millon, 1996). By reframing BPD drug studies to focus on psychotherapeutic process and outcome, researchers may uncover important new information about the interaction of biological and psychological processes in the etiology and dynamics of borderline conditions. A combined psychotherapeutic-psychopharmacological treatment approach will not only help clinicians develop more effective BPD treatments, but might also provide information that will allow borderline symptoms to be arrested before they develop into a full-blown, treatment-resistant Axis II disorder.

1980; Weisz & Weiss, 1993), numerous investigations confirm that a moderate level of symptom severity is associated with the strongest motivation to engage in productive therapeutic work over the long term (e.g., Clementer et al., 1990; Weisz et al., 1995).

REFERENCES

Akiskal, H. S., Djenderedjian, A. H., Rosenthal, T. L., & Khani, M. K. (1977). Cyclothymic disorder: Validating criteria for inclusion in the bipolar affective group. *American Journal of Psychiatry, 134,* 1227–1233.

American Psychiatric Association. (1980). *Diagnostic and statistical manual of mental disorders* (3rd ed.). Washington, DC: Author.

American Psychiatric Association. (1994). *Diagnostic and statistical manual of mental disorders* (4th ed.). Washington, DC: Author.

Blatt, S. J. (1990). Interpersonal relatedness and self-definition: Two personality configurations and their implications for psychopathology and psychotherapy. In J. L. Singer (Ed.), *Repression and dissociation* (pp. 299–335). Chicago: University of Chicago Press.

Blatt, S. J. (1991). A cognitive morphology of psychopathology. *Journal of Nervous and Mental Disease, 179,* 449–458.

Blatt, S. J., & Auerbach, J. S. (1988). Differential cognitive disturbances in three types of borderline patients. *Journal of Personality Disorders, 2,* 198–211.

Bornstein, R. F. (1995). Comorbidity of dependent personality disorder and other psychological disorders: An integrative review. *Journal of Personality Disorders, 9,* 286–303.

Bornstein, R. F., & Bowen, R. F. (1995). Dependency in psychotherapy: Toward an integrated treatment approach. *Psychotherapy, 32,* 520–534.

Brinkley, J. R. (1993). Pharmacotherapy of borderline states. *Psychopharmacology, 16,* 853–884.

Brinkley, J. R., Beitman, B. D., & Friedel, R. O. (1979). Low-dose neuroleptic regimens in the treatment of borderline patients. *Archives of General Psychiatry, 36,* 319–326.

Cashdan, S. (1973). *Interactional psychotherapy.* New York: Grune & Stratton.

Cashdan, S. (1988). *Object relations therapy.* New York: Norton.

Clarke, G. N. (1995). Improving the transition from basic efficacy research to effectiveness studies: Methodological issues and procedures. *Journal of Consulting and Clinical Psychology, 63,* 718–725.

Clementer, C., Malan, D., & Trauer, T. (1990). A retrospective follow-up study of 84 patients treated with individual psychoanalytic psychotherapy: Outcome and predictive factors. *British Journal of Psychotherapy, 6,* 363–374.

Coccaro, E. F., Astill, J. L., & Herbert, J. L. (1990). Fluoxetine treatment of impulsive aggression in *DSM-III-R* borderline personality disorder patients. *Journal of Clinical Psychopharmacology, 10,* 373–375.

Coen, S. J. (1992). *The misuse of persons: Analyzing pathological dependency.* Hillsdale, NJ: Erlbaum.

Cornelius, J. R., Soloff, P. H., George, A., Ulrich, R. F., & Perel, J. M. (1993). Haloperidol versus phenelzine in continuation therapy of borderline personality disorder. *Psychopharmacology Bulletin, 29,* 333–337.

Cornelius, J. R., Soloff, P. H., & Perel, J. M. (1990). Fluoxetine trial in borderline personality disorder. *Psychopharmacology Bulletin, 26,* 151–154.

Cornelius, J. R., Soloff, P. H., & Perel, J. M. (1991). A preliminary trial of fluoxetine in refractory borderline patients. *Journal of Clinical Psychopharmacology, 11,* 116–120.

Cornelius, J. R., Soloff, P. H., Perel, J. M., & Ulrich, R. F. (1993). Continuation pharmacotherapy of borderline personality disorder with haloperidol and phenelzine. *American Journal of Psychiatry, 150,* 1843–1848.

Cowdry, R. W., & Gardner, D. L. (1988). Pharmacotherapy of borderline personality disorder: Alprazolam, carbamezapine, trifluoperazine, and tranylcypromine. *Archives of General Psychiatry, 45,* 111–119.

Cowdry, R. W., Pickar, D., & Davies, R. (1986). Symptoms and EEG findings in the borderline syndrome. *International Journal of Psychiatry in Medicine, 15,* 201–211.

De la Fuente, J. M., & Lotstra, F. (1994). A trial of carbamazepine in borderline personality disorder. *European Neuropsychopharmacology, 4,* 479–486.

Dewan, M. J., & Koss, M. (1989). The clinical impact of the side effects of psychotropic drugs. In S. Fisher & R. P. Greenberg (Eds.), *The limits of biological treatments for psychological distress* (pp. 189–233). Hillsdale, NJ: Erlbaum.

Dyrud, J. E. (1972). The treatment of borderline syndrome. In E. Offer & D. X. Freedman (Eds.), *Modern psychiatry and clinical research* (pp. 159–173). New York: Basic Books.

Egan, J. (1986). Etiology and treatment of borderline personality disorder in adolescents. *Hospital and Community Psychiatry, 37,* 613–618.

Faltus, F. J. (1984). The positive effect of alprozalam in the treatment of three patients with borderline personality disorder. *American Journal of Psychiatry, 141,* 802–803.

Fisher, S., & Greenberg, R. P. (1989a). *The limits of biological treatments for psychological disorders.* Hillsdale, NJ: Erlbaum.

Fisher, S., & Greenberg, R. P. (1989b). A second opinion: Rethinking the claims of biological psychiatry. In S. Fisher & R. P. Greenberg (Eds.), *The limits of biological treatments for psychological distress* (pp. 309–336). Hillsdale, NJ: Erlbaum.

Freeman, A., & Leaf, R. C. (1989). Cognitive therapy applied to personality disorders. In A. Freeman, K. M. Simon, L. E. Beutler, & H. Arkowitz (Eds.), *Comprehensive handbook of cognitive therapy* (pp. 403–434). New York: Plenum Press.

Freinhar, J. P., & Alvarez, W. A. (1985). Clonazepam: A novel therapeutic adjunct. *International Journal of Psychiatry in Medicine, 15,* 321–328.

Goldberg, S. C., Schulz, C., Schulz, P. M., Resnick, R. J., Hamer, R. M., & Friedel, R. O. (1986). Borderline and schizotypal personality disorders treated with low-dose thiothixene versus placebo. *Archives of General Psychiatry, 43,* 680–686.

Goldstein, W. N. (1995). The borderline patient: Update on the diagnosis, theory, and treatment from a psychodynamic perspective. *American Journal of Psychotherapy, 49,* 317–336.

Greenberg, R. P., Bornstein, R. F., Greenberg, M. D., & Fisher, S. (1992a). A meta-analysis of antidepressant outcome under "blinder" conditions. *Journal of Consulting and Clinical Psychology, 60,* 664–669.

Greenberg, R. P., Bornstein, R. F., Greenberg, M. D., & Fisher, S. (1992b). As for the kings: On depressant subtypes and antidepressant response. *Journal of Consulting and Clinical Psychology, 60,* 675–677.

Greenberg, R. P., Bornstein, R. F., Zborowski, M. J., Fisher, S., & Greenberg, M. D. (1994). A meta-analysis of fluoxetine outcome in the treatment of depression. *Journal of Nervous and Mental Disease, 182,* 547–551.

Greenberg, R. P., & Fisher, S. (1989). Examining antidepressant effectiveness: Findings, ambiguities, and some vexing puzzles. In S. Fisher & R. P. Greenberg (Eds.), *The limits of biological treatments for psychological distress* (pp. 1–38). Hillsdale, NJ: Erlbaum.

Greenberg, R. P., Fisher, S., & Riter, J. A. (1995). Placebo washout is not a meaningful part of antidepressant drug trials. *Perceptual and Motor Skills, 81,* 688–690.

Greene, L. R., Rosenkrantz, J., & Muth, D. Y. (1985). Splitting dynamics, self-representations and boundary phenomena in the group psychotherapy of borderline personality disorders. *Psychiatry, 48,* 234–245.

Grinker, R. R., Werble, B., & Drye, R. C. (1968). *The borderline syndrome: A behavioral study of ego functions.* New York: Basic Books.

Gunderson, J. (1989). Borderline personality disorder. In A. Tasman, R. E. Hales, & A. J. Frances (Eds.), *The American Psychiatric Press review of psychiatry* (Vol. 8, pp. 3–125). Washington, DC: American Psychiatric Press.

Gunderson, J., & Phillips, K. A. (1991). A current view of the interface between borderline personality disorder and depression. *American Journal of Psychiatry, 148,* 967–975.

Gunderson, J., & Zanarini, M. (1987). Current overview of the borderline diagnosis. *Journal of Clinical Psychiatry, 48,* 5–11.

Havens, L. L. (1968). Some difficulties in giving schizophrenic and borderline patients medications. *Psychiatry, 31,* 44–50.

Hoch, P., & Polatin, P. (1949). Pseudoneurotic forms of schizophrenia. *Psychoanalytic Quarterly, 23,* 248–276.

Hughes, C. H. (1884). Moral (affective) insanity: Psycho-sensory insanity. *Alienist and Neurologist, 5,* 296–315.

Hull, J. W., Clarkin, J. F., & Alexopoulos, G. S. (1993). A time series analysis of intervention effects: Fluoxetine therapy as a case illustration. *Journal of Nervous and Mental Disease, 181,* 48–53.

Jacobson, N. S., & Hollon, S. D. (1996). Cognitive-behavior therapy versus pharmacotherapy: Now that the jury's returned its verdict, it's time to present the rest of the evidence. *Journal of Consulting and Clinical Psychology, 64,* 74–80.

Kendler, K. S., Gruenberg, A. M., & Strauss, J. S. (1981). An independent analysis of the Copenhagen sample of the Danish Adoption Study of schizophrenia: 2. The relationship between schizotypal personality disorder and schizophrenia. *Archives of General Psychiatry, 38,* 982–984.

Kernberg, O. F. (1968). The treatment of patients with borderline personality organization. *International Journal of Psychoanalysis, 49,* 600–619.

Kernberg, O. F. (1970). A psychoanalytic classification of character pathology. *Journal of the American Psychoanalytic Association, 18,* 800–822.

Kernberg, O. F. (1975). *Borderline conditions and pathological narcissism.* New York: Aronson.

Kernberg, O. F. (1984). *Severe personality disorders.* New Haven, CT: Yale University Press.

Kernberg, O. F., Selzer, M. A., Koenigsberg, H. W., Carr, A. C., & Appelbaum, A. H. (1989). *Psychodynamic psychotherapy of borderline patients.* New York: Basic Books.

Klein, D. F. (1975). Psychopharmacology and the borderline patient. In J. E. Mack (Ed.), *Borderline states in psychiatry* (pp. 75–92). New York: Grune & Stratton.

Klein, D. F. (1977). Psychopharmacological treatment and delineation of borderline disorders. In P. Hortocollis (Ed.), *Borderline personality disorders* (pp. 365–383). New York: International Universities Press.

Klein, D. F. (1996). Preventing hung juries about therapy studies. *Journal of Consulting and Clinical Psychology, 64,* 81–87.

Kohut, H. (1971). *The analysis of the self.* New York: International Universities Press.

Kohut, H. (1977). *The restoration of the self.* New York: International Universities Press.

Kraepelin, E. (1915). *Psychiatrie: Ein lehrbuch* (8th ed.). Leipzig: Barth.

Kretschmer, E. (1925). *Physique and character.* London: Kegan Paul.

Kutcher, S., Blackwood, D., & St. Clair, D. (1987). Auditory P300 in borderline personality disorder and schizophrenia. *Archives of General Psychiatry, 44,* 645–650.

Kutcher, S., Papatheodorou, G., Reiter, S., & Gardner, D. (1995). The successful pharmacological treatment of adolescents and young adults with borderline personality disorder: A preliminary open trial of flupenthixol. *Journal of Psychiatry and Neuroscience, 20,* 113–118.

Langley, M. H. (1994). *Self-management therapy for borderline personality disorder: A therapist-guided approach.* New York: Springer.

LaWall, J. S., & Wesselius, C. L. (1982). The use of lithium carbonate in borderline patients. *Journal of Psychiatric Treatment Evaluation, 4,* 265–267.

Lazarus, A. R. (1982). *The practice of multimodal therapy.* New York: McGraw-Hill.

Leibovich, M. A. (1983). Why short-term therapy for borderlines? *Psychotherapy and Psychosomatics, 39,* 1–9.

Leone, N. F. (1982). Response of borderline patients to loxapine and chlorpromazine. *Journal of Clinical Psychiatry, 43,* 148–150.

Liebowitz, M. R., & Klein, D. F. (1981). Inter-relationship of hysteroid dysphoria and borderline personality disorder. *Psychiatric Clinics of North America, 4,* 67–87.

Linehan, M. M., Tutek, D. A., Heard, H. L., & Armstrong, H. E. (1994). Interpersonal outcome of cognitive behavioral treatment for chronically suicidal borderline patients. *American Journal of Psychiatry, 151,* 1771–1776.

Links, P. S., Mitton, J. E., & Steiner, M. (1990). Predicting outcome for borderline personality disorder. *Comprehensive Psychiatry, 31,* 490–498.

Links, P. S., Steiner, M., Boiago, I., & Irwin, D. (1990). Lithium therapy for border-line patients: Preliminary findings. *Journal of Personality Disorders, 4*, 173–181.

Luborsky, L., & Crits-Christoph, P. (1990). *Understanding transference: The core conflictual relationship theme method.* New York: Basic Books.

Markowitz, P. J., Calabrese, J. R., & Schulz, S. C. (1991). Fluoxetine in the treat-ment of borderline and schizotypal personality. *American Journal of Psychia-try, 148*, 1064–1067.

McCann, J. T. (1991). Convergent and discriminant validity of the MCMI-II and MMPI personality disorder scales. *Psychological Assessment, 3*, 9–18.

Millon, T. (1969). *Modern psychopathology: A biosocial approach to maladaptive learn-ing and functioning.* Philadelphia: Saunders.

Millon, T. (1981). *Disorders of personality.* New York: Wiley.

Millon, T. (1996). *Disorders of personality: DSM-IV and beyond.* New York: Wiley.

Murray, E. J. (1989). Measurement issues in the evaluation of psychopharmaco-logical therapy. In S. Fisher & R. P. Greenberg (Eds.), *The limits of biological treatments for psychological distress* (pp. 39–68). Hillsdale, NJ: Erlbaum.

Nace, E. P. (1992). Alcoholism and the borderline patient. In D. Silver & M. Rosenbluth (Eds.), *Handbook of borderline disorders* (pp. 677–722). Madison, CT: International Universities Press.

Norden, M. J. (1989). Fluoxetine in borderline personality disorder. *Progress in Neuro-Psychopharmacology and Biological Psychiatry, 13*, 885–893.

Paris, J. (1994). *Borderline personality disorder: A multidimensional approach.* Wash-ington, DC: American Psychiatric Press.

Parloff, M. B. (1984). Psychotherapy research and its incredible credibility crisis. *Clinical Psychology Review, 4*, 95–109.

Parsons, B., Quitkin, F. M., McGrath, P. J., Stewart, J. W., Tricamo, E., Ocepek-Welikson, K., Harrison, W., Rabkin, J. G., Wager, S. C., & Nunes, E. (1989). Phenelzine, imipramine and placebo in borderline patients meeting crite-ria for atypical depression. *Psychopharmacology Bulletin, 25*, 524–534.

Perry, J. C., & Klerman, G. L. (1978). The borderline patient. *Archives of General Psychiatry, 35*, 141–150.

Perry, S. (1989). Treatment time and the borderline patient: An underappreciated strategy. *Journal of Personality Disorders, 3*, 230–239.

Reinherr, F. W., Ward, M. F., & Byerly, W. F. (1989). The introductory placebo washout: A retrospective evaluation. *Psychiatry Research, 30*, 191–199.

Russ, M. W., Roth, S. D., Kakuma, T., Harrison, K., & Hull, J. W. (1994). Pain per-ception in self-injurious borderline patients: Naloxone effects. *Biological Psy-chiatry, 35*, 207–209.

Salzman, C., Wolfson, A. N., Schatzberg, A., Looper, J., Henke, R., Albanese, M., Schwartz, J., & Miyawaki, E. (1995). Effect of flouxetine on anger in sympto-matic volunteers with borderline personality disorder. *Journal of Clinical Psy-chopharmacology, 15*, 23–29.

Serban, G., & Siegel, S. (1984). Response of borderline and schizotypal patients to small doses of thiothixene and haloperidol. *American Journal of Psychiatry, 141*, 1455–1458.

Shea, M. T., Widiger, T. A., & Klein, M. H. (1992). Comorbidity of personality disorders and depression: Implications for treatment. *Journal of Consulting and Clinical Psychology, 60,* 857–868.

Sheard, M. H., Marini, J. L., & Bridges, C. I. (1976). The effects of lithium on impulsive aggressive behavior in man. *American Journal of Psychiatry, 133,* 1409–1413.

Silk, K. R. (1994). *Biological and neurobehavioral studies of borderline personality disorder.* Washington, DC: American Psychiatric Press.

Smith, M. L., Glass, G. V., & Miller, T. L. (1980). *The benefits of psychotherapy.* Baltimore, MD: Johns Hopkins University Press.

Smith, T. E., Koenigsberg, H. W., Yeomans, F. E., & Clarkin, J. F. (1995). Predictors of dropout in psychodynamic psychotherapy of borderline personality disorder. *Journal of Psychotherapy Practice and Research, 4,* 205–213.

Soloff, P. H., Cornelius, J., & George, A. (1991). The depressed borderline: One disorder or two? *Psychopharmacology Bulletin, 27,* 23–30.

Soloff, P. H., George, A., & Nathan, R. S. (1987). Behavioral dyscontrol in borderline patients treated with amitriptyline. *Psychopharmacology Bulletin, 23,* 177–181.

Soloff, P. H., George, A., Nathan, R. S., Schulz, P. M., & Perel, J. M. (1986). Paradoxical effects of amitriptyline on borderline patients. *American Journal of Psychiatry, 143,* 1603–1605.

Soloff, P. H., George, A., Nathan, R. S., Schulz, P. M., Ulrich, R. F., & Perel, J. M. (1986). Progress in pharmacotherapy of borderline disorders. *Archives of General Psychiatry, 43,* 691–697.

Soloff, P. H., & Millward, J. W. (1983). Psychiatric disorders in the families of borderline patients. *Archives of General Psychiatry, 40,* 37–48.

Sommers-Flanagan, J., & Sommers-Flanagan, R. (1996). Effect of antidepressant medication with depressed youth: What psychologists should know. *Professional Psychology, 27,* 145–153.

Stein, D. J., Simeon, D., Frenkel, M., Islam, M. N., & Hollander, E. (1995). An open trial of valproate in borderline personality disorder. *Journal of Clinical Psychiatry, 56,* 506–510.

Stein, K. F. (1996). Affect instability in adults with a borderline personality disorder. *Archives of Psychiatric Nursing, 10,* 32–40.

Stern, A. (1938). Psychoanalytic investigation of and therapy in the border line group of neuroses. *Psychoanalytic Quarterly, 7,* 467–489.

Stevenson, J., & Meares, R. (1992). An outcome study of psychotherapy for patients with borderline personality disorder. *American Journal of Psychiatry, 149,* 358–362.

Trivedi, M. H., & Rush, J. (1994). Does a placebo run-in or a placebo treatment cell affect the efficacy of antidepressant medications? *Neuropsychopharmacology, 11,* 33–43.

Tucker, L., Bauer, S. F., Wagner, S., Harlam, D., & Sher, I. (1987). Long-term hospital treatment of borderline patients: A descriptive outcome study. *American Journal of Psychiatry, 144,* 1443–1448.

Tuinier, S., & Verhoeven, W. M. A. (1995). Dimensional classification and behavioral pharmacology of personality disorders: A review and hypothesis. *European Neuropsychopharmacology, 5,* 135–146.

Weiss, J., & Sampson, H. (1986). *The psychoanalytic process: Theory, observations and clinical research.* New York: Guilford Press.

Weissman, M. M. (1993). The epidemiology of personality disorders: An update. *Journal of Personality Disorders, 7,* 44–62.

Weisz, J. R., & Weiss, B. (1993). *Effects of psychotherapy with children and adolescents.* Newbury Park, CA: Sage.

Weisz, J. R., Weiss, B., Han, S. S., & Granger, D. A. (1995). Effects of psychotherapy with children and adolescents revisited: A meta-analysis of treatment outcome studies. *Psychological Bulletin, 117,* 450–468.

Westen, D. (1991). Cognitive-behavioral interventions in the psychoanalytic psychotherapy of borderline personality disorders. *Clinical Psychology Review, 11,* 211–230.

Wilcox, J. (1994). Divalproex sodium in the treatment of aggressive behavior. *Annals of Clinical Psychiatry, 6,* 17–20.

PART THREE

EFFICACIES OF PSYCHOACTIVE DRUGS FOR CHILDREN

CHAPTER 8

Are We Justified in Treating Children with Psychotropic Drugs?

RHODA L. FISHER and SEYMOUR FISHER

P SYCHOTROPIC DRUGS NOW play a prominent role in the treatment of psychological disturbance in children and adolescents. Pediatricians and child psychiatrists dispense large quantities of psychotropic medications to the youth segment of the population. In 1992, there were multiple millions of prescriptions for such drugs. Even in the age range 0 to 4 years, prescriptions exceeding a million were reported (Jensen, Vitiello, Leonard, & Loughren, 1994). Practitioners claim drugs can ameliorate such diverse symptoms as depression, mania, anxiety, and obsession-compulsion. In fact, psychotropic drugs are often also prescribed for numerous other symptom categories (e.g., poorly controlled aggression, school failure, enuresis, phobias, eating difficulties, antisocial activities). Additionally, a remarkable percentage of children (largely boys) is also being treated with drugs for that amorphous state known as attention-deficit/hyperactivity disorder (ADHD; see Chapter 9).

DEPRESSION

This appraisal of the literature concerned with the efficacy of psychotropic treatments for psychological disturbance in children and adolescents will begin with the use of antidepressants to banish depression in

307

the youth population. Literally millions of depressed children are being managed with drugs like imipramine and fluoxetine. Goleman (1993) states that 4 to 6 million prescriptions for desipramine and related medications were written in 1992 for depressed children under 18 years of age. In most locales, it is standard practice to put depressed children on a psychotropic regimen. Many textbooks (e.g., Green, 1991) routinely advise such use of antidepressants.

However, a probe of the available scientific reservoir of pertinent studies does not reveal any serious evidence that antidepressants do more for childhood depression than do placebos. We found 13 double-blind, placebo-controlled studies that have evaluated the therapeutic power of antidepressants for children and adolescents, as follows: Boules et al., 1991; Geller, Cooper, Graham, Marsfeller, and Bryant, 1990; Geller et al., 1992; Hughes et al., 1990; Kashani, Shekim, and Reid, 1994; Kramer and Feiguine, 1981; Kutcher, Boulos, Ward, and Marton, 1994; Lucas, Lockett, and Grimm, 1965; Petti and Law, 1982; Preskorn, Weller, Hughes, Weller, and Bolte, 1987;[1] Puig-Antich et al., 1979; Puig-Antich et al., 1987; Simeon, DiNicola, Phil, Ferguson, and Copping, 1990.

No one has really shown a therapeutic advantage for drug over placebo in samples of depressed children, with the possible exception of a few marginal instances. Actually, two studies (Geller et al., 1990; Puig-Antich et al., 1987) have provided examples of placebo exceeding active drug in power. The failure of antidepressants to demonstrate therapeutic efficacy has been recognized by numerous scholars.[2] Gadow (1991) stated: "To date, none of the placebo-controlled, double-blind studies of tricyclics in depressed prepubertal children have found drug therapy to be superior to placebo . . . Equally discouraging are the findings from drug studies of depressed adolescents" (pp. 843–844).

Green (1991) remarked: "A literature review of the use of tricyclic antidepressants in children and adolescents with major depression found them to be clinically effective in several open studies, but no double-blind

---

[1] Although Preskorn et al. (1987) stated in one phase of their report that an antidepressant was more effective than a placebo in treating depressed prepubertal children, one finds, upon closer examination, that not only was the actively treated sample reduced to an N of 9, but also the statistical analysis was seriously deficient insofar as no attempt was made to ascertain if there were differences in baseline depression levels between the drug-treated and placebo samples.

[2] Thurber, Ensign, Punnett, and Welter (1995) surveyed a large spectrum of the open and also blind studies that have evaluated the efficacy of antidepressants for children and adolescents. One of their particularly interesting findings was an inverse relationship between apparent efficacy and the presence of adequate experimental controls.

placebo controlled study reported that tricyclics were superior to placebo" (p. 115).[3]

In a review of studies published between 1985 and 1994 concerned with the efficacy of antidepressants for children and adolescents, Sommers-Flanagan and Sommers-Flanagan (1996) came to a similar negative conclusion: "Results indicate that (anti-depressants) have not demonstrated greater efficacy than placebo in alleviating depressive symptoms in children and adolescents, despite the use of research strategies designed to give anti-depressants an advantage over placebo" (p. 145). Relatedly, Hazell, O'Connell, Heathcote, Robertson, and Henry (1995), after completing a meta-analysis of 12 controlled studies of the efficacy of tricyclic drugs for children and adolescents, concluded: "Tricyclic antidepressants appear to be no more effective than placebo in the treatment of depression in children and adolescents" (p. 897).

A medley of findings converge in affirming that antidepressants are no more effective than placebos in alleviating depression in children. Such findings have gradually stirred uneasiness in practitioners who continue to distribute antidepressants widely. This uneasiness has been further reinforced because several children have died suddenly, and unexplainably while taking desipramine (Riddle, Geller, & Ryan, 1993; Zimnitzky & Popper, 1995). Probably there is some increased cardiac risk associated with treating children with psychotropic agents like desipramine (Biederman, Thisted, Greenhill, & Ryan, 1995; Waslick, 1995).

The tension aroused by the contradiction between research findings and widespread clinical practices relative to treating depression in children was officially addressed in an editorial written by Charles Popper (1992) in the *Journal of Child and Adolescent Psychopharmacology*. The editorial declared:

> But there is no escaping the fact that research studies certainly have not supported the efficacy of tricyclic antidepressants in treating depressed adolescents. There are critical questions about this treatment which, simply

---

[3] Other investigators have made similar comments. Thus, Ambrosini, Bianchi, Rabinovish, and Ella (1993) concluded: "The empirical data reviewed does not support antidepressant efficacy in child and adolescent Major Depressive Disorder, neither when results are collated nor when the few double-blind placebo-controlled studies are reviewed empirically" (p. 3).

Further, Conners (1992) stated: "Widespread use of tricyclic antidepressant (TCA) drug treatment for depressed adolescents reflects a momentum continuing from early uncontrolled trials in adolescents and children, as well as the apparent success of controlled trials of TCA therapy among adults. The results of more recent controlled trials in youths, however, are uniformly negative" (p. 11).

put, appear to have been demonstrated to be ineffective. Yet clinicians have come to use antidepressants to treat adolescent depression on such a wide scale that it has become essentially a standard of practice in many locales. Even many of the researchers who have found negative findings in their studies continue to use tricyclic antidepressants in treating adolescents in their clinical practice.

What is going on here? What has become of the tradition of research in laying the groundwork and leading the way to improved clinical care? (p. 1)

The editorial further offers reasons why clinicians may be wiser than the published research conclusions about antidepressant effectiveness with children. Illustratively, the editorial asserts that the clinician's definition of depression may be more realistic than the *DSM-III-R* criteria utilized by researchers; that clinical treatment is more flexible; that individual patient outcome patterns are appraised in a more detailed fashion clinically than is typical of the research mode; and so forth. In addition, the editorial suggests: "At present, clinicians must again use their professional judgment when making treatment recommendations, bearing in mind the uncertainties. Among the uncertainties regarding antidepressant treatment of adolescents, we have to ask whether the clinicians are ahead of the researchers, or whether the handwriting on the wall is just hard to believe" (p. 3).

What we see here is an editorial telling clinicians to feel free to continue to prescribe antidepressants for children despite the tide of research data indicating that they are no more therapeutic than placebos. Presumably, since research enterprises have flaws they can, in good conscience, be bypassed. One finds analogous postures taken in various textbooks. Consider a recent publication, *Handbook of Depression in Children and Adolescents*, by Johnson and Fruehling (1994). After analyzing the usual repertoire of studies indicating that antidepressants are no more therapeutic than placebos for children, they inform the reader that it is premature to portray antidepressants as not being a valid form of treatment for children. To rationalize their conclusion, they state:

Perhaps the most persuasive reason is the widespread clinical use of these medications in depressed children. *It seems unlikely that clinicians would continue to prescribe these medications if no clinical benefit were being realized.* Second, the studies completed thus far are all methodologically compromised, yet many of them show trends toward efficacy that are not statistically significant [italics added]. (p. 388)

Apparently, Johnson and Fruehling assume that if the scientific data go the wrong way, it is fair to switch to a different set of justifying criteria. It is also a bit disconcerting to be informed that a treatment is probably valid because numerous clinicians are using it. The history of many therapeutic descriptions is replete with examples of treatments that were widely popular but eventually proved to have no value.

Others have empathized with the right of clinicians to ignore research findings if they find individual reasons to do so. The question is what limits should be placed on such individual intuitions? One justification for clinicians to ignore research data is that formal scientific studies of therapeutic efficacy state their results in terms of probabilities of success in composites of patients, whereas clinicians are concerned with the single patient. Clinicians are said to have to judge whether group findings apply to the individual in question. Wulff (1986) commented on this point in the *Journal of Medicine and Philosophy,* which devoted an issue to the process of decision making in medicine. He noted the ambiguity often surrounding therapeutic and diagnostic judgments about single cases, and suggested it is this ambiguity that probably invites going beyond what is scientifically known.

Actually, it is an old tradition in medicine to regard the practitioner as having the "final authority." This has fed opposition to defining physician judgments as synonymous with the scientific facts. Pellegrino and Thomasma (1981) comment:

> A large part of the physician's specific activity . . . depends upon skills outside of the traditional scientific paradigm. Whenever the physician resorts to experience or empirical data, he or she must use the scientific canon, but once the data are in, the physician's internal dialogue conforms more closely to the canons of the liberal arts. This does not mean that these canons are not susceptible to explicit analysis, but only that any unitary theory of medicine which identifies it exclusively with science is doomed to failure. (p. 147)

They point to a "tension between the scientific-actuarial and the artist-intuitionist models of clinical judgment" (p. 120).

Somewhat more self-disciplining ideas are expressed by other medical ethicists. Lynoe (1992) states: "For a physician with an academic medical education it would be unethical and irreconcilable with the tenets of science and proven experience to provide a treatment, the effect of which is indistinguishable from the placebo effect" (p. 221).

Similarly, Roy (1986) remarks: "When there is uncertainty or definite doubt about the safety or efficacy of an innovative or established treatment, there *is,* not simply *may* be a higher moral obligation to test it critically than to prescribe it year-in, year-out with the support of custom or of wishful thinking" (p. 286).

In surveying the current scene, it becomes obvious that clinicians frequently fashion treatment regimens that are not justified by what is known scientifically. The volume of antidepressants directed toward children exemplifies how the practitioners of disciplines (e.g., psychiatrists and pediatricians) can choose to pursue procedures that are opposed by the research facts and construct rationalizations for their actions. What limits should be placed on the license to outflank scientific cautions? How can practitioners be better motivated and prepared to use scientific findings?

The medical establishment periodically confronts such questions, as exemplified in publications by Banta and Thacker (1990) and Grimes (1993). Blame has been directed at the failure of medical schools to encourage a skeptical, appraising stance based on filtering information in the context of scientific networks. It has been proposed (Bishop, 1984; Grimes, 1993) that medical students be instructed in the essentials of experimental design and statistical theory so that they will acquire the tools for evaluating the validities of new treatments, drugs, and technologies offered to them. The problem that child psychiatrists have apparently had in assimilating the implications of the research bearing on treating children with antidepressants is not unique. Similar problems have surfaced with reference to such treatments and procedures as episiotomy, fetal monitoring, and electroencephalography (Banta & Thacker, 1990).

In any case, our central specific concern is whether any psychotropic drug should be prescribed for children or others in the absence of solid information that it is effective. Can it be at least agreed that no therapeutic mode should be recommended that has been shown empirically not to be more effective than a placebo?

In another context (Fisher & Fisher, 1996), we raised the very issues just reviewed and two discussants with medical ethicist credentials were asked to comment.

One of the commentators (Eisenberg, 1996) noted:

> The reason child psychiatrists and pediatricians continue to prescribe antidepressants is not far to seek. They are consulted by distressed patients and families. Yet, they have no reliable treatment. Not only is there no evidence to support drug use, but the other treatment modes that work for adults, cognitive behavior therapy (CBT) and interpersonal psychotherapy (ITP) have not been validated for adolescents. . . .
>
> Given this situation, what are doctors to do? After all, there is no obvious physiological reason why these treatments shouldn't work and there are no validated therapeutic alternatives . . . depression is associated with considerable morbidity. . . . Under these circumstances, few practitioners will feel they can dismiss the patient without an attempt at treatment. The fact that

clinicians continue to prescribe drugs in the face of negative research reports hardly establishes that clinicians "know" something researchers
don't; it reflects their limited options. (p. 103)

A second commentary was contributed by Pellegrino (1996):

> With most everyday treatments, there may be no evidence for benefit, but
> definitive evidence for ineffectiveness is lacking as well. . . . This is not the
> case, however, with the use of tricyclic antidepressants in children and
> adolescents. . . . Here there is substantial evidence of ineffectiveness in
> thirteen double-blind, placebo-controlled trials. In addition, there is some
> suggestion that they may be associated with sudden deaths which are oth-
> erwise unexplained. . . .
>   Despite these negative results, these agents are widely used, even by
> some of the same investigators whose published studies indicate there is no
> measurable therapeutic effect. (p. 106)

The energy for child psychiatry clinicians to disregard scientific standards came to a significant degree from early published reports of open
trials of antidepressants in youthful samples and also from letters to
editors that claimed great results. Such trials and letters are typically
pumped up, wishful reports that lack factual solidity. However, reputable
journals accept and propagate them and, in so doing, give them an aura
of scholarly authority. We seriously question whether scientific journals
should publish the results of open therapeutic trials. Such communications are typically misleading and set the stage for years of trying to sell
ineffective forms of therapy.

BIPOLAR DISORDERS

Lithium carbonate is by far the drug most frequently used to treat
manic-depressive children and adolescents. What is the state of the literature concerned with the efficacy of lithium in youthful populations?
Our searches indicate that a scientific literature is really nonexistent.
Goodwin and Jamison (1990) came to a similar conclusion: "Although
lithium has been used in all age groups since the initial prophylactic trials, studies of efficacy in the very young . . . are for the most part uncontrolled" (p. 691). A similar perspective is taken by Greenhill and
Setterberg (1993) and Lapierre and Raval (1989). Scattered studies (e.g.,
DeLong & Nieman, 1983; Strober, Morrell, Lampert, & Burroughs, 1990)
have sought to introduce some blindness and other controls into their designs, but one cannot take them seriously because they are based on very
small numbers and leave blatant opportunities for clinical judgment to

be contaminated by bias. At this point, not a single one of these studies deserves to be considered as properly controlled. There is also the usual quota of open and retrospective studies touting exaggerated therapeutic results (e.g., DeLong, 1978; DeLong & Aldershof, 1987; McGlashan, 1988).

Overall, there is no scientific evidence that would support the use of lithium for treating children and adolescents with manic-depressive symptomatology.[4]

ANXIETY DISORDERS

Anxiety disorders[5] are among the most prevalent forms of psychopathology in children and adolescents (Bernstein, 1994). The effectiveness of psychotropic drugs for most of the anxiety syndromes has been only meagerly appraised. Bernstein (1994) states: "There are a limited number of studies evaluating the efficacy of antianxiety medications in children and adolescents. Moreover, because many of these studies have methodological shortcomings, the results are often equivocal or difficult to interpret" (p. 440). Mirza, Michael, and Divan (1994) concluded, after surveying the pertinent literature, that actual controlled research findings concerning drug efficacy were available for only three of the anxiety categories—separation anxiety disorder, overanxiety disorder, and obsessive-compulsive disorder.

Four double-blind studies have been published involving the use of antidepressants to treat anxious children who have difficulty attending school (presumably reflecting underlying separation anxiety). Of these four studies (Berney, Kolvin, & Bhate, 1981; Bernstein, Garfinkel, & Borchardt, 1990; Gittelman-Klein & Klein, 1971; Klein, Koplewicz, & Kanner, 1992) only one (Gittelman-Klein & Klein, 1971) demonstrated that the antidepressant was more effective than placebo in improving school attendance. All these studies involve relatively small numbers of patients, and it would be a bold act to conclude that they add up to anything more than uncertainty.

For overanxious disorder, one finds a single double-blind, placebo-controlled endeavor (Simeon et al., 1992) that involved the use of alprazolam versus placebo in a small sample. The active drug did not significantly exceed the placebo's effectiveness in reducing anxiety levels.

---

[4] The findings are inconclusive concerning the short-term and long-term side effects of lithium in children and adolescents (Campbell, Perry, & Green, 1994). However, such side effects as the following have been observed: weight gain, decreased motor activity, irritability, tremor, vomiting, stomachache, EEG changes.

[5] Child and adolescent anxiety disorders embrace simple phobia, social phobia, avoidant disorder, separation anxiety, overanxious disorder, panic disorder, posttraumatic stress disorder, and obsessive-compulsive disorder.

The pharmacotherapy of avoidant disorders seems to have been formally studied in only one instance (Simeon et al., 1992), in a sample of 9 patients. The active drug was not superior to the placebo. Mention should also be made of the one placebo-controlled study (Kutcher, Reiter, Gardner, & Klein, 1992) of the pharmacotherapy of panic disorder. It reported that in a sample of 12 adolescent patients clonazepam was therapeutically superior to placebo. However, prudence dictates that one not take seriously this isolated finding based on so few patients.

The virtual drought prevailing in the literature dealing with the pharmacotherapies of the anxiety syndromes just described contrasts with the accumulated findings bearing on the treatment of obsessive-compulsive (OCD) disturbance in children and adolescents. A number of double-blind, placebo-controlled studies of OCD in youthful samples have been published (DeVeaugh-Geiss et al., 1992; Flament et al., 1985; Leonard et al., 1991; Leonard, Swedo, Rapaport, Coffey, & Cheslow, 1988; Leonard et al., 1989; Riddle et al., 1992). As a group, these studies indicate a definite trend for pharmacotherapies to provide some relief for OCD symptomatology in children and adolescents. It is also true however, that most of these studies have limitations because they are based on small numbers of patients; are in some instances clearly vulnerable to penetration of the double-blind; and typically report only partial relief of discomforting symptoms. In commenting on such limitations in the series of OCD studies, Geller, Biederman, Reed, Spencer, and Wilens (1995) noted:

> Despite highly statistically significant results, the overall role of improvement was not larger than 60%, with an effect size of up to 40%. Although encouraging, these results also indicate that clomipramine (CMI) treatment of juveniles with OCD leaves many subjects unimproved and that those who improve may continue to have substantial residual symptomatology. In addition, treatment with CMI was associated with a variety of adverse effects including anticholinergic symptoms (i.e., dry mouth . . . , tremor . . . , dizziness . . .) and sedation . . . making it difficult to tolerate for some patients even in the context of a robust clinical response. (pp. 36–37)

Most of the double-blind OCD studies have involved the use of clomipramine as the therapeutic agent. The drug trial paradigm was usually based on random assignment to either active drug or placebo. However, one study (Leonard et al., 1989) used random assignment to clomipramine or desipramine (instead of placebo). Another (Leonard et al., 1991) called for 3 months of clomipramine treatment. Then, half the patients continued on clomipramine and half had desipramine blindly substituted. One investigation by Riddle et al. (1992) utilized fluoxetine instead of clomipramine; and called for random assignment to either fluoxetine or placebo. A number of the studies also arranged for a crossover after the initial drug and placebo divisions.

Although, as already indicated, the findings generally demonstrated a certain amount of therapeutic power for clomipramine and fluoxetine (compared with placebo or desipramine) one is impressed with multiple weaknesses in the drug trial designs and sometimes the borderline quality of the results.

Two of the studies (Leonard et al., 1991; Riddle et al., 1992) ultimately ended up with extremely small numbers of patients in the comparison groups. The analysis of the Riddle et al. data was based on 6 patients in the active treatment and 7 in the placebo groups.

In all the studies, a significant number of the patients were concomitantly receiving psychotherapeutic treatments. This is a confounding variable, since there is no way of knowing what differences existed between active drug and placebo patients with reference to the types or frequencies of their psychotherapy sessions. The concomitant psychotherapy is simply an uncontrolled variable exerting undefined and unpredictable effects on the outcome data.

Also, the side effects of the active drug versus control substances (placebo, desipramine) were in several instances documented to be quite different raising serious possibilities that the double-blind was penetrated. The side effect differences would provide obvious cues as to which patients were receiving active drug or placebo. This possibility was so apparent that the researchers in two instances directly addressed the issue (Flament et al., 1985; Leonard et al., 1991).

The reported differences between measures of active drug and placebo (control) effects were in some instances quite ephemeral and inconsistent. In the Riddle et al. (1992) study, which claimed that "fluoxetine is an . . . effective short-term treatment for children with OCD" (p. 1062), the following contradictory information appears: "Changes from baseline scores for the fluoxetine group significantly exceeded the change scores for the placebo group on the CGI-OCD (a clinical global impression rating of severity of OCD symptoms) . . . *The magnitude of change on all other symptom severity measures did not differ significantly across the two groups* [italics added]" (p. 1066). Actually, there were 5 measures in the category of those not demonstrating significant differences between fluoxetine and placebo. Thus, only 1 of 6 indices indicated superiority of fluoxetine over placebo. This hardly justifies the Riddle et al. conclusion that fluoxetine is "effective." Similarly, Leonard et al. (1991) report that when patients remaining on clomipramine were compared with patients who were taken off clomipramine and put on desipramine (which was predicted to be ineffective and treated basically as a placebo), only 1 of 4 major measures of symptomatology showed a significant advantage for clomipramine.

Such discrepancies and design defects do not generate real confidence in the OCD pharmacotherapy literature. By way of balance, though, it should be indicated that the DeVeaugh-Geiss et al. (1992) study that showed a clear advantage for clomipramine over placebo was well designed. It was a multicenter project; involved relatively substantial numbers of patients (27 in the clomipramine and 27 in the placebo samples) and found that whereas only 8% of the placebo patients improved significantly in their obsessive-compulsive symptomatology during the trial, 37% of these on clomipramine did so. The only potentially serious defect in the design was that some of the patients received concomitant psychotherapy with their drug treatment.[6]

INTEGRATIVE COMMENTS

Our explorations of a number of the major uses of psychotropic drugs for psychologically distressed children and adolescents have brought into view a wasteland. There is no consistent scientific evidence that the major drugs widely prescribed for depressive, manic-depressive, and anxiety symptoms are superior to placebos. In a review of studies published between 1985 and 1994 concerned with the efficacy of antidepressants for children and adolescents, Sommers-Flanagan and Sommers-Flanagan (1996) came to a similar negative conclusion. Incidentally, there is also little dependable research concerning the efficacy of neuroleptics for treating psychosis in children and adolescents (Whitaker & Rao, 1992). It is not an exaggeration to assert that, by and large, the psychopharmacotherapy of the youth segment of the population is scientifically unjustified.[7] Individual practitioners who insist, in increasing numbers, on prescribing psychotropic drugs for depressive and anxiety symptomatology are doing so without rational support. Moved by pressures emanating from their patients and patients' parents who want relief and also by their own internal pressures to prove they are participants in the new biological psychiatry, they either implacably oppose the contrary facts or pretend that such facts do not exist. As Eisenberg (1996) and also Pellegrino (1996) have commented, this amounts to unethical action.

---

[6] There were also sizable differences in several side effects between the clomipramine and placebo patients; and this raises the possibility that the double-blind was breached.
[7] Some evidence exists (e.g., Kazdin, 1991) that psychotherapeutic approaches are more effective for various forms of disturbance in children and adolescents than is no treatment although the studies involved have rarely, if ever, been blind.

How can physicians prescribe drugs for children even though these drugs have never been shown to be effective? How is this possible legally? Popper (1993) describes the restrictions Food and Drug Administration imposed:

> Under the Federal Food, Drug, and Cosmetic Act a drug approved for marketing may be labeled, promoted, and advertised by the manufacturer only for those uses for which the drug's safety and efficacy have been established and which the FDA has approved.

Popper further explains:

> The Act does not, however, limit the manner in which a physician may use an approved drug. Once a product has been approved for marketing a physician may prescribe it for uses (disorders) or in treatment regimens (doses) or patient populations (ages) that are not included in approved labeling. . . . Accepted medical practice often includes drug use that is not reflected in approved drug labeling. (p. 52)

He adds:

> The court system has always concurred that it is appropriate for physicians to use commercially released drugs according to the physician's best judgment. (pp. 52–53)

In other words, because psychotropic drugs have been approved by the FDA for treating various symptoms in adults, physicians may use them for children in any way they see fit. They are authorized to apply such drugs to children without reasonable scientific grounds for doing so.

REFERENCES

Ambrosini, P. J., Bianchi, M. D., Rabinovish, H., & Ella, J. (1993). Antidepressant treatments in children and adolescents: 1. Affective disorders. *Journal of the American Academy of Child and Adolescent Psychiatry, 32,* 1–5.

Banta, H. D., & Thacker, S. B. (1990). The case for reassessment of health care technology: Once is not enough. *Journal of the American Medical Association, 264,* 235–246.

Berney, T., Kolvin, I., & Bhate, S. R. (1981). School phobia: A therapeutic trial of clomipramine and short-term outcome. *British Journal of Psychiatry, 138,* 110–118.

Bernstein, G. A. (1994). Psychopharmacological interventions. In T. H. Ollendick, N. J. King, & W. Yule (Eds.), *International handbook of phobic and anxiety disorders in children and adolescents* (pp. 439–451). New York: Plenum Press.

Bernstein, G. A., Garfinkel, B. D., & Borchardt, C. M. (1990). Comparative studies of pharmacotherapy for school refusal. *Journal of the American Academy of Child and Adolescent Psychiatry, 29,* 773–781.

Biederman, J., Thisted, R. A., Greenhill, L. L., & Ryan, N. D. (1995). Estimation of the association between desipramine and the risk for sudden death in 5- to 14-year-old children. *Journal of Clinical Psychiatry, 56,* 87–93.

Bishop, J. M. (1984). Infuriating tensions: Science and the medical student. *Journal of Medical Education, 59,* 91–102.

Boules, C., Kutcher, S., Marton, P., Simeon, J., Ferguson, B., & Roberts, N. (1991). Response to desipramine treatment in adolescent major depression. *Psychopharmacology Bulletin, 27,* 59–65.

Campbell, M., Perry, R., & Green, W. H. (1994). Use of lithium in children and adolescents. *Psychosomatics, 105,* 95–101.

Conners, C. K. (1992). Methodology of antidepressant drug trials for treating depression in adolescents. *Journal of Child and Adolescent Psychopharmacology, 2,* 11–22.

DeLong, G. R. (1978). Lithium carbonate treatment of select behavior disorders in children suggesting manic-depressive illness. *Journal of Pediatrics, 93,* 689–694.

DeLong, G. R., & Aldershof, A. L. (1987). Long-term experience with lithium treatment in childhood: Correlation with clinical diagnosis. *Journal of the American Academy of Child and Adolescent Psychiatry, 26,* 389–394.

DeLong, G. R., & Nieman, G. W. (1983). Lithium-induced behavior changes in children with symptoms suggesting manic-depressive illness. *Psychopharmacology Bulletin, 19,* 258–265.

DeVeaugh-Geiss, J., Moroz, G., Biederman, J., Cantwell, D., Fontaine, R., Greist, J. H., Reichler, R., Katz, R., & Landau, P. (1992). Clomipramine hydrochloride in childhood and adolescent obsessive-compulsive disorder—A multicenter trial. *Journal of the American Academy of Child and Adolescent Psychiatry, 31,* 45–49.

Eisenberg, L. (1996). What should doctors do in the face of negative evidence? *Journal of Nervous and Mental Disease, 184,* 99–108.

Fisher, R. L., & Fisher, S. (1996). Antidepressants for children: Is scientific support necessary? *Journal of Nervous and Mental Disease, 184,* 99–108.

Flament, M. F., Rapaport, J. L., Berg, C. J., Scerry, W., Kilts, C., Mellstrom, B., & Linnoila, M. (1985). Clomipramine treatment of childhood obsessive-compulsive disorder. *Archives of General Psychiatry, 42,* 977–983.

Gadow, K. D. (1991). Clinical issues in child and adolescent psychopharmacology. *Journal of Consulting and Clinical Psychology, 59,* 842–852.

Geller, D. A., Biederman, J., Reed, E. D., Spencer, T., & Wilens, T. E. (1995). Similarities in response to fluoxetine in the treatment of children and adolescents with obsessive-compulsive disorder. *Journal of the American Academy of Child and Adolescent Psychiatry, 34,* 36–44.

Geller, B., Cooper, T. B., Graham, D. L., Fetner, H. H., Marsfeller, F. A., & Wells, J. (1992). Pharmacokinetically designed double-blind placebo-controlled study of nortriptyline in 6 to 12 year olds with major depressive disorder. *Journal of the American Academy of Child and Adolescent Psychiatry, 31,* 34–44.

Geller, B., Cooper, T. B., Graham, D. L., Marsfeller, F. A., & Bryant, D. M. (1990). Double-blind placebo-controlled study of nortriptyline in depressed adolescents using a "fixed plasma level" design. *Psychopharmacology Bulletin, 26,* 85–90.

Gittelman-Klein, R., & Klein, D. F. (1971). Controlled imipramine treatment of school phobia. *Archives of General Psychiatry, 25,* 204–207.

Goleman, D. (1993, December 15). Use of antidepressants in children at issue. *The New York Times,* p. 7.

Goodwin, F. K., & Jamison, K. R. (1990). *Manic-depressive illness.* New York: Oxford University Press.

Green, W. H. (1991). *Child and adolescent clinical psychopharmacology.* Baltimore: Williams & Wilkins.

Greenhill, L. L., & Setterberg, S. (1993). Pharmacotherapy of disorders of adolescents. *Psychiatric Clinics of North America, 16,* 793–814.

Grimes, D. A. (1993). Technology follies: The uncritical acceptance of medical innovation. *Journal of the American Medical Association, 269,* 3030–3033.

Hazell, P., O'Connell, D., Heathcote, D., Robertson, J., & Henry, D. (1995). Efficacy of tricyclic drugs in treating child and adolescent depression: A meta-analysis. *British Medical Journal, 310,* 897–901.

Hughes, C. W., Preskorn, S. H., Woller, E., Woller, R., Hassamein, R., & Tucker, S. (1990). The effect of concomitant disorders in childhood depression on predicting treatment response. *Psychopharmacological Bulletin, 26,* 235–238.

Jensen, P. S., Vitiello, B., Leonard, H., & Loughren, T. P. (1994). Design and methodology issues for clinical treatment trials in children and adolescents. *Psychopharmacology Bulletin, 1,* 3–8.

Johnson, H. F., & Fruehling, J. J. (1994). Pharmacological therapy for depression in children and adolescents. In W. M. Reynolds & H. R. Johnston (Eds.), *Handbook of depression in children and adolescents* (pp. 145–160). New York: Plenum Press.

Kashani, J. H., Shekim, W. O., & Reid, J. C. (1994). Amitriptyline in children with major depressive disorder: A double-blind crossover pilot study. *Journal of the American Academy of Child and Adolescent Psychiatry, 23,* 348–351.

Kazdin, A. E. (1991). Effectiveness of psychotherapy with children and adolescents. *Journal of Consulting and Clinical Psychology, 59,* 785–798.

Klein, R. G., Koplewicz, H. S., & Kanner, A. (1992). Imipramine treatment of children with separation anxiety disorder. *Journal of the American Academy of Child and Adolescent Psychiatry, 31,* 21–28.

Kramer, A., & Feiguine, R. (1981). Clinical effects of amitriptyline in adolescent depression: A double-blind crossover pilot study. *Journal of the Academy of Child and Adolescent Psychiatry, 20,* 36–44.

Kutcher, S., Boulos, C., Ward, B., & Marton, P. (1994). Response to desipramine treatment in adolescent depression: A fixed-dose placebo controlled trial. *Journal of the American Academy of Child and Adolescent Psychiatry, 33,* 686–694.

Kutcher, S. P., Reiter, S., Gardner, D. M., & Klein, R. G. (1992). The pharmacotherapy of anxiety disorders in children and adolescents. *Pediatric Psychopharmacology, 15,* 41–67.

Lapierre, Y. D., & Raval, K. J. (1989). Pharmacotherapy of affective disorders in children and adolescents. *Psychiatric Clinics of North America, 12,* 951–961.

Leonard, H. L., Swedo, S. E., Levane, M. C., Rettew, D. C., Cheslow, D. L., Hamburger, S. D., & Rapaport, J. L. (1991). A double-blind desipramine substitution during long-term clomipramine treatment in children and adolescents with obsessive-compulsive disorder. *Archives of General Psychiatry, 48,* 922–927.

Leonard, H. L., Swedo, S. E., Rapaport, J. L., Coffey, M., & Cheslow, D. (1988). Treatment of childhood obsessive-compulsive disorder with clomipramine and desmethylimipramine: A double-blind crossover comparison. *Psychopharmacology Bulletin, 24,* 93–95.

Leonard, H. L., Swedo, S. E., Rapaport, J. L., Koby, E. V., Lenane, M. C., Cheslow, D. L., & Hamburger, S. D. (1989). Treatment of obsessive-compulsive disorder with clomipramine and desipramine in children and adolescents. *Archives of General Psychiatry, 46,* 1088–1092.

Lucas, A., Lockett, H., & Grimm, F. (1965). Amitriptyline in childhood depressions. *Disease of the Nervous System, 26,* 105–110.

Lynoe, V. (1992). Ethical and professional aspects of practice of alternative medicine. *Scandinavian Journal of Social Medicine, 4,* 217–225.

McGlashan, T. (1988). Adolescent versus adult onset mania. *American Journal of Psychiatry, 145,* 221–223.

Mirza, K. A. H., Michael, A., & Divan, T. G. (1994). Recent advances in pediatric psychopharmacology: A brief overview. *Human Psychopharmacology, 9,* 13–24.

Pellegrino, E. D. (1996). Clinical judgment, scientific data, and ethics: Antidepressant therapy in adolescents and children. *Journal of Nervous and Mental Disease, 184,* 99–108.

Pellegrino, E. D., & Thomasma, D. C. (1981). *A philosophical basis of medical practice.* New York: Oxford University Press.

Petti, T., & Law, W. (1982). Imipramine treatment of depressed children: A double-blind pilot study. *Journal of Clinical Psychopharmacology, 2,* 107–110.

Popper, C. W. (1992). Editorial: Are clinicians ahead of researchers in finding a treatment for adolescent depression? *Journal of Child and Adolescent Psychopharmacology, 2,* 1–3.

Popper, C. W. (1993). Psychopharmacologic treatment of anxiety disorders in adolescents and children. *Journal of Clinical Psychiatry, 54,* 52–63.

Preskorn, S. H., Weller, E. B., Hughes, C., Weller, R. A., & Bolte, K. (1987). Depression in prepubertal children: Dexamethasone nonsuppression predicts differential response to imipramine vs. placebo. *Psychopharmacological Bulletin, 23,* 265–268.

Puig-Antich, J., Perel, J. M., Lupatkin, W., Chambers, W., Shea, C., Tabrize, M. A., & Stiller, R. (1979). Plasma levels of imipramine and desmethylimipramine

(DMI) and clinical response in prepubertal major depressive disorders. *Journal of the American Academy of Child and Adolescent Psychiatry, 18,* 616–627.

Puig-Antich, J., Perel, J. M., Lupatkin, W., Chambers, W. J., Tabrizi, M. A., King, J., Goetz, R., Davies, M., & Stiller, R. L. (1987). Imipramine in prepubertal major depressive disorders. *Archives of General Psychiatry, 44,* 81–89.

Riddle, M. A., Geller, B., & Ryan, N. (1993). Another sudden death in a child treated with desipramine. *Journal of the American Academy of Child and Adolescent Psychiatry, 9,* 283–289.

Riddle, M. A., Scahill, L., King, R. A., Harding, M. T., Anderson, G. M., Ort, S. I., Smith, J. C., Leckman, J. F., & Cohen, D. J. (1992). Double-blind, crossover trial of fluoxetine and placebo in children and adolescents with obsessive-compulsive disorder. *Journal of the American Academy of Child and Adolescent Psychiatry, 31,* 1062–1069.

Roy, D. J. (1986). Ethics in clinical research and clinical practice. *Clinical and Investigative Medicine, 9,* 283–289.

Simeon, J., DiNicola, V., Phil, M., Ferguson, H., & Copping, W. (1990). Adolescent depression: A placebo-controlled fluoxetine treatment study and follow-up. *Progress in Neuropsychopharmacological Biology Psychiatry, 14,* 791–795.

Simeon, J. G., Ferguson, B., Knott, V., Roberts, N., Gauthier, B., Dubois, C., & Wiggins, D. (1992). Clinical, cognitive, and neurophysiological effects of alprazolam in children with overanxious and avoidant disorders. *Journal of the American Academy of Child and Adolescent Psychiatry, 31,* 29–33.

Sommers-Flanagan, J., & Sommers-Flanagan, R. (1996). Efficacy of antidepressant medication with depressed youth: What psychologists should know. *Professional Psychology: Research and Practice, 27,* 145–153.

Strober, M., Morrell, W., Lampert, C., & Burroughs, J. (1990). Relapse following discontinuation of lithium maintenance therapy in adolescents with bipolar I illness: A naturalistic study. *American Journal of Psychiatry, 147,* 457–461.

Thurber, S., Ensign, J., Punnett, A. F., & Welter, K. (1995). A meta-analysis of antidepressant outcome studies that involved children and adolescents. *Journal of Clinical Psychology, 51,* 340–345.

Waslik, B. (1995). Cardiac effects of desipramine. *Journal of the American Academy of Child and Adolescent Psychiatry, 34,* 125.

Whitaker, A., & Rao, U. (1992). Neuroleptics in pediatric psychiatry. *Psychiatric Clinics of North America, 15,* 243–276.

Wulff, H. R. (1986). Rational diagnoses and treatment. *Journal of Medicine and Philosophy, 11,* 123–134.

Zimnitzky, B., & Popper, C. (1995). *A fifth case of sudden death in a child taking desipramine* (Abstract NR478-A, 181). In New Research Program and Abstracts of 147th Annual Meeting of the American Psychiatric Association, Philadelphia, PA.

CHAPTER 9

Stimulant Pharmacotherapy for Attention-Deficit/Hyperactivity Disorders: An Analysis of Progress, Problems, and Prospects

CAROL K. WHALEN and BARBARA HENKER

ALMOST ANYONE TODAY has personal knowledge and a ready opinion about hyperactivity and stimulant drugs. A coworker describes how Ritalin® kept her 10-year-old son in school, after she had tried everything else she could think of. A neighbor tells you that if mothers would stay home with their children, we wouldn't be having a hyperactivity epidemic. A hairstylist asserts that if we put more teachers in the classroom and police officers on the streets, there would be no need for Ritalin. A scout leader describes the difficulties he has ensuring the safety of young charges on field trips and in the workshop, adding that his job would be impossible if it weren't that two of the boys in his group take Ritalin. A young teen complains that it's not fair to restrict Ritalin to hyperactive kids; she, too, could use some help concentrating and getting high scores on the SATs. A mother is concerned that giving stimulants to school-age children teaches them that drugs are the way to solve problems. A pharmacist confides his suspicion that the father who has just filled a prescription for his daughter is actually taking the pills himself.

Stimulant pharmacotherapy for attention-deficit/hyperactivity disorder (ADHD) is arguably the most prominent, best documented, and most economical intervention for any psychological disorder of childhood. It is also the most controversial. In this chapter, we examine two fundamental aspects of this treatment modality that seem inextricably enmeshed: its scientific respectability and its widespread notoriety. We begin by examining the empirical justification for stimulant pharmacotherapy. Next, we identify complications and causes for concern, followed by an exploration of current developments in combination treatments. The chapter concludes with an attempt to integrate the science and the rhetoric in a discussion of pharmacotherapy in multiple contexts: child and family systems, professional and institutional forces, and societal trends.

THE CASE FOR STIMULANT PHARMACOTHERAPY FOR ADHD

For any therapeutic modality, the most vital issue is accountability, or what is more commonly called efficacy. There are two interwoven aspects of accountability: the desirability and potency of the outcomes, and the quality of the research methodologies used to generate data on these outcomes. Stimulant pharmacotherapy scores high in both of these realms. Not surprisingly, early studies often lacked adequate experimental control and methodological rigor. Over two decades ago, Sulzbacher (1973) reviewed studies of psychotropic medication with children and concluded that there was an inverse relationship between the degree of rigorousness in methodology and the positivity of the findings. If a similar analysis of stimulant treatment effects for ADHD were repeated today, the opposite would obtain: Rigorous studies yield strongly positive treatment effects. In fact, many studies of pharmacotherapy for ADHD conducted over the past 20 years can serve as models of scientific method; this research arena has been a staging ground for innovative and ever-more sophisticated approaches to the design and analysis of treatment studies.

Research density in the area of stimulant pharmacotherapy for ADHD is high and seems to be increasing. A brief computerized literature search illustrates the mushrooming numbers of published studies over the past few decades, from 410 between 1965 and 1974, to 1,963 between 1975 and 1984, to 3,779 between 1985 and 1994. Given the large numbers of studies and the heterogeneity of settings, samples, and procedures, the consistency of the findings is compelling. The results converge on the conclusion that stimulants result in rapid and often marked behavioral improvements in between 60% and 90% of children with ADHD (Rapport, Denney, DuPaul, & Gardner, 1994; Spencer et al., 1996). Particularly noteworthy is that these improvements remain robust over and beyond a relatively large positive placebo response that can be found in up to 30% of cases (Swanson, McBurnett, Christian, & Wigal, 1995).

The extensive effects of stimulants are welcome and highly salient, meaningful in a clinical as well as a statistical sense. In study after study, noticeable and even dramatic improvements emerge in focal symptom domains such as attentional patterns, disruptiveness, and impulsivity. Many of these changes are apparent immediately, in the first day or two of treatment, unlike the more delayed effects of many other pharmacological or psychosocial treatments. Another major advantage is that stimulant pharmacotherapy is a practical intervention. Typically costing between $1.00 and $2.00 per day, it is readily available and easily administered. Careful medical monitoring is required to detect untoward effects, to encourage adherence, and to ensure that the medication continues to be needed. But once a stable regimen has been implemented, subsequent visits to a physician's office often become routine consultations dictated by the dual needs to uncover any adverse effects and renew the prescription.

In an article comparing ADHD treatments, Whalen and Henker (1991b) summarized the multiple facets of treatment decisions and practices in a set of therapeutic ". . . abilities" (see Table 9.1). This baker's dozen list of abilities forms a useful and comprehensive set of criteria for designing, evaluating, and comparing therapeutic interventions. When these criteria are applied in the service of contrasting stimulant pharmacotherapy to other approaches for managing ADHD, the relative advantages of pharmacotherapy are cast in sharp relief. As noted earlier, stimulant therapy receives its highest marks in the areas related to accountability. It is an effective, practical, and readily available tool. It is applicable across a wide range of problems and ages. In these days of managed care and empirically validated treatments for psychological problems, the standards of service delivery are easier to establish, teach, and maintain for this therapy than for any other major mode. Incontestably, stimulant therapy has the most impressive track record to date, yet it continues to be burdened by a mantle of misgivings. Table 9.1 provides a comprehensive set of criteria for comparing and evaluating interventions. This slate of criteria also serves to highlight a host of complications, qualifiers, and concerns.

COMPLICATIONS, CAUTIONS, AND CAUSES FOR CONCERN

Just as there is no definitive diagnostic indicator for identifying ADHD, there is no magic bullet for "treating" it. ADHD is a pervasive, multiproblem, and chronic disorder, and the effects of pharmacotherapy—as

Table 9.1
Comparing and Contrasting Treatment Modalities:
An Array of Therapeutic ". . . abilities"

Accountability. What desired changes does treatment produce?

Adaptability. How readily can the treatment be tuned or tailored to meet particular clinical and developmental requirements?

Applicability. What is the bandwidth or scope of problems that can be treated, and what is the developmental range of effectiveness?

Availability. Once the initial research and demonstration projects conclude, how readily can the treatment be provided by community practitioners under real-life conditions?

Communicability/Teachability. How readily can the basic therapeutic skills and ingredients be identified and taught?

Compatibility. How readily can the treatment be combined with other necessary or desirable interventions?

Constrainability. How widespread and serious are the unintended side effects and undesirable emanative effects of the treatment?

Controllability. How readily can standards of delivery be ensured across administratively, philosophically, and geographically diverse treatment settings?

Durability. What is the stability or predictability of improvement during the course of treatment, and how long are treatment-generated gains maintained once treatment is discontinued?

Feasibility. How manageable is the sum total of temporal, psychological, economic, and other burdens imposed on the child and his or her significant others?

Generalizability. How well do positive outcomes generalize beyond the treatment targets and settings? What is the range and quality of positive emanative effects?

Palatability. How good is the match between client goals, values, and proclivities and therapeutic philosophies and tactics?

Visibility. How likely is the child to be stigmatized because of participation in treatment?

Adapted from "Therapies for Hyperactive Children: Comparisons, Combinations, and Compromises," by C. K. Whalen and B. Henker, 1991, *Journal of Consulting and Clinical Psychology, 59,* 126–137. Copyright, 1991, by American Psychological Association. Used with permission.

well as those of any other treatment—are limited in both scope and duration. The challenge is amplified by the heterogeneity that pervades both the disorder and the treatment outcomes. No two children with ADHD have the identical profile of problems, and all treatment modalities have variable effects, leading to improvement in different domains for different youngsters (Forness, Swanson, Cantwell, Guthrie, & Sena, 1992; Rapport et al., 1994). As noted by Conners et al. (1994), heterogeneity is not itself a problem, but ignoring its influence is. In the following paragraphs, we review the major implications of the many faces of heterogeneity and the unanswered questions that result.

UNSUBSTANTIATED LONG-TERM BENEFITS

Stimulant pharmacotherapy is often construed as an aid to help children and families negotiate rough spots and potholes in the developmental terrain, or as a means of modulating arousal and self-control so that children with ADHD can benefit, like their peers, from everyday opportunities to acquire cognitive skills and adaptive coping strategies. But if stimulants actually facilitate skill acquisition, wouldn't one expect the gains to maintain after treatment ends? One of the most nettlesome enigmas surrounding stimulant pharmacotherapy is the difficulty of documenting long-term advantage despite reliable evidence of short-term gain. It is often disheartening to observe how rapidly behavior deteriorates when medication is discontinued. Apparently, whether a child is medicated for 5 days, 5 months, or 5 years, many problems return the day after the last pill is taken.

The dearth of extended treatment studies (Jacobvitz, Sroufe, Stewart, & Leffert, 1990; Schachar & Tannock, 1993) stands in marked contrast to the plethora of acute, short-term studies, thereby rendering tentative any generalizations about long-term outcomes. This is not surprising given the constraints on research funding along with the difficulty of maintaining experimental or even quasi-experimental control over extended time intervals. Welcome as well as undesirable effects may erode or expand over time in natural environments, as individuals mature, undergo a host of salutary and stressful experiences, and continue to engage more or less actively in problem-solving and treatment-seeking activities. Based on the glaring gap between short- and long-term effects, some specialists are recommending that stimulant pharmacotherapy continue throughout the life cycle, but neither the safety nor the efficacy of lifetime treatment has been documented. Needed now are studies of the natural course of ADHD that use field rather than laboratory methodologies. These studies need to focus not only on long-term functioning but also on the type, timing, and quality of therapeutic interventions and other environmental experiences that may be linked to positive versus negative outcomes.

In discussing the large-scale *Consumer Reports* survey of psychotherapy outcome, Seligman (1995) draws the useful distinction between efficacy and effectiveness studies. The former use random assignment, systematic controls, operationalized targets, and the other rigors of laboratory methodologies. In so doing, they inexorably omit many crucial elements of the natural course of disorder and treatment, including that—in the real world—treatment types and amounts are selected rather than assigned randomly, treatment durations are individualized and idiosyncratic rather than fixed, problems are often much broader than specific diagnostic criteria acknowledge, and perceived outcome is based on overall functioning as well as on symptom relief. Seligman (1995) argues persuasively that credible empirical validation requires both types of studies. Whereas rigorous laboratory methodologies are appropriate for efficacy studies, other methods such as large-scale surveys are more appropriate for evaluating treatment effectiveness in the natural environment.

Adverse Outcomes and Dissociated Dose Effects

Some children with ADHD do not respond positively to stimulant medication, and there are also reliable indications of deterioration in a minority of treated children. Rapport et al. (1994), for example, reported deterioration rates ranging from 9% to 16% in attention, academic efficiency, and teacher-rated classroom behavior at one or more dosage levels of methylphenidate. When dosage was increased, the majority of these children improved, often to the point of normalization, but some failed to show gains at any dosage level, especially in the domain of academic efficiency. Attempts to identify a consistent subgroup of adverse responders continue but thus far have had little success (Douglas, Barr, Desilets, & Sherman, 1995).

Another possibility is that positive behavioral changes in one realm may be accompanied by undesirable changes in related realms. An ironic example of such a pattern emerged in a study of covert antisocial behavior in which methylphenidate decreased stealing and property destruction but seemed to increase cheating on an academic task, perhaps because, when medicated, boys with ADHD become more engaged in assignments and more motivated to succeed (Hinshaw, Heller, & McHale, 1992).

Questions about the possibility of cognitive toxicity have also surfaced, beginning with Sprague and Sleator's (1977) landmark study suggesting that the optimal dose for learning may be lower than that for social behavior. The concern is, in essence, that doses that yield optimal improvements in everyday behaviors, as indexed by parent and teacher ratings, may adversely affect cognitive performance and academic achievement. Especially worrisome has been the suggestion that the unsalutary effects occur in the realm of complex, higher-order cognitive functions such as flexible problem-solving or divergent thinking. The typical research paradigm uses dosage levels around 0.3 mg/kg as low, 0.6 mg/kg as medium or moderate, and 0.9 or 1.0 mg/kg as high. Systematic tests of dose-response curves within this typically prescribed range have failed to substantiate the earlier concerns about cognitive toxicity (Douglas et al., 1995; Solanto & Wender, 1989; Tannock, Schachar, & Logan, 1995). In fact, Douglas et al. (1995) reported that, when significant dosage differences were found, they indicated linear functions, with higher doses yielding greater improvement.

Whereas there is scant evidence of cognitive toxicity per se, dissociated or discordant dose effects across domains and measures are quite common. With some measures, dose-response curves appear to be linear. For example, Tannock et al. (1995) found that increasing dosage yielded incremental improvement in behavior ratings and motor restlessness as well as linear increases in heart rate. With other measures, most notably those tapping cognitive functioning, the dose-response function may be U-shaped, with optimal performance emerging at moderate dose levels. The empirical results do not fit into neat domain × dosage categories, however; these varying dose-response curves have been documented within as well as between performance domains (Tannock et al., 1995). Rapport et al. (1994) suggested that domain discordance may characterize only a subset of children with ADHD. Many youngsters show parallel dose-response effects across behavioral, attentional, and academic functioning domains.

The findings on dissociated dose-response curves and performance deterioration illustrate the need for further research on individual differences as well as careful monitoring of treatment effects across a broad range of performance parameters. The varying dose-response curves also underscore the difficulty of determining optimal doses and the need for practitioners to base dosage determinations on a combination of indicators rather than relying on a single measure such as parent or teacher ratings.

After the drug wears off or is discontinued, a minority of children may show *behavioral rebound,* a general worsening of behavior (e.g., increased excitability, impulsivity, or talkativeness) over baseline or placebo levels (Cantwell, 1996). In a systematic study of evening behavior following daytime doses of methylphenidate versus placebo, Johnston, Pelham, Hoza, and Sturges (1988) found only limited indications of rebound, concluding that these effects were not clinically significant and did not warrant any changes in medication regimen. The considerable variability across children, however, along with other reports of rebound (e.g., Porrino, Rapoport, Behar, Ismond, & Bunney, 1983; Rapoport et al., 1978), suggests the need for more extensive investigation.

Remaining Concerns about Treatment-Emergent Side Effects

Any drug must be expected to have some untoward effects—in at least a few individuals and circumstances. The most common side effects of the stimulants are appetite and sleep disturbances. Anecdotal reports of social disengagement and dysphoria also abound, and these effects have been documented in well-controlled studies (e.g., Buhrmester, Whalen, Henker, MacDonald, & Hinshaw, 1992; Whalen & Henker, 1991a; Whalen, Henker, & Granger, 1989). In most instances, side effects are mild, short-lived, and readily reversible with dosage reduction or a change to a different but similar medication (Elia, Borcherding, Rapoport, & Keysor, 1991).

Many of the side effects reported in controlled studies show comparable or even higher rates under placebo than under active drug conditions (Barkley, McMurray, Edelbrock, & Robbins, 1990; Fine & Johnston, 1993; Pelham, Swanson, Furman, & Schwindt, 1995; Rapoport, Quinn, Bradbard, Riddle, & Brooks, 1974). Because medication provides a ready attributional anchor, in some cases symptoms due to other causes may be falsely identified as side effects. In addition, parents may report as treatment-emergent side effects problems such as restlessness or irritability that are actually associated with the disorder rather than with the treatment; in fact, severity of disorder appears to be associated with severity of perceived side effects (Fine & Johnston, 1993). For example, Pelham et al. (1995) noted that restlessness was reported as a side effect 50% of the time in the placebo condition but only 12% to 30% of the time in active drug conditions. These findings raise questions not about the safety of the medication, but rather about the attributional processes involved when people reason about cause-and-effect relationships. Whether incorrectly labeling behavior problems as side effects interferes with treatment acceptance and adherence is an important question for further study.

More serious side effects have also been noted, including rare reports of psychotic symptoms such as hallucinations or thought disorders (Klein & Bessler, 1992). Abnormal motor movements or tics have received considerable attention because of the possibility that stimulants may induce or trigger Tourette syndrome or other tic disorders. Although a recent systematic study did not support earlier concerns about the use of stimulant treatment when there is a family or individual history of tic disorder (Gadow, Sverd, Sprafkin, Nolan, & Ezor, 1995), scattered reports of stimulant-related tics dictate continued caution, especially with prolonged treatment at higher dosages.

The concerns about long-term effects on growth (height suppression) have been reduced by studies comparing stimulant-treated adolescents and young adults with their peers (Spencer et al., 1996). There is evidence that prepubertal children show catchup growth during drug holidays and following drug discontinuation (Klein & Mannuzza, 1988), and customary doses of methylphenidate do not seem to affect growth velocity during adolescence (Vincent, Varley, & Leger, 1990). Whereas some studies show no enduring medication effects on cardiovascular functioning, others show small increases in heart rate or blood pressure that are statistically significant, but their clinical significance is unclear (Safer, 1992; Zeiner, 1995). Cardiovascular changes that persist over several years during active developmental periods should not be ignored, however, nor should the possibility that African American youth may be at particular risk for such medication-induced changes (Brown & Sexson, 1989).

Another frequently mentioned concern is that stimulant treatment may encourage concurrent or later substance abuse. Some long-term studies fail to find elevated rates of substance problems in young people with ADHD (Weiss & Hechtman, 1993). Others have documented a link between childhood ADHD and later substance use, but this link appears to be mediated by conduct or antisocial disorder (Mannuzza, Klein, Bessler, Malloy, & LaPadula, 1993). There is no evidence that stimulant pharmacotherapy itself contributes to substance problems (Henker, Whalen, Bugental, & Barker, 1981; Mannuzza et al., 1991; Weiss & Hechtman, 1993). In terms of stimulant addiction or abuse per se, only isolated cases have been reported. Even so, practitioners need to remain alert to the possibility that adolescents or adults may save and sell their own pills, or those prescribed for a child or younger sibling, for abusive use (Jaffe, 1991).

In summary, the most common side effects are mild, and the most serious ones are rare. Many stimulant-related side effects diminish after the first week or two of treatment or respond to dosage reductions or discontinuation. Because the several stimulants have different side effects for different people, in many instances switching to a second stimulant ameliorates whatever problem was caused by the first. There is no doubt that these drugs are among the safest in use today for childhood disorders. It is far too early, however, to be sanguine about possible untoward effects from extended treatments that span childhood and may continue into late adolescence and adulthood. The jury is still out on whether such extended treatment may result in long-term growth impairment, cardiovascular problems, or other untoward physiological effects for a minority of individuals with ADHD. The inadvertent effects of stimulants may be as widely variable as the targeted effects, and thus careful medical monitoring is needed even with short-term treatment. Careful monitoring is especially important when two or three doses per day are prescribed because the effects may overlap and thus the actual drug levels may be higher than intended during some periods of the day (Ahmann et al., 1993; Douglas et al., 1995). There are also indications that some children, such as those with comorbid ADHD and anxiety, may be at particular risk for intolerable stimulant side effects such as obsessive-compulsive behaviors or dysphoria (Tannock, in press).

Emanative Effects on Social Perceptions and Attributional Reasoning

A third class of intervention effects, in addition to direct behavioral outcomes and the so-called side effects, are the social sequelae and cognitive interpretations that attend any treatment regimen. These changes, sometimes called emanative or ripple effects (Whalen & Henker, 1976, 1991a, in press) take many forms and can be seen in many realms of the individual's life. These effects are sometimes positive, sometimes negative, and often both.

Positive ripple effects can be seen when drug-induced behavioral improvement in a child with ADHD reduces disruptiveness among peers, strengthens peer relations, or decreases criticism from a teacher. Concomitant negative effects may also be apparent, as when a child is teased by peers for daily trips to the nurse's office or told, after giving an incorrect answer in class or interrupting a game on the playground, that "It's time to take your hyper pill." A good example of a decidedly mixed effect can be seen when a successful medication trial relieves a mother's sense of anxiety and guilt by pointing to a biochemical explanation, rather than a parenting deficit, for a child's school failure. At the same time, the behavioral improvement and parental relief may combine to reduce efforts toward academic remediation or more skillful parenting.

Often these ripple effects operate through attributional processes, as seen in the preceding example. All treatments carry attributional messages, and stimulant medication is a particularly likely candidate to act as an attributional anchor. A positive drug response is often interpreted, by physicians and teachers as well as by parents and children, as confirming a biochemical or genetic dysfunction and indicating that the child's behavior is not under personal control. The net effects of such attributional baggage may be quite significant in the life of a child, yet the consequences, particularly in the long term, have received little study.

The hypothesis that medication treatment may have unwelcome effects on causal reasoning and perceived self-efficacy in some children and parents (Whalen & Henker, 1976) has received a modicum of empirical support (Borden & Brown, 1989; Pelham et al., 1992; Whalen, Henker, Hinshaw, Heller, & Huber-Dressler, 1991). Yet there is also some evidence that medication may exert a positive effect on attributional reasoning and self-confidence (Milich, Carlson, Pelham, & Licht, 1991), most likely mediated by welcome behavioral improvements. Empirical reports of either positive or negative effects are few. Valid assessments of how people form interpretations of treatment processes and outcomes are extremely difficult to obtain, given the susceptibility of self-report data to the effects of social desirability biases and measurement or interview contexts. The overt changes brought about by medication may overshadow the more subtle and covert attitudinal changes in terms of visibility and "researchability." But they may not so overshadow them in long-term impact or durability.

REMAINING GAPS IN KNOWLEDGE ABOUT WHO BENEFITS, WHEN, AND FOR HOW LONG

Despite the vast body of literature on ADHD and stimulant pharmacotherapy, serious gaps in knowledge remain. The vast majority of studies focus on the most prevalent and accessible subgroup, school-age boys, resulting in a dearth of information on females, ethnic minorities, and adults. As noted earlier, most of the methodologically sound studies are brief, often lasting only a few weeks. There are continuing concerns about the possibility of drug tolerance, or the attenuation of stimulant effects and resultant need for stronger doses as treatment continues over months and years (Jacobvitz et al., 1990; Schachar & Tannock, 1993). Research investigations tend not to target tolerance per se, and thus there is little empirical evidence either documenting or disconfirming the phenomenon. Interdose behavioral rebound is also poorly understood. Another constellation of questions in need of systematic study concerns the links between ADHD and depression as well as stimulant-related dysphoria and disengagement (Spencer et al., 1996; Whalen & Henker, 1992).

Perhaps one of the biggest remaining puzzles concerns person × treatment × target domain interactions. Although some factors such as family stability and motivation may be global predictors of treatment responsiveness, there are likely to be specific mediators and moderators for different therapeutic modalities. Some child characteristics, settings, and family variables may portend a more optimal response to pharmacological and others to psychosocial interventions. The list of potential predictors is long, including child characteristics such as comorbid disorders or IQ; family characteristics such as medication attitudes or ability to implement a behavioral system in the home; and setting characteristics such as social support or teacher involvement.

Inconsistencies in medication responsiveness across *and even within* domains are the rule rather than the exception. A positive responder on a measure of task attention or oral reading, for example, may be a nonresponder or even an adverse responder on measures of reading comprehension or academic efficiency (Forness et al., 1992; Rapport et al., 1994). For any medication and any domain, there is still little basis for predicting who will respond positively, adversely, or not at all and who will improve on placebo. Some encouraging hints are emerging from the research literature, however. Several investigators have found that children with both ADHD and internalizing problems (especially anxiety) are less likely than other children with ADHD to respond positively, although the empirical literature is somewhat inconsistent (Buitelaar, van der Gaag, Swaab-Barneveld, & Kuiper, 1995; DuPaul, Barkley, & McMurray, 1994; Pliszka, 1989; Tannock, in press; Tannock, Ickowicz, & Schachar, 1995). Not surprisingly, youngsters with more serious problems or more dysfunctional families are also less likely to benefit. In terms of target domains, problems with disinhibition and oppositionality are especially treatment-responsive, whereas gains in cognitive functioning, academic performance, and peer relations are both more elusive and more variable (Forness et al., 1992; Hinshaw, Henker, Whalen, Erhardt, & Dunnington, 1989; Rapport et al., 1994; Whalen, Henker, Buhrmester, et al., 1989; Whalen, Henker, & Granger, 1989).

Beyond these relatively global distinctions, specialists have had little success predicting whether, how, and to what extent an individual child will respond to stimulant pharmacotherapy. In practice, this information gap is counteracted to a certain extent because stimulants produce their effects quickly, with improvement often apparent within a half-hour following ingestion, and the effects typically diminish after 4 to 6 hours. This means that clinical questions about how an individual child will respond can be answered, at least for the short run, by a brief medication trial; behavioral improvement and deterioration following the first few doses may be a particularly valid predictor of long-term treatment responsiveness. Whereas behavioral treatments may enjoy a similar advantage, most psychosocial treatments do not: Their effects—either positive or negative—may take more time to surface.

There is a need for more information about placebo responses, negative as well as positive (Campbell & Cueva, 1995). This need is even greater in the realm of psychosocial than pharmacological treatments, most likely because it is difficult to design credible placebo therapy. Better understanding of placebo processes is needed for both scientific and clinical purposes. When treatments are being evaluated and compared, it is important to recognize the ways in which nonspecific effects may compromise the validity or interpretation of the findings (Whalen & Henker, 1986b). And when treatment programs are being designed for individual children, it is important to identify those who may benefit from nonspecific interventions that can be briefer, less intensive, and less risky than full-scale therapeutic programs.

EVER-EXPANDING ELIGIBILITY

Although stimulant pharmacotherapy is viewed as appropriate and has been tested primarily for the behavioral symptoms of ADHD, the array of problems and individuals being treated is expanding. Children and adolescents who may be viewed as candidates for stimulant pharmacotherapy include not only those diagnosed as having ADHD, but also those who (a) show symptoms of ADHD superimposed on another primary disorder such as mental retardation, autism, or bipolar disorder (Aman, Kern, McGhee, & Arnold, 1993; Birmaher, Quintana, & Greenhill, 1988; Handen, Janosky, McAuliffe, Breaux, & Feldman, 1994; Strayhorn, Rapp, Donina, & Strain, 1988); (b) do not have ADHD but show some of the same types of behavior problems such as aggression or oppositionality (e.g., Brown, Jaffe, Silverstein, & Magee, 1991); and (c) do not appear to have problems serious enough to merit the diagnosis but may have a subsyndromal variant of ADHD and could use some help focusing and performing academically. There are also discussions about the merits of prescribing stimulants for nondiagnosed individuals who show few if any problems but would like to improve their grades or maximize their test scores.

The range of applicability appears even broader in adults. Wender (1995) has proposed an ADHD spectrum of disorders, suggesting that stimulants may be helpful when relatives of patients with ADHD show suggestive signs or symptoms but do not meet diagnostic criteria for ADHD. Stimulants have also been used to treat severe depression, depression that accompanies medical illnesses such as AIDS, apathy or withdrawal in the elderly, and bipolar disorders. In addition, stimulants have been prescribed for schizophrenia when neuroleptics improve positive symptoms (e.g., hallucinations) but leave negative symptoms (e.g., poverty of speech) unchanged (Chiarello & Cole, 1987; Klein & Wender, 1995). The marked heterogeneity of response and rapidity of action seem to encourage some to recommend a stimulant trial for almost any psychological problem in adults when conventional pharmacotherapy is limited or ineffective.

The temporal window for treatment onset is also expanding. Traditionally, stimulant pharmacotherapy was prescribed for school-age children. Preschoolers have also been treated with stimulants, however, a pattern that may be spurred by the trend toward teaching academic fundamentals during the preschool and kindergarten years. It is no longer rare for adolescents to be started on this treatment even though they were never identified or treated during childhood, and a similar process is occurring with young and even middle-aged adults, some of whom first come to clinical attention when they bring their children to a physician for diagnosis and treatment. Indeed, some specialists consider ADHD in adults to be an underdiagnosed and undertreated disorder (Ferdinand, Verhulst, & Wiznitzer, 1995; Spencer et al., 1995).

In addition to the expanding age range for treatment initiation, the duration of treatment is increasing. When stimulant pharmacotherapy was in its infancy, it was often viewed as useful for short-term crisis management or as a "starter" treatment that makes the child (as well as the teacher and family) more amenable to psychosocial interventions or academic remediation. It soon became standard practice to continue the regimen through the school-age years, terminating treatment either at puberty or graduation from elementary school. It is now relatively common to see treatment continuing throughout an individual's academic career and even beyond. Changes over the past two decades are illustrated by Safer and Krager's (1994) recent summary of results from biennial surveys in Baltimore County: In the 1990s, 30% of all students who were taking stimulants for ADHD were adolescents attending secondary schools, whereas this rate was only 11% in 1975, the first year the survey was conducted. The average duration of treatment for middle school students was 4 to 5 years and for high school students, 7 to 8 years. As noted earlier, ADHD is beginning to be viewed as a chronic rather than a self-limiting disorder, and stimulant pharmacotherapy is becoming a lifetime regimen rather than a short-term intervention.

In summary, three types of slippery slopes have emerged in the practice of stimulant pharmacotherapy, most likely resulting from the success of this modality. People of almost any age and with an ever-widening array of disorders are seen as appropriate candidates for treatment, and the temporal window is expanding in both directions, toward earlier initiation and later discontinuation. In other words, more and more individuals are being treated with stimulants for longer and longer periods of time. Often overlooked is that most of the data on safety and efficacy are based on a much narrower range of individuals, disorders, developmental levels, and treatment durations than found in contemporary clinical practice.

INCREASING PRESCRIPTION RATES

Drug prescription rates and sales information have been tracked for a good number of years, and the trends tell an intriguing tale. In Safer and Krager's (1992) ongoing survey, the rate of stimulant medication for the treatment of ADHD doubled every 4 to 7 years between 1971 and 1987. Then, a spate of lawsuits were filed and there were numerous media warnings of dire consequences and hidden agendas behind the "drugging of schoolchildren." Despite the notable lack of success of the lawsuits, surveys conducted during 1989 and 1991 indicated a marked (39%) decline in methylphenidate prescription rates, and the decreases were most dramatic in the cities where the lawsuits were filed (Safer, 1994). There is every indication, however, that this dip between 1989 and 1991 has been reversed and that office visits and prescription rates are again on the rise, and sharply so (Swanson, Lerner, & Williams, 1995; Swanson et al., 1996).

The temporary decrease demonstrates the impact that notoriety and fear appeals can have on treatment acceptability, regardless of scientific facts. But whatever the reason, the more recent mushrooming of prescription rates attests to the vitality of this treatment modality. Its salient primacy in the armamentarium of treatment options has no doubt been strengthened by the recent bevy of celebrities and respected professionals disclosing their ADHD diagnoses and successful treatment on national television and in the popular literature (e.g., Hallowell & Ratey, 1994, 1996). Unknown at this time is the extent to which these increasing prescription rates are attributable to increases in the rate of diagnosed ADHD, the willingness to prescribe stimulants for children given this diagnosis, the duration of treatment, or the range of disorders and developmental levels for which stimulant therapy is considered appropriate. Swanson, Lerner, and Williams (1995) report dramatic increases from 1990 to 1993 in both the amount of methylphenidate manufactured and the annual number of outpatient visits for ADHD, the vast majority of which resulted in a prescription for methylphenidate. These authors suggest that these changes result not from increased prevalence of ADHD, but rather from heightened public awareness due to parent advocacy groups coupled with regulatory changes in the education system that obligate schools to serve students with ADHD.

NECESSARY VERSUS SUFFICIENT TREATMENTS

It would not be difficult to substantiate the assertion that stimulant pharmacotherapy is a necessary treatment for many children with ADHD if these youngsters are to achieve their full potential. The immediately apparent gains that attend this treatment often suggest that the problem has been solved, allowing overburdened parents and professionals to turn to other pressing matters. The limitations of this treatment—or of any other single approach—often take longer to surface and thus may be overlooked.

One issue, discussed earlier, is that the gains are often temporary and may not enhance long-term adjustment. A second issue concerns the degree of improvement and questions about whether behavior and performance are actually "normalized." Often the changes appear to be both desirable and meaningful but insufficient, and the likelihood of normalization remains an open question (DuPaul & Rapport, 1993; Granger, Whalen, Henker, & Cantwell, 1996; Rapport et al., 1994).

A third issue concerns the problem domains that respond to treatment. Children with ADHD are multiproblem youngsters, often experiencing not only the core symptoms of ADHD such as disinhibition and disorganization, but also many related difficulties such as academic failure, peer rejection, and low self-efficacy. In most instances, the problems exist for several years before treatment begins, and thus by the time a child comes to professional attention he or she may already show delays or deficits in several areas of functioning. After beginning stimulant pharmacotherapy, Shannon may now be able to listen to the teacher, focus on the task at hand, and complete one task before beginning another. But she may not have mastered the fundamental reading or mathematics skills needed to complete assignments at her grade level, and she may lag far behind her peers in her capacity to organize task components, plan successive problem-solving stages, and monitor her own progress. Michael may now talk rather than shout, request rather than grab, and wait his turn when playing a game with peers. But he may not know how to initiate a conversation, join an ongoing group activity, or provide social support to a friend. Jason's mother and father may now be able to tolerate and even enjoy their child, but they may not know how to set age-appropriate goals, gauge the optimal level of challenge, provide reasonable incentives and consequences, and deal with the inevitable mishaps or relapses in ways that promote growth and family harmony.

We know that pills don't teach skills, that stimulants lead to improvements in only some performance realms, and that there are broad individual differences in medication responsiveness. Thus it is more the rule than the exception that adjunctive interventions focused on academic skills, peer relations, or parenting competence will also be needed.

COMBINATION TREATMENTS

The well-documented limitations of stimulant pharmacotherapy have fostered two types of combination treatments. One combines two or more psychoactive drugs, and the other adds psychosocial treatments such as classroom behavioral intervention or parent training to the medication regimen.

COMBINATION DRUG REGIMENS

Combination drug regimens are used for three main purposes. When a stimulant medication generates improvement that is viewed as insufficient, a second drug may be added to boost the effects, perhaps even in an interactive rather than merely an additive manner (e.g., Pataki, Carlson, Kelly, Rapport, & Biancaniello, 1993). To achieve both immediate and enduring effects, it has even been suggested that two forms of methylphenidate be used simultaneously: the standard and the sustained-release preparations (Fitzpatrick, Klorman, Brumaghim, & Borgstedt, 1992; Fried, 1991). Another rationale for adding a second drug is to treat the side effects of the first drug, such as using clonidine to alleviate the sleep disturbances attributed to methylphenidate (Prince, Wilens, Biederman, Spencer, & Wozniak, 1996). A third reason for combination drug treatments involves comorbidity, a remarkably common phenomenon in child psychiatry (Bird, Gould, & Staghezza, 1993; Caron & Rutter, 1991; Cohen et al., 1993; Hammen & Compas, 1994; Loeber & Keenan, 1994; Wolraich, Hannah, Pinnock, Baumgaertel, & Brown, 1996). When a child is diagnosed with comorbid ADHD and depression, he or she may be treated with methylphenidate and a tricyclic antidepressant such as desipramine (Carlson, Rapport, Kelly, & Pataki, 1995; Pataki et al., 1993) or a serotonin reuptake blocker such as fluoxetine (Gammon & Brown, 1993); children diagnosed with both ADHD and bipolar disorder have been given a trial of methylphenidate combined with lithium (Carlson, Rapport, Kelly, & Pataki, 1992); and a child with ADHD who has serious problems with aggression may receive both methylphenidate and imipramine, clonidine, or guanfacine (Hunt, Lau, & Ryu, 1991; Wilens, Spencer, Biederman, Wozniak, & Conner, 1995). To cite one more example, children who meet diagnostic criteria for ADHD and also show possible childhood schizophrenia have been treated with risperidone in combination with methylphenidate (Sternlicht & Wells, 1995).

The practice of combination drug treatments seems to be expanding faster than the empirical justification, and there is often little indication that the combination increases overall efficacy. The results tend to be both modest and mixed, and they vary across response domain and measure (G. A. Carlson et al., 1992, 1995; Fitzpatrick et al., 1992). There is reason to doubt whether antidepressants have reliably positive effects with children beyond those obtained using placebo (see Chapter 8, this volume). Moreover, serious side effects have been noted. The combination of methylphenidate and imipramine may cause blood dyscrasias, presumably because methylphenidate seems to slow down the metabolism of imipramine, thereby increasing its effective "dose" to potentially harmful levels (Burke, Josephson, & Lightsey, 1995; Markowitz & Patrick, 1996). Still more alarming are the sudden deaths that have been reported in children taking what is probably the most common drug combination: clonidine and a stimulant (Dulcan & American Academy of Child and Adolescent Psychiatry Work Group, in press; Swanson, Flockhart, et al., 1995), even though the causal link has not been established. Needless to say, the strong possibility of biochemical interactions, especially when each drug produces cardiovascular effects, dictates considerable caution and careful monitoring when drugs are combined.

Combination Psychosocial and Pharmacological Packages

Of all the psychosocial approaches, family and school-based behavioral interventions have achieved the most notable success with children with ADHD. Studies of an array of behavioral procedures have generated much useful information. It has been shown, for example, that home-based contingency programs can be both successful and cost-effective, generating gains in academic performance as well as in social behaviors at school, and decreasing demands on already overburdened teachers (Pfiffner & O'Leary, 1993). Behavioral studies have demonstrated that programs using response cost may be more effective than those relying exclusively on positive reinforcement (Sullivan & O'Leary, 1990), and that comprehensive behavioral packages have a more consistent impact on disruptive and inattentive behavior in the classroom than on academic productivity (Pelham et al., 1993). Particularly promising are approaches that use prescriptive behavioral consultation with the classroom teachers who are on the firing line day after day (Conners et al., 1994).

Although knowledge has been gained and improvements documented, the results of behavioral programs have been disappointing thus far. The changes are often transient and circumscribed, failing to generalize to natural settings or to persist beyond the period of active treatment. Not all children respond to these programs, and some may require hefty doses of negative consequences before noticeable improvements occur. And cognitive-mediational approaches, which appeared initially to be the most promising for treating self-regulation deficits, have been the most disappointing (Abikoff, 1991; Whalen & Henker, 1986a). There seems to be sufficient indication of improvement and promise to justify continued study of behavioral approaches but insufficient evidence of efficacy to recommend widespread application.

Despite the uneven and limited outcomes to date, there are multiple justifications for the frequent recommendation that pharmacotherapy be combined with behavioral or psychosocial treatments:

- Comorbidity is the rule rather than the exception, and optimal treatments differ across disorders and problem domains.
- The range of problems shown by most children with ADHD is broad, and the scope of any one treatment modality is limited. As noted earlier, medication appears to have more robust effects on behavioral than on cognitive targets (Conners et al., 1994), and behavioral interventions aimed at improving academic or social skills cannot be expected to generalize broadly. And given the long-standing nature of ADHD-related problems, these youngsters may need help not only with self-regulation and skill acquisition, but also with understanding their problems, coping with peer rejection, and enhancing perceived self-efficacy. Abikoff and Hechtman (1996) have developed a comprehensive multimodal treatment package that includes a psychotherapy component focused on these realms.
- Children with ADHD often have adverse or dysfunctional family environments (Biederman et al., 1995). Adjunctive treatment may be needed to teach parenting competency, support parents in their attempts to deal with difficult children, reduce marital discord, and help parents obtain needed resources, to cite just a few examples. Cunningham, Bremmer, and Boyle (1995) have developed a promising community-based program for preschoolers at risk for disruptive behavior disorders. Parents meet in groups, collaborate in the formulation of child management strategies, share their successes, and provide feedback to each other. By using low-threat and high-participation techniques in a group setting, this program appears to reduce both the psychological and the logistic barriers to clinic-based treatment programs often found in low-income populations.
- Even when the family is functioning well, a child with ADHD can be a chronic stressor, and parents (especially mothers) often have or are at risk for developing serious problems, most notably in the realm of depression and low self-esteem (Brown & Pacini, 1989; Cunningham, Benness, & Siegel, 1988; Mash & Johnston, 1990). Involving parents in their child's treatment can have direct and beneficial effects on parent functioning and well-being (Anastopoulos, Shelton, DuPaul, & Guevremont, 1993), and these effects may have a positive impact on the child that extends beyond the changes targeted directly by the intervention.
- Psychosocial or behavioral approaches may facilitate pharmacotherapy, perhaps by encouraging adherence to medication regimens,

enhancing the maintenance of behavioral improvements after medication is discontinued, or reducing the required dosage of medication. Carlson, Pelham, Milich, and Dixon (1992) found that when behavior therapy was combined with a low dose of methylphenidate (0.3 mg/kg), the positive effects on classroom performance were roughly equivalent to those obtained when a higher (0.6 mg/kg) dose of methylphenidate was used alone. The facilitation may also occur in the opposite direction. When parents observe and benefit from the early success of a medication regimen, they may become more willing to devote the time, effort, and energy needed to implement an effective behavioral management program.

Although studies completed to date show no clear advantage of such multimodal treatment packages over medication alone (e.g., Abikoff & Hechtman, 1996), definitive tests of multimodal treatments have not yet been completed. A number of logistic and methodological obstacles plague comparative treatment studies, including the difficulty of implementing treatments that are at once intensive and comprehensive enough and that continue for a sufficient length of time under controlled experimental conditions. Designing credible placebos for psychosocial treatments that allow variations in intensity or "dosage" is a daunting task (Conners et al., 1994; Whalen & Henker, 1991b). Additional dilemmas surface in the realm of subject selection and sample size, given the heterogeneity of ADHD and the range of comorbid conditions and associated characteristics that may influence course and outcome (Conners et al., 1994). With the objective of providing conclusive answers to questions about multimodal treatments, the NIMH is in the midst of a collaborative, multisite study of pharmacological and psychosocial approaches for ADHD (Greenhill et al., 1996; Richters et al., 1995). This major undertaking, the first such large-scale cooperative treatment study in the United States that focuses on child mental health, promises to fill many existing gaps in our knowledge about the nature and treatment of ADHD.

PHARMACOTHERAPY IN CONTEXT: A SOCIAL ECOLOGICAL PERSPECTIVE

A valid understanding of stimulant pharmacotherapy requires a multipronged focus that extends beyond specific problems and solutions. There is no adequate formula for deciding whether to begin a medication trial, nor can measures of changes in the child portray the comprehensive nature of treatment process and outcome. A number of years ago, we proposed a social ecological model of medication effects, based on a set of concentric circles of bidirectional influence, that bears some resemblance to Bronfenbrenner's (1977) seminal model of human development. The inner circle focuses on observable changes—both targeted and inadvertent—in individual children with ADHD. The next circle considers more subtle and elusive attitudinal processes in these children and their significant others that affect, and are affected by, stimulant pharmacotherapy. The outer two circles, which we can mention only briefly here, widen the scope to involve more macrolevels of analysis, including ways that the availability and efficacy of medication influence diagnostic practices and decision making, educational strategies, and societal views of deviance and remediation (Whalen & Henker, 1980).

The bidirectional nature of these processes is paramount, as stimulant pharmacotherapy both influences and is influenced by multiple facets of social and institutional environments. Once one journeys beyond observable changes in individual children, the processes become more elusive and less amenable to scientific inquiry. But the importance of considering treatment contexts as well as tactics and targets is increasingly recognized. Two examples of this broader perspective are described in the following paragraphs. The first considers the immediate sociocognitive environment, illustrating the role of attitudes and values; the second reaches to more distal contexts, focusing on innovative models of service delivery.

ATTITUDES, EXPECTATIONS, AND TREATMENT ACCEPTABILITY

One of the advantages of stimulant pharmacotherapy is that a pill ingested is a treatment delivered. But attitudes can have a profound impact on treatment delivery and outcome, even when the treatment appears to be largely routine and mechanical, as is the case with medication. Earlier, we mentioned that ripple effects, both good and bad, can emanate from the child's drug response. Here we turn briefly to the evaluative context that surrounds the use of stimulants.

Adults are generally reluctant to medicate children. This reluctance has been found not only in psychiatric realms but also in medical arenas such as the management of postoperative pain (Brown, Dreelin, & Dingle, 1997; Tarnowski, Gavaghan, & Wisniewski, 1989). When parents and teachers are asked about preferred treatments for behavioral problems, they generally rank behavioral, educational, and psychosocial approaches positively and place medication at the bottom of the acceptability list (Epstein, Singh, Luebke, & Stout, 1991; Liu, Robin, Brenner, & Eastman, 1991; Mittl & Robin, 1987). Self-regulation procedures fare particularly well in these palatability judgments, perhaps because of their humanistic connotations and the focus on development of internal control. Drug treatments, by contrast, have connotations and raise concerns that may operate independently of the observable outcomes. Some people are fundamentally opposed to what they view as chemical coping, fearing that such treatments may ameliorate superficial rather than true problems, undermine a child's intrinsic motivation, or encourage future substance abuse.

Negative or ambivalent attitudes can affect treatment directly by decreasing adherence to the prescribed regimen or leading to premature discontinuation. Such attitudes can also exert unsalutary indirect effects by devaluing the child's medication-related behavior changes. In some instances, a child is placed in the middle of parental disagreements and given conflicting messages when one parent feels strongly that medication is needed and the other attempts to terminate or sabotage the treatment. It is not unusual to find that only 50% of children for whom pharmacotherapy is recommended enter and complete a short-term trial, and even the completers may skip more than 25% of their pills (Brown, Borden, Wynne, Spunt, & Clingerman, 1987; Firestone, 1982). An analysis in New York revealed that over half of the 1-month prescriptions for methylphenidate were not renewed during a 12-month period (Sherman & Hertzig, 1991). Although there are several possible contributors to this "single-prescription phenomenon," including questionable prescribing practices, it seems likely that nonadherence plays a major role. These high nonadherence rates underscore the need to attend to attitudinal dimensions; the finding that mothers who know more about ADHD are more likely to accept pharmacotherapy (Liu et al., 1991) indicates the potential value of considering beliefs and attitudes when launching a treatment plan. The increasingly compelling evidence of a genetic basis for ADHD (e.g., Gjone, Stevenson, & Sundet, 1996; LaHoste et al., 1996) may relieve parental burdens of guilt and perceived inadequacy and provide parents with the justification they need to embrace a biological treatment for a disorder that surfaces in behavioral and psychological realms (Faraone, 1996; Whalen & Henker, 1976).

Models of Service Delivery

Greene, Marchant, and Siperstein (1996) have attempted to translate the social ecological model into a framework for classroom interventions that focuses on the match or mismatch between the child and multiple aspects of the environment. These authors describe several "compatibility equations" designed to enhance the goodness-of-fit between the child with ADHD and his or her teachers, peers, settings, and treatments. The importance of teacher-treatment compatibility is also emphasized, given the heterogeneity in teachers' backgrounds, personal styles, and proclivities as well as the need to understand how such factors mediate treatment delivery and outcomes (Greene, 1995).

Other social ecological perspectives extend beyond schools, teachers, and students with ADHD. One example is the comprehensive initiative formulated by Adelman and Taylor (in press; Adelman, 1996; Taylor & Adelman, 1996) that is aimed at preventing or ameliorating the vast array of learning, behavior, emotional, and health problems confronted by today's children and adolescents. This model proposes to address a comprehensive array of barriers to teaching and learning by integrating the education, health, community, and social service systems into a single functional unit. A core concept is the enabling component, a flexible compendium of interventions that includes not only classroom-focused activities, but also family assistance programs, crisis coping, support for transitions, and community outreach.

Adelman and Taylor present an ambitious and promising proposal for systemic reform in education and mental health services. Although feasibility and efficacy remain to be demonstrated, the model provides a sharp contrast to the current piecemeal, uncoordinated forms of service delivery wherein the needs of the individual with ADHD fall between the slots of the educational and medical systems, and any therapies beyond the drug therapies are often unaffordable or simply unavailable. But merely shifting the emphasis from individual services to system reform is unlikely to improve either costs or outcomes. Bickman's (1996) detailing of the disappointing outcomes of a comprehensive continuum-of-care demonstration project provides a sobering reminder of the need for a simultaneous focus on system and individual levels of intervention. The union of such reform initiatives and the current insistence on empirically validated psychological treatments may guide the development of multimodal approaches that work.

A GLIMPSE AHEAD

As the twenty-first century draws near, it seems an apt time not only to take stock, as in this chapter, but also to take a brief glance at the immediate future. By the time this book appears in print, distinct progress will have been made in the race to map the genetic markers for the heterogeneous behavioral components of ADHD. On the one hand, the search to unlock the genetic codes will inevitably bring or accompany progress in pinpointing and assessing different subtypes of ADHD. Improved identification and delineation, in turn, should lead the way to more specific and effective therapies, both pharmacologic and nonpharmacologic. These advances may also lead to truly preventive interventions. On the other hand, improved technologies for identifying disorders and predicting outcomes will also confront professionals and parents with a host of ethical dilemmas and value conflicts in their search to prevent and ameliorate the set of problems we now know as ADHD.

ALL THINGS CONSIDERED: BALANCING PROS, CONS, AND UNKNOWNS

If one merely counts the number of words in this chapter devoted to the positive versus the negative or uncertain aspects of stimulant pharmacotherapy, one might conclude that this is a risky treatment that should be considered only as a last resort. But nothing could be further from the truth. As noted at the outset, no other treatment modality for childhood behavior problems has the documented success record of stimulant pharmacotherapy. The research database for this treatment is unique in both its extensiveness and its methodological rigor. Multiple studies across heterogeneous populations, procedures, and settings converge on a positive conclusion: The vast majority of school-age boys with ADHD-type problems benefit from stimulant medication in ways that are clinically meaningful to the children themselves as well as to their families, peers, and others with whom they interact. Although the evidence is far less extensive, there are also indications that school-age girls and adolescents of both genders show similar gains, and many adults seem to benefit as well, despite a somewhat less predictable course during the adult years.

But several limitations and problems were also described. The identification of ADHD always requires a degree of subjectivity, and many of the behavior problems that characterize ADHD are also found in individuals with other disorders or with no diagnosable disorder. When the diagnostic boundaries are elastic and the treatment markedly effective, it is not surprising to find expanding eligibility criteria and increasing prescription rates. Despite a dearth of empirical justification, slippery slopes are apparent as stimulant pharmacotherapy is being recommended for an increasing range of daily discomforts, clinical disorders, and developmental levels. Even within the ADHD population, heterogeneity is endemic, both in the problem domains seen in different individuals diagnosed with ADHD, and in treatment responsiveness. Dosage changes have different effects on different domains in different individuals, and improvement in one area may be accompanied by no change or even deterioration in another. Some areas such as academic performance and peer relations appear to be particularly resistant to treatment.

Although serious side effects have been relatively rare, they are always possible, as are more subtle untoward effects on self-perceptions and social impressions. There is little empirical basis for predicting either who will benefit or who might be at risk for unsalutary consequences. And finally, most of the well-controlled outcome studies are based on brief treatment durations; there are few studies documenting long-term improvements, either with continuing treatment or after treatment has been discontinued.

These conclusions lead ineluctably to questions about how to balance the impressive track record against the host of unknowns. Our own view is that the limitations raised throughout this chapter neither can nor should detract from the strongly positive bottom line. They were delineated not to discourage the treatment, but rather to identify important research directions and to detail inherent complexities that may be overlooked when a treatment is so convenient to administer and often so dramatic in its effects. It is unreasonable to expect a single treatment to ameliorate the multiplicity and chronicity of the problems that define ADHD. Yet the relief that results from rapid gains in some areas may obscure difficulties that prove treatment-resistant and others that improve but fail to normalize. The attractiveness of the treatment compels continuing vigilance and systematic cost/benefit analyses to ensure that stimulant pharmacotherapy is given only when and for as long as it is needed and beneficial. The heterogeneous, limited, and at times inconsistent results, along with the paucity of evidence of long-term gains, mandate multimodal treatment approaches and careful attention to the framing and sequencing of treatment components. These considerations also underscore the need to monitor an array of behavioral domains that extends far beyond specific therapeutic targets.

In sum, the scientific database provides sturdy support for those making clinical decisions to use stimulant medication in appropriate cases. The knowledgeable prescriber will be well aware of both the limitations of these drugs and the fact that they are most effective in helping to manage problems, not to remediate them.

REFERENCES

Abikoff, H. (1991). Cognitive training in ADHD children: Less to it than meets the eye. *Journal of Learning Disabilities, 24,* 205–209.

Abikoff, H., & Hechtman, L. (1996). Multimodal therapy and stimulants in the treatment of children with ADHD. In P. Jensen & T. Hibbs (Eds.), *Psychosocial treatment for child and adolescent disorders: Empirically based approaches* (pp. 341–369). Washington, DC: American Psychological Association.

Adelman, H. S. (1996). *Restructuring education support services: Toward the concept of an enabling component.* Kent, OH: American School Health Association.

Adelman, H. S., & Taylor, L. (in press). System reform to address barriers to learning: Beyond school-linked services and full service schools. *American Journal of Orthopsychiatry.*

Ahmann, P. A., Waltonen, S. J., Olson, K. A., Theye, F. W., Van Erem, A. J., & LaPlant, R. (1993). Placebo-controlled evaluation and Ritalin side effects. *Pediatrics, 91,* 1101–1106.

Aman, M. G., Kern, R. A., McGhee, D. E., & Arnold, L. E. (1993). Fenfluramine and methylphenidate in children with mental retardation and ADHD: Clinical and side effects. *Journal of the American Academy of Child and Adolescent Psychiatry, 32,* 851–859.

Anastopoulos, A. D., Shelton, T. L., DuPaul, G. J., & Guevremont, D. C. (1993). Parent training for attention-deficit hyperactivity disorder: Its impact on parent functioning. *Journal of Abnormal Child Psychology, 21,* 581–596.

Barkley, R. A., McMurray, M. B., Edelbrock, C. S., & Robbins, K. (1990). Side effects of methylphenidate in children with attention deficit hyperactivity disorder: A systemic (sic), placebo-controlled evaluation. *Pediatrics, 86,* 184–192.

Bickman, L. (1996). A continuum of care. More is not always better. *American Psychologist, 51,* 689–701.

Biederman, J., Milberger, S., Faraone, S. V., Kiely, K., Guite, J., Mick, E., Ablon, J. S., Warburton, R., Reed, E., & Davis, S. G. (1995). Impact of adversity on functioning and comorbidity in children with attention-deficit hyperactivity disorder. *Journal of the American Academy of Child and Adolescent Psychiatry, 34,* 1495–1503.

Bird, H. R., Gould, M. S., & Staghezza, B. M. (1993). Patterns of diagnostic comorbidity in a community sample of children aged 9 through 16 years. *Journal of the American Academy of Child and Adolescent Psychiatry, 32,* 361–368.

Birmaher, B., Quintana, H., & Greenhill, L. L. (1988). Methylphenidate treatment of hyperactive autistic children. *Journal of the American Academy of Child and Adolescent Psychiatry, 27,* 248–251.

Borden, K. A., & Brown, R. T. (1989). Attributional outcomes: The subtle messages of treatments for attention deficit disorder. *Cognitive Therapy Research, 13,* 147–160.

Bronfenbrenner, U. (1977). Toward an experimental ecology of human development. *Child Development, 32,* 513–531.

Brown, R. T., Borden, K. A., Wynne, M. E., Spunt, A. L., & Clingerman, S. R. (1987). Compliance with pharmacological and cognitive treatments for attention deficit disorder. *Journal of the American Academy of Child and Adolescent Psychiatry, 26,* 521–526.

Brown, R. T., Dreelin, E., & Dingle, A. D. (1997). Neuropsychological effects of stimulant medication on children's learning and behavior. In C. R. Reynolds & E. Fletcher-Janzen (Eds.), *Handbook of clinical child neuropsychology* (2nd ed., pp. 539–572). New York: Plenum Press.

Brown, R. T., Jaffe, S. L., Silverstein, J., & Magee, H. (1991). Methylphenidate and adolescents hospitalized with conduct disorder: Dose effects on classroom behavior, academic performance, and impulsivity. *Journal of Clinical Child Psychology, 20,* 282–292.

Brown, R. T., & Pacini, J. N. (1989). Perceived family functioning, marital status, and depression in parents of boys with attention deficit disorder. *Journal of Learning Disabilities, 22,* 581–587.

Brown, R. T., & Sexson, S. B. (1989). Effects of methylphenidate on cardiovascular responses in attention deficit hyperactivity disordered adolescents. *Journal of Adolescent Health Care, 10,* 179–183.

Buhrmester, D., Whalen, C. K., Henker, B., MacDonald, V., & Hinshaw, S. P. (1992). Prosocial behavior in hyperactive boys: Effects of stimulant medication and comparison with normal boys. *Journal of Abnormal Child Psychology, 20,* 103–121.

Buitelaar, J. K., van der Gaag, R. J., Swaab-Barneveld, H., & Kuiper, M. (1995). Prediction of clinical response to methylphenidate in children with attention-deficit hyperactivity disorder. *Journal of the American Academy of Child and Adolescent Psychiatry, 34,* 1025–1032.

Burke, M. S., Josephson, A., & Lightsey, A. (1995). Combined methylphenidate and imipramine complication. *Journal of the American Academy of Child and Adolescent Psychiatry, 34,* 403–404.

Campbell, M., & Cueva, J. E. (1995). Psychopharmacology in child and adolescent psychiatry: A review of the past seven years. Part I. *Journal of the Academy of Child and Adolescent Psychiatry, 34,* 1124–1132.

Cantwell, D. P. (1996). Attention deficit disorder: A review of the past 10 years. *Journal of the Academy of Child and Adolescent Psychiatry, 35,* 978–987.

Carlson, C. L., Pelham, W. E., Milich, R., & Dixon, J. (1992). Single and combined effects of methylphenidate and behavior therapy on the classroom performance of children with attention-deficit hyperactivity disorder. *Journal of Abnormal Child Psychology, 20,* 213–231.

Carlson, G. A., Rapport, M. D., Kelly, K. L., & Pataki, C. S. (1992). The effects of methylphenidate and lithium on attention and activity level. *Journal of the American Academy of Child and Adolescent Psychiatry, 31,* 262–270.

Carlson, G. A., Rapport, M. D., Kelly, K. L., & Pataki, C. S. (1995). Methylphenidate and desipramine in hospitalized children with comorbid behavior and mood disorders: Separate and combined effects on behavior and mood. *Journal of Child and Adolescent Psychopharmacology, 5,* 191–204.

Caron, C., & Rutter, M. (1991). Comorbidity in child psychopathology: Concepts, issues and research strategies. *Journal of Child Psychology and Psychiatry, 32,* 1063–1080.

Chiarello, R. J., & Cole, J. O. (1987). The use of psychostimulants in general psychiatry. A reconsideration. *Archives of General Psychiatry, 44,* 286–295.

Cohen, P., Cohen, J., Kasen, S., Velez, C. N., Hartmark, C., Johnson, J., Rojas, M., Brook, J., & Streuning, E. L. (1993). An epidemiological study of disorders in late childhood and adolescence—I. Age- and gender-specific prevalence. *Journal of Child Psychology and Psychiatry, 34,* 851–867.

Conners, C. K., Wells, K. C., Erhardt, D., March, J. S., Schulte, A., Osborne, S., Fiore, C., & Butcher, A. T. (1994). Multimodality therapies. Methodologic issues in research and practice. *Child and Adolescent Psychiatric Clinics of North America, 3,* 361–377.

Cunningham, C. E., Benness, B. B., & Siegel, L. S. (1988). Family functioning, time allocation, and parental depression in the families of normal and ADDH children. *Journal of Clinical Child Psychology, 17,* 169–177.

Cunningham, C. E., Bremmer, R., & Boyle, M. (1995). Large group community-based parenting programs for families of preschoolers at risk for disruptive behaviour disorders: Utilization, cost effectiveness, and outcome. *Journal of Child Psychology and Psychiatry, 36,* 1141–1160.

Douglas, V. I., Barr, R. G., Desilets, J., & Sherman, E. (1995). Do high doses of stimulants impair flexible thinking in attention-deficit hyperactivity disorder? *Journal of the American Academy of Child and Adolescent Psychiatry, 34,* 877–885.

Dulcan, M. K., & American Academy of Child and Adolescent Psychiatry Work Group. (in press). Practice parameters for the assessment and treatment of attention-deficit/hyperactivity disorder. *Journal of the American Academy of Child and Adolescent Psychiatry.*

DuPaul, G. J., Barkley, R. A., & McMurray, M. B. (1994). Response of children with ADHD to methylphenidate: Interaction with internalizing symptoms. *Journal of the American Academy of Child and Adolescent Psychiatry, 33,* 894–903.

DuPaul, G. J., & Rapport, M. D. (1993). Does methylphenidate normalize the classroom performance of children with attention deficit disorder? *Journal of the American Academy of Child and Adolescent Psychiatry, 32,* 190–198.

Elia, J., Borcherding, B. G., Rapoport, J. L., & Keysor, C. S. (1991). Methylphenidate and dextroamphetamine treatments of hyperactivity: Are there true nonresponders? *Psychiatry Research, 36,* 141–155.

Epstein, M. H., Singh, N. N., Luebke, J., & Stout, C. E. (1991). Psychopharmacological intervention. II: Teacher perceptions of psychotropic medication for students with learning disabilities. *Journal of Learning Disabilities, 24,* 477–483.

Faraone, S. V. (1996). Discussion of "Genetic influence on parent-reported attention-related problems in a Norwegian general population twin sample." *Journal of the American Academy of Child and Adolescent Psychiatry, 35,* 596–598.

Ferdinand, R. F., Verhulst, F. C., & Wiznitzer, M. (1995). Continuity and change of self-reported problem behaviors from adolescence into young adulthood. *Journal of the American Academy of Child and Adolescent Psychiatry, 34,* 680–690.

Fine, S., & Johnston, C. (1993). Drug and placebo side effects in methylphenidate-placebo trial for attention deficit hyperactivity disorder. *Child Psychiatry and Human Development, 24,* 25–30.

Firestone, P. (1982). Factors associated with children's adherence to stimulant medication. *American Journal of Orthopsychiatry, 52,* 447–457.

Fitzpatrick, P. A., Klorman, R., Brumaghim, J. T., & Borgstedt, A. D. (1992). Effects of sustained-release and standard preparations of methylphenidate on attention deficit disorder. *Journal of the Academy of Child and Adolescent Psychiatry, 31,* 226–234.

Forness, S. R., Swanson, J. M., Cantwell, D. P., Guthrie, D., & Sena, R. (1992). Response to stimulant medication across six measures of school-related performance in children with ADHD and disruptive behavior. *Behavioral Disorders, 18,* 42–53.

Fried, J. E. (1991). Use of Ritalin in the practice of pediatrics. In L. L. Greenhill & B. B. Osman (Eds.), *Ritalin: Theory and patient management* (pp. 131–139). New York: Mary Ann Liebert.

Gadow, K. D., Sverd, J., Sprafkin, J., Nolan, E. E., & Ezor, S. N. (1995). Efficacy of methylphenidate for attention-deficit hyperactivity disorder in children with tic disorder. *Archives of General Psychiatry, 52*, 444–455.

Gammon, G. D., & Brown, T. E. (1993). Fluoxetine augmentation of methylphenidate for attention deficit and comorbid disorders. *Journal of Child and Adolescent Psychopharmacology, 3*, 1–10.

Gjone, H., Stevenson, J., & Sundet, J. M. (1996). Genetic influence on parent-reported attention-related problems in a Norwegian general population twin sample. *Journal of the American Academy of Child and Adolescent Psychiatry, 35*, 588–596.

Granger, D. A., Whalen, C. K., Henker, B., & Cantwell, C. (1996). ADHD boys' behavior during structured classroom social activities: Effects of social demands, teacher proximity, and methylphenidate. *Journal of Attention Disorders, 1*, 16–30.

Greene, R. W. (1995). Students with ADHD in school classrooms: Teacher factors related to compatibility, assessment, and intervention. *School Psychology Review, 24*, 81–93.

Greene, R. W., Marchant, C., & Siperstein, G. N. (1996). *Responding to the social needs of students with ADHD: Compatibility equations to guide classroom interventions.* Manuscript submitted for publication.

Greenhill, L. L., Abikoff, H. B., Arnold, L. E., Cantwell, D. P., Conners, C. K., Elliott, G., Hechtman, L., Hinshaw, S. P., Hoza, B., Jensen, P. S., March, J. S., Newcorn, J., Pelham, W. E., Severe, J. B., Swanson, J. M., Vitiello, B., & Wells, K. (1996). Medication treatment strategies in the MTA study: Relevance to clinicians and researchers. *Journal of the American Academy of Child and Adolescent Psychiatry, 35*, 1304–1313.

Hallowell, E. M., & Ratey, J. J. (1994). *Driven to distraction.* New York: Pantheon.

Hallowell, E. M., & Ratey, J. J. (1996). *Answers to distraction.* New York: Bantam.

Hammen, C., & Compas, B. E. (1994). Unmasking unmasked depression in children and adolescents: The problem of comorbidity. *Clinical Psychology Review, 14*, 585–603.

Handen, B. L., Janosky, J., McAuliffe, S., Breaux, A. M., & Feldman, H. (1994). Prediction of response to methylphenidate among children with ADHD and mental retardation. *Journal of the American Academy of Child and Adolescent Psychiatry, 33*, 1185–1193.

Henker, B., Whalen, C. K., Bugental, D. B., & Barker, C. (1981). Licit and illicit drug use patterns in stimulant treated children and their peers. In K. D. Gadow & J. Loney (Eds.), *Psychosocial aspects of drug treatment for hyperactivity* (pp. 443–462). Boulder, CO: Westview Press.

Hinshaw, S. P., Heller, T., & McHale, J. P. (1992). Covert antisocial behavior in boys with attention-deficit hyperactivity disorder: External validation and effects of methylphenidate. *Journal of Consulting and Clinical Psychology, 60*, 274–281.

Hinshaw, S. P., Henker, B., Whalen, C. K., Erhardt, D., & Dunnington, R. E., Jr. (1989). Aggressive, prosocial, and nonsocial behavior in hyperactive boys: Dose effects of methylphenidate in naturalistic settings. *Journal of Consulting and Clinical Psychology, 57,* 636–643.

Hunt, R. D., Lau, S., & Ryu, J. (1991). Alternative therapies for ADHD. In L. L. Greenhill & B. B. Osman (Eds.), *Ritalin: Theory and patient management* (pp. 75–95). New York: Mary Ann Liebert.

Jacobvitz, D., Sroufe, L. A., Stewart, M., & Leffert, N. (1990). Treatment of attentional and hyperactivity problems in children with sympathomimetic drugs: A comprehensive review. *Journal of the American Academy of Child and Adolescent Psychiatry, 29,* 677–688.

Jaffe, L. L. (1991). Intranasal abuse of prescribed methylphenidate by an alcohol and drug abusing adolescent with ADHD. *Journal of the American Academy of Child and Adolescent Psychiatry, 30,* 773–775.

Johnston, C., Pelham, W. E., Hoza, J., & Sturges, J. (1988). Psychostimulant rebound in attention deficit disordered boys. *Journal of the American Academy of Child and Adolescent Psychiatry, 27,* 806–810.

Klein, R. G., & Bessler, A. W. (1992). Stimulant side effects in children. In J. M. Kane & J. A. Lieberman (Eds.), *Adverse effects of psychotropic drugs* (pp. 470–496). New York: Guilford Press.

Klein, R. G., & Mannuzza, S. (1988). Hyperactive boys almost grown up. III. Methylphenidate effects on ultimate height. *Archives of General Psychiatry, 45,* 1131–1134.

Klein, R. G., & Wender, P. (1995). The role of methylphenidate in psychiatry. *Archives of General Psychiatry, 52,* 429–433.

LaHoste, G. J., Swanson, J. M., Wigal, S. B., Glabe, C., Wigal, T., King, N., & Kennedy, J. L. (1996). Dopamine D4 receptor gene polymorphism is associated with attention deficit hyperactivity disorder. *Molecular Psychiatry, 1,* 121–124.

Liu, C., Robin, A. L., Brenner, S., & Eastman, J. (1991). Social acceptability of methylphenidate and behavior modification for treating attention deficit hyperactivity disorder. *Pediatrics, 88,* 560–565.

Loeber, R., & Keenan, K. (1994). Interaction between conduct disorder and its comorbid conditions: Effects of age and gender. *Clinical Psychology Review, 14,* 497–523.

Mannuzza, S., Klein, R. G., Bessler, A., Malloy, P., & LaPadula, M. (1993). Adult outcome of hyperactive boys: Educational achievement, occupational rank, and psychiatric status. *Archives of General Psychiatry, 50,* 565–576.

Mannuzza, S., Klein, R. G., Bonagura, N., Malloy, P., Giampino, T. L., & Addalli, K. A. (1991). Hyperactive boys almost grown up. V. Replication of psychiatric status. *Archives of General Psychiatry, 48,* 77–83.

Markowitz, J., & Patrick, K. (1996). Polypharmacy side effects [letter to the editor]. *Journal of the American Academy of Child and Adolescent Psychiatry, 35,* 842.

Mash, E. J., & Johnston, C. (1990). Determinants of parenting stress: Illustrations from families of hyperactive children and families of physically abused children. *Journal of Clinical Child Psychology, 19,* 313–328.

Milich, R., Carlson, C. K., Pelham, W. E., & Licht, B. G. (1991). Effects of methylphenidate on the persistence of ADHD boys following failure experiences. *Journal of Abnormal Child Psychology, 19,* 519–536.

Mittl, V. F., & Robin, A. (1987). Acceptability of alternative interventions for parent-adolescent conflict. *Behavioral Assessment, 9,* 417–428.

Pataki, C. S., Carlson, G. A., Kelly, K. L., Rapport, M. D., & Biancaniello, T. M. (1993). Side effects of methylphenidate and desipramine alone and in combination in children. *Journal of the American Academy of Child and Adolescent Psychiatry, 32,* 1065–1072.

Pelham, W. E., Carlson, C., Sams, S. E., Vallano, G., Dixon, M. J., & Hoza, B. (1993). Separate and combined effects of methylphenidate and behavior modification on boys with attention deficit-hyperactivity disorder in the classroom. *Journal of Consulting and Clinical Psychology, 61,* 506–515.

Pelham, W. E., Murphy, D. A., Vannatta, K., Milich, R., Licht, B. G., Gnagy, E. M., Greenslade, K. E., Greiner, A. R., & Vodde-Hamilton, M. (1992). Methylphenidate and attributions in boys with attention-deficit hyperactivity disorder. *Journal of Consulting and Clinical Psychology, 60,* 282–292.

Pelham, W. E., Swanson, J. M., Furman, M. B., & Schwindt, H. (1995). Pemoline effects on children with ADHD: A time-response by dose-response analysis on classroom measures. *Journal of the American Academy of Child and Adolescent Psychiatry, 34,* 1504–1413.

Pfiffner, L. J., & O'Leary, S. G. (1993). School-based psychological treatments. In J. L. Matson (Ed.), *Handbook of hyperactivity in children* (pp. 234–255). Boston: Allyn & Bacon.

Pliszka, S. R. (1989). Effect of anxiety on cognition, behavior, and stimulant response in ADHD. *Journal of the American Academy of Child and Adolescent Psychiatry, 28,* 882–887.

Porrino, L. J., Rapoport, J. L., Behar, D., Ismond, D. R., & Bunney, W. E., Jr. (1983). A naturalistic assessment of the motor activity of hyperactive boys. II. Stimulant drug effects. *Archives of General Psychiatry, 40,* 688–693.

Prince, J. B., Wilens, T. E., Biederman, J., Spencer, T. J., & Wozniak, J. R. (1996). Clonidine for sleep disturbances associated with attention-deficit hyperactivity disorder: A systematic chart review of 62 cases. *Journal of the American Academy of Child and Adolescent Psychiatry, 35,* 599–605.

Rapoport, J. L., Buchsbaum, M. S., Zahn, T. P., Weingartner, H., Ludlow, C., & Mikkelsen, E. J. (1978). Dextroamphetamine: Cognitive and behavioral effects in normal prepubertal boys. *Science, 199,* 560–562.

Rapoport, J. L., Quinn, P. O., Bradbard, G., Riddle, K. D., & Brooks, E. (1974). Imipramine and methylphenidate treatments of hyperactive boys: A double-blind comparison. *Archives of General Psychiatry, 30,* 789–793.

Rapport, M. D., Denney, C., DuPaul, G. J., & Gardner, M. J. (1994). Attention deficit disorder and methylphenidate: Normalization rates, clinical effectiveness, and response prediction in 76 children. *Journal of the American Academy of Child and Adolescent Psychiatry, 33,* 882–893.

Richters, J. E., Arnold, L. E., Jensen, P. S., Abikoff, H., Conners, C. K., Greenhill, L. L., Hechtman, L., Hinshaw, S. P., Pelham, W. E., & Swanson, J. M. (1995). NIMH collaborative multisite multimodal treatment study of children with ADHD: 1. Background and rationale. *Journal of the American Academy of Child and Adolescent Psychiatry, 34,* 987–1000.

Safer, D. J. (1992). Relative cardiovascular safety of psychostimulants used to treat attention-deficit hyperactivity disorder. *Journal of Child and Adolescent Psychopharmacology, 2,* 279–290.

Safer, D. J. (1994). The impact of recent lawsuits on methylphenidate sales. *Clinical Pediatrics, 33,* 166–168.

Safer, D. J., & Krager, J. M. (1992). Effect of a media blitz and a threatened lawsuit on stimulant treatment. *Journal of the American Medical Association, 268,* 1004–1007.

Safer, D. J., & Krager, J. M. (1994). The increased rate of stimulant treatment for hyperactive/inattentive students in secondary schools. *Pediatrics, 94,* 462–464.

Schachar, R., & Tannock, R. (1993). Childhood hyperactivity and psychostimulants: A review of extended treatment studies. *Journal of Child and Adolescent Psychopharmacology, 3,* 81–97.

Seligman, M. E. P. (1995). The effectiveness of psychotherapy: The *Consumer Reports* survey. *American Psychologist, 50,* 965–974.

Sherman, M., & Hertzig, M. E. (1991). Prescribing practices of Ritalin: The Suffolk County, New York Study. In L. L. Greenhill & B. B. Osman (Eds.), *Ritalin: Theory and patient management* (pp. 187–193). New York: Mary Ann Liebert.

Solanto, M. V., & Wender, E. H. (1989). Does methylphenidate constrict cognitive functioning? *Journal of the American Academy of Child and Adolescent Psychiatry, 28,* 897–902.

Spencer, T. J., Biederman, J., Harding, M., O'Donnell, D., Faraone, S. V., & Wilens, T. E. (1996). Growth deficits in ADHD children revisited: Evidence for disorder-associated growth delays? *Journal of the American Academy of Child and Adolescent Psychiatry, 35,* 1460–1469.

Spencer, T., Biederman, J., Wilens, T., Harding, M., O'Donnell, D., & Griffin, S. (1996). Pharmacotherapy of attention-deficit hyperactivity disorder across the life cycle. *Journal of the American Academy of Child and Adolescent Psychiatry, 35,* 409–432.

Spencer, T., Wilens, T., Biederman, J., Faraone, S. V., Ablon, J. S., & Lapey, K. (1995). A double-blind, crossover comparison of methylphenidate and placebo in adults with childhood-onset attention-deficit hyperactivity disorder. *Archives of General Psychiatry, 52,* 434–443.

Sprague, R. L., & Sleator, E. K. (1977). Methylphenidate in hyperkinetic children: Differences in dose effects on learning and social behavior. *Science, 198,* 1274–1276.

Sternlicht, H. C., & Wells, S. R. (1995). Risperidone in childhood schizophrenia [letter to the editor]. *Journal of the American Academy of Child and Adolescent Psychiatry, 34,* 540.

Strayhorn, J. M., Jr., Rapp, N., Donina, W., & Strain, P. S. (1988). Randomized trial of methylphenidate for an autistic child. *Journal of the American Academy of Child and Adolescent Psychiatry, 27*, 244–247.

Sullivan, M. A., & O'Leary, S. G. (1990). Maintenance following reward and cost token programs. *Behavior Therapy, 21*, 139–149.

Sulzbacher, S. I. (1973). Psychotropic medication with children: An evaluation of procedural biases in results of reported studies. *Pediatrics, 51*, 513–517.

Swanson, J. M., Flockhart, D., Udrea, D., Cantwell, D., Connor, D., & Williams, L. (1995). Clonidine in the treatment of ADHD: Questions about safety and efficacy [letter to the editor]. *Journal of Child and Adolescent Psychopharmacology, 5*, 301–304.

Swanson, J. M., Lerner, M., & Williams, L. (1995). More frequent diagnosis of attention deficit-hyperactivity disorder [letter to the editor]. *New England Journal of Medicine, 333*, 944.

Swanson, J. M., McBurnett, K., Christian, D. L., & Wigal, T. (1995). Stimulant medications and the treatment of children with ADHD. In T. H. Ollendick & R. J. Prinz (Eds.), *Advances in clinical child psychology* (Vol. 17, pp. 265–322). New York: Plenum Press.

Swanson, J., Udrea, D., Cantwell, D., Connor, D., Wigal, S., Crowley, K., Lerner, M., Williams, L., Wigal, T., Elliot, G., March, J., Greenhill, L., Perel, J., Vitiello, B., Arnold, G., & Jensen, P. (1996). *Clonidine in the treatment of children with ADHD: 1. Efficacy.* Manuscript submitted for publication.

Tannock, R. (in press). Attention deficit disorders with anxiety disorders. In T. E. Brown (Ed.), *Attention deficit disorders and comorbidities in children, adolescents and adults.* New York: American Psychiatric Press.

Tannock, R., Ickowicz, A., & Schachar, R. (1995). Differential effects of methylphenidate on working memory in ADHD children with and without comorbid anxiety. *Journal of the American Academy of Child and Adolescent Psychiatry, 34*, 886–896.

Tannock, R., Schachar, R., & Logan, G. (1995). Methylphenidate and cognitive flexibility: Dissociated dose effects in hyperactive children. *Journal of Abnormal Child Psychology, 23*, 235–266.

Tarnowski, K. J., Gavaghan, M. P., & Wisniewski, J. J. (1989). Acceptability of interventions for pediatric pain management. *Journal of Pediatric Psychology, 14*, 463–472.

Taylor, L., & Adelman, H. S. (1996). Mental health in the schools: Promising directions for practice. In L. Juszcak & M. Fisher (Eds.), *Health care in schools.* Philadelphia: Hanley & Belfus.

Vincent, J., Varley, C. K., & Leger, P. (1990). Effects of methylphenidate on early adolescent growth. *American Journal of Psychiatry, 147*, 501–502.

Weiss, G., & Hechtman, L. T. (1993). *Hyperactive children grown up. ADHD in children, adolescents, and adults* (2nd ed.). New York: Guilford Press.

Wender, P. H. (1995). *Attention-deficit hyperactivity disorder in adults.* New York: Oxford University Press.

Whalen, C. K., & Henker B. (1976). Psychostimulants and children: A review and analysis. *Psychological Bulletin, 83,* 1113–1130.

Whalen, C. K., & Henker, B. (1980). The social ecology of psychostimulant treatment: A model for conceptual and empirical analysis. In C. K. Whalen & B. Henker (Eds.), *Hyperactive children: The social ecology of identification and treatment* (pp. 3–51). New York: Academic Press.

Whalen, C. K., & Henker, B. (1986a). Cognitive behavior therapy for hyperactive children: What do we know? *Journal of Children in Contemporary Society, 19,* 123–141.

Whalen, C. K., & Henker, B. (1986b). Group designs in applied psychopharmacology. In K. D. Gadow & A. Poling (Eds.), *Advances in learning and behavioral disabilities (Suppl. 1): Methodological issues in human psychopharmacology* (pp. 137–222). Greenwich, CT: JAI Press.

Whalen, C. K., & Henker, B. (1991a). The social impact of stimulant treatment for hyperactive children. *Journal of Learning Disabilities, 24,* 231–241.

Whalen, C. K., & Henker, B. (1991b). Therapies for hyperactive children: Comparisons, combinations, and compromises. *Journal of Consulting and Clinical Psychology, 59,* 126–137.

Whalen, C. K., & Henker, B. (1992). The social profile of attention-deficit hyperactivity disorder: Five fundamental facets. *Child and Adolescent Psychiatric Clinics of North America, 1,* 395–410.

Whalen, C. K., & Henker, B. (in press). Attention-deficit/hyperactivity disorders. In T. H. Ollendick & M. Hersen (Eds.), *Handbook of child psychopathology* (3rd ed.). New York: Plenum Press.

Whalen, C. K., Henker, B., Buhrmester, D., Hinshaw, S. P., Huber, A., & Laski, K. (1989). Does stimulant medication improve the peer status of hyperactive children? *Journal of Consulting and Clinical Psychology, 57,* 545–549.

Whalen, C. K., Henker, B., & Granger, D. A. (1989). Ratings of medication effects in hyperactive children: Viable or vulnerable? *Behavioral Assessment, 11,* 179–199.

Whalen, C. K., Henker, B., Hinshaw, S. P., Heller, T., & Huber-Dressler, A. (1991). The messages of medication: Effects of actual versus informed medication status on hyperactive boys' expectancies and self-evaluations. *Journal of Consulting and Clinical Psychology, 59,* 602–606.

Wilens, T. E., Spencer, T., Biederman, J., Wozniak, J., & Connor, D. (1995). Combined pharmacotherapy: An emerging trend in pediatric psychopharmacology. *Journal of the American Academy of Child and Adolescent Psychiatry, 34,* 110–112.

Wolraich, M. L., Hannah, J. N., Pinnock, T. Y., Baumgaertel, A., & Brown, J. (1996). Comparison of diagnostic criteria for attention-deficit hyperactivity disorder in a county-wide sample. *Journal of the American Academy of Child and Adolescent Psychiatry, 35,* 319–324.

Zeiner, P. (1995). Body growth and cardiovascular function after extended treatment (1.75 years) with methylphenidate in boys with attention-deficit hyperactivity disorder. *Journal of Child and Adolescent Psychopharmacology, 5,* 129–138.

Part Four

OVERVIEW

CHAPTER 10

What Are We to Conclude about Psychoactive Drugs? Scanning the Major Findings

SEYMOUR FISHER and ROGER P. GREENBERG

T HE CONTRIBUTORS TO this book have probed and discussed a widely inclusive spectrum of the research pertinent to judging and thinking about the psychoactive drugs. In this chapter, we will scan the core information that emerged from each chapter concerned with drug efficacies for the presumed categories of psychopathology.

First, to provide a framework for interpreting the multiple specific findings that emerged, it will be helpful to consider two broad theoretical issues initially taken up in Chapters 1–3. Chapter 1 focuses on the nature of the placebo, the overlap between placebo and active drug, and the psychosocial conditions mediating both drug and placebo responses; Chapters 2 and 3 appraise matters related to the meaning and reliabilities of the *DSM* categories.

The writings concerned with the *Diagnostic and Statistical Manual of Mental Disorders (DSM)* analyze the logic and credibility of the *DSM* scheme. This is directly relevant to the present work because so frequently drug treatments are portrayed as if they target specific syndromes. Presumably, antidepressants are specific for depressive symptomatology; anxiolytics are directed at defined anxiety clusters; and so forth. Psychopathology is conceptualized as a series of disorders that can be reliably differentiated and traced to separate origins or causations. The *DSM* portrays a schema in which clear formal boundaries can be spelled out among the various categories of pathology. The apparent existence of such boundaries rationalizes the notion of constructing a drug treatment for each category.[1] The *DSM* is presumably a reliable map of basic symptom domains that require targeted therapeutic drugs.

In Chapter 3, Carson raises trenchant questions about the rationality of the *DSM*. He asserts that not only is the *DSM* based on vague, tautological definitions of psychopathology, but also that most of the ever-increasing categories lack reliability. The categories often overlap making it difficult to obtain consistent clinical judgments concerning where individual symptom clusters belong. Especially important, says Carson, is that no one has demonstrated the validity of the *DSM*. There is little scientific evidence that classifying an individual within the *DSM* schema predicts much of significance about future course or prognosis. This implies that there are deficiencies of some consequence in the schema and perhaps in the therapies that, in part, derive their rationale from it.

M. Greenberg, in Chapter 2, persuasively provides affirmation of such doubt. He cites dramatic data consistently indicating that high rates of comorbidity characterize psychiatric patients—at least 50% of such patients display symptoms indicating that they do not fall simply into one *DSM* category but rather into two or more. This fluidity in the *DSM* boundaries leads to the conclusion that the *DSM* only pretends to the existence of a credibly functional diagnostic structure. Kirk and Kutchins reached a similar conclusion (1992) after their detailed review of the pertinent literature. M. Greenberg also presents provocative evidence that patients with comorbid diagnoses probably obtain significantly less benefit from psychotropic drugs than do those who are non-comorbid. The importance of this likelihood can be illustrated in the context of persons diagnosed as depressed. Since the rate of positive therapeutic response of the depressed to psychotropic drugs usually cited for controlled trials is based on the study of "pure" depressed samples (with all comorbid individuals eliminated), this represents an exaggeration of what is actually true in real life where comorbidity is highly prevalent. This is another reason to doubt the claims about how well antidepressants work. Similar illustrations of such exaggeration seem to be in the offing for persons with other diagnoses.

A second major theoretical issue, highlighted in Chapter 1, has to do with the difference between active drug and placebo. It also concerns the

---

[1] Hudson and Pope (1990) have, in fact, documented that such psychotropic drugs as the antidepressants lack specificity for depression and are actually used for a gamut of syndromes.

question of how to conceptualize the difference between what is called biological versus psychological. Biological psychiatry typically seeks to portray the effects of psychotropic drugs as due to alterations in brain function, whereas placebo effects are attributed to another realm, the psychological. This distinction is a relic of old Cartesian assumptions. Placebo responses are just as "biological," in the sense that they occur in tissue, as responses to "active" drugs. But further, both are significantly influenced by psychosocial variables. Thus, as indicated by data from the NIMH Depression Collaborative Research Program (Krupnick et al., 1996), the goodness of the therapeutic alliance (between patient and practitioner) seems to contribute as much variance to positive therapeutic outcome in the case of an antidepressant as it does in the case of psychotherapy or placebo. Reviews of earlier studies indicate that both drug and placebo agents are mediated not only by attitudes of administrants but also the verbal labels applied to them, the expectations of those ingesting them, and even personality variables (e.g., acquiescence). It is often difficult to differentiate, with any scientific certainty, the apparent therapeutic effects of each presumably separate class of agents. One can only describe as dramatic the degree to which contextual variables can drastically influence responses to "active" as well as "inactive" substances. Both placebo and drug may mobilize attitudes, intentions, compensatory defenses, and self-repairing maneuvers only tangentially linked to the chemical properties of the original substances. All the old concepts that nicely delineated the separate domains of psyche and brain as well as the disparate therapeutic agents that presumably targeted the domains are now slippery and merging.

Indeed, if one synthesizes the Fisher and Greenberg perspective with that of Carson and also M. Greenberg concerning the fluidity of the *DSM* classes, it is evident that the original landmarks of the psychopharmacology terrain are disappearing. Where once there was a clear map of the psychoactive drug enterprise divided into "real" and "not real therapeutic effects," with nicely parallel protocols for testing how much better the real is than the unreal, ambiguity now prevails. To ignore this ambiguity is to engage in illusion. As will be noted, the ambiguity presages a pan-uncertainty that keeps emerging in multiple studies of psychoactive drug efficacy.

More specific findings concerning individual treatments have been appraised in several chapters. Greenberg and Fisher focused on the treatment of unipolar depression and bipolar disorder. In Chapter 4, they presented a sweeping review of both the drug and psychotherapeutic approaches to such treatment. It is amazing how much energy has gone into testing the various antidepressants. The very mass of this work renders analysis a redoubtable project. However, a fairly reasonable story has emerged concerning the power of antidepressants compared with placebos. In essence, the conventional claims for the superior potency of the antidepressants have been grossly exaggerated. A number of meta-analyses have shown that the effect sizes for the antidepressants fall at the lower end of the potential range. This applies also to the supposed wonder drug, fluoxetine (Prozac®). But the most telling point is that the apparent potency of any antidepressant is typically inverse to the degree to which the drug trial in which it was tested was adequately controlled. Trials that do not include a placebo reference point almost always demonstrate greater therapeutic power than do placebo-controlled trials. Inadequate controls invite bias that exaggerates presumed therapeutic power. Since drug trials are typically carried out by persons highly motivated to prove the drug works, lack of controls facilitates fictitious claims.

If one considers this point in conjunction with comorbidity and the evidence that the double-blind, as a control, was seriously flawed and probably breached in most studies (Fisher & Greenberg, 1993), the genuine possibility exists that even the relatively small advantages of antidepressants over placebo reported in the literature are not dependable. This view is strongly reinforced by two sets of findings. First, there is Thomson's (1982) report that the use of active placebos (generating body sensations mimicking those aroused by an active drug) in studies of antidepressants eliminates a significant difference between the efficacies of drug and placebo.

Second, one is confronted with the findings of Greenberg, Bornstein, Greenberg, and Fisher (1992) concerning what happens to the apparent efficacy of an antidepressant when evaluated by experimenters who are no longer in a position to focus their bias knowledgeably. Greenberg et al. located a series of studies that sought primarily to test a new antidepressant but included both a placebo and an older antidepressant (imipramine or amitriptyline) for comparison purposes. It was hypothesized that because two active drugs rather than one were involved, this would introduce a new higher level of complexity that would make it more difficult to penetrate the double-blind and this would, in turn, interfere with any underlying intent to enhance any one agent's effectiveness compared with others (e.g., placebo). The hypothesis was strongly supported. Imipramine and amitriptyline were judged not to be significantly more therapeutic than placebo. This was especially true when therapeutic effectiveness was defined in terms of the patients' self-ratings of depression rather than psychiatrists' ratings. Basically, this study dramatized the likelihood that an opportunity for researchers to focus their bias is necessary to arrive at results apparently showing that an antidepressant is therapeutically much better than a placebo. This is a central finding with wide-ranging importance.

It is paradoxical that while the role of such extraneous bias in therapeutic outcome is noteworthy, no one has convincingly shown that parameters more closely linked to the drug itself can be related to therapeutic impact. Neither the dose size of the antidepressant nor its measured blood plasma level usually predicts therapeutic outcome with any reasonable consistency.

Another important observation that emerged is that nondrug modes of treatment (e.g., cognitive therapy) for depression produce as good or better results than the antidepressants. Also, the benefits of combining nondrug and drug treatments have been exaggerated; it has yet to be demonstrated that combined treatments are consistently better than specific psychotherapeutic modes alone. Further, there is a suggestion that the psychotherapeutic approaches may affect a wider range of the depressed individual's behavior repertoire than do the antidepressants and, therefore, may be more preventive of relapse.

A final issue taken up by Greenberg and Fisher concerns the power of lithium in treating persons with bipolar symptoms. Questions are raised about the logic and scientific rigor of the early studies usually cited as witness that lithium is an effective agent. Special criticism is directed at early studies that judged therapeutic efficacy on the basis of how much more quickly stabilized patients required hospitalization when they were removed from lithium and placed on placebo than when stabilized patients remained on lithium. It was noted that not only are judgments of when patients need rehospitalization likely to be unreliable and shaped by bias but also significantly mediated by how abruptly placebos are substituted for lithium. Gradual rather than abrupt withdrawal reduces the probability of relapse. In the early studies, withdrawal was almost always done abruptly. Overall, it has become clear that lithium is considerably less effective than touted by many enthusiasts. Actually, until better controlled studies are done, one cannot reasonably define the level of effectiveness.

Cohen, in his perusal of the drug treatment literature pertinent to schizophrenia (Chapter 5), presents a largely skeptical picture. He notes, somewhat satirically, that after decades of use there is still no clear definition of optimum dose levels for the various standard neuroleptic agents. He offers a rather unique review of the early history of the development of the neuroleptics and points out that initially the effects of chlorpromazine were likened to the residual symptoms of encephalitis. These effects were perceived not as "antipsychotic" but rather as creating a state of indifference to the psychotic turmoil. In reviewing the therapeutic efficacies of the neuroleptic drugs, Cohen leaves us with a strong sense of uncertainty. He points out that while many studies indicate that the neuroleptics produce about one-third greater rates of therapeutic improvement in schizophrenics than do placebos, the basic design of such studies is often one in which patients who have been taking neuroleptics for extended periods are taken off their medications (with placebo substituted) and their subsequent course is compared with that of patients not removed from medication. Cohen considers this design faulty because typically the patients were taken off their medication quite abruptly, and it has been shown (e.g., Baldessarini & Viguera, 1995) that such abrupt discontinuation, in contrast to a more gradual mode, artificially increases psychological disturbance. This means that many studies of schizophrenics have probably exaggerated the advantage of being maintained on drug versus shifting to placebo. Cohen also contends that in the few really well-controlled studies in which neuroleptic efficacy was compared in a serial fashion over time with that of an active placebo (e.g., sedative) capable of producing a feeling of having ingested a real drug, the difference between drug and placebo was not significant. He adds to this negative portrayal by citing data indicating high rates of nonresponse to neuroleptics and the absence of solid evidence that they result in much improvement in ability to cope with social complexities. Finally, he highlights the multiple troubling side effects (e.g., tardive dyskinesia, tardive dementia) triggered by the toxic brain effects of neuroleptics and criticizes the psychiatric community for minimizing and even ignoring them.

Danton and Antonuccio (Chapter 6) provide an appraisal of drugs designed to alleviate a medley of anxiety symptoms (e.g., generalized anxiety disorder, panic disorder, obsessive-compulsive disorder). The multiple *DSM* defined anxiety categories considered have a pseudo-exact quality, as do widely recommended specific medications for these categories. Actually, the research literature concerned with the anxiolytics has been quite uneven. While some benzodiazepines and antidepressants seem to be more therapeutic than inert placebos in the short run, this is probably less true in the longer run. Incidentally, the antidepressant drugs seem generally to be more therapeutically effective for anxiety symptoms than do specifically designated "antianxiety agents."

There is mounting evidence that various psychological therapies (cognitive, behavioral) achieve considerably higher therapeutic effect sizes than do the pharmacotherapies and, even more importantly, lower rates of long-term relapse. Another consideration is that the psychological therapies do not produce the often serious side effects linked especially with the benzodiazepines (but also the antidepressants). Danton and Antonuccio also cite data suggesting that treatment with psychotherapies is generally not more expensive than the pharmacotherapies. Actually, it is dizzying to attempt to integrate the observations in Chapter 6 because the authors deal with such an anfractuous array of variables (e.g., therapeutic agents, settings, diagnostic types of patients, time intervals, combinations of therapies).

One cannot easily or comfortably arrive at solid general impressions. It is doubtful that any confident long-term therapeutic claims can be made about the repertoire of drugs currently widely employed in the battle against anxiety.

The largely negative picture presented by Danton and Antonuccio with reference to the power of the anxiolytics fits well with Lipman's (1989) overall evaluation based on a thorough analysis of an earlier literature:

> Although it seems natural to assume that the anxiolytic medications would be the most effective psychotropic medications for the treatment of the anxiety disorders . . . the evidence does not support this assumption . . . the benzodiazepines are the most frequently prescribed psychotropic medications for the anxiety disorders . . . , but their efficacy, except for the short term treatment of GAD . . . and alprazolam for the treatment of agoraphobia/panic . . . is not supported by well-controlled studies. (pp. 95–96)

Bornstein, in Chapter 7, describes how drugs have been applied to the treatment of persons identified as "borderline," a diagnosis that is quite unreliable. Most of the studies of the power of psychotropic drugs to help borderlines have been poorly constructed—not infrequently lacking random assignment and placebo markers. Occasional trials come up with results indicating positive therapeutic possibilities for antipsychotic agents and lithium. Basically, however, no dependable scientific data exist indicating any advantage in treating borderlines with lithium or other agents variously designated as antidepressant, anxiolytic, antipsychotic, or anticonvulsant.

In Chapter 8, R. Fisher and S. Fisher assess the state of the art in treating psychologically disturbed children and adolescents with psychoactive drugs. They concentrated their review on how well antidepressants achieve results with depression in the younger segment of the population. Thirteen double-blind studies were located that put this matter to the test; and they unanimously indicated that the active drugs were no more efficacious than the placebo controls. In addition, some evidence was uncovered that antidepressants (particularly tricyclics) may have the potential to create serious (perhaps even life-threatening) side effects in children.[2]

Fisher and Fisher examined too the literature concerned with the efficacies of anxiolytics, lithium, and antipsychotics for children with anxiety symptoms, manic-depressive cycles, and psychotic disturbance respectively. Controlled studies (based on adequate samples) were difficult to

---

[2] Two prominent medical commentators (Eisenberg, 1996; Pellegrino, 1996) who were asked to evaluate the implications of these data, concluded it would be unethical to prescribe antidepressants for depressed children or adolescents.

find for any of these symptom areas, and the authors concluded that no consistent scientific verification exists that the major drugs used for such symptoms are superior to placebo.

Quite contrastingly, Whalen and Henker, in Chapter 9, assert that stimulant drugs show considerable efficacy in treating children and adolescents with attention-deficit/hyperactivity disorder (ADHD) features. They state that stimulant drugs produce significantly more improvement than placebos in "focal symptom domains such as attentional patterns, disruptiveness, and impulsivity." They feel that the scientific data are unequivocal in this respect and that practitioners should feel free to prescribe stimulant medications for ADHD symptomatology.

However, this apparently confident message is presented in a context of multiple reservations and uncertainties. Whalen and Henker conclude their positively toned chapter in the following modest voice: "The knowledgeable prescriber will be well aware of both the limitations of these drugs (stimulants) and the fact that they are most effective in *helping to manage problems, not to remediate them*" (italics added). It is a real shift from asserting that the stimulant drugs represent an effective treatment for ADHD to casting such drugs as "helping to manage problems, not to remediate them."

If one reviews the Whalen and Henker analysis one finds the following limiting comments with regard to stimulant treatment of ADHD:

- The ADHD syndrome is vaguely defined and difficult to diagnose reliably. Further, it has been pushed beyond its defined boundaries and many individuals are now considered candidates for ADHD treatment who only remotely fit with the original category.
- Only the short-term therapeutic efficacy of the stimulant drugs has been demonstrated. After 6,000 published studies, no reliable statement can be made about long-term efficacy. Further, somewhere between 9% and 16% of children treated with stimulants may actually show a "deterioration" in some of their symptoms.
- The therapeutic efficacy of the stimulant drugs is largely confined to the improvement of problems with disinhibition and oppositionality and does relatively little for gains in "cognitive functioning, academic performance, and peer relations."
- Various side effects (some quite serious) are associated with the stimulant drugs. Although it is now an accepted practice to assign children to take such drugs for extended periods: "The jury is still out on whether . . . extended treatment may result in long-term growth impairment, cardiovascular problems, or other untoward physiological effects" for some undefined minority segment.

These considerable reservations are even further complicated by issues raised by Whalen and Henker relating to comorbidity, the rarity with which "normalization" of the child is achieved, the probable need (if consistent success is to be attained) to have coordinated psychosocial treatment efforts, and the low rate (50%) of treatment completion.

We would urge caution with respect to the sometimes enthusiastic position that Whalen and Henker adopt about stimulant treatment for ADHD. This highlights again the subjectivity and the ultimate uncertainty that prevails in arriving at decisions about any of the psychotropic drug treatments. One can perhaps best illustrate the uncertainty that exists by comparing the Whalen and Henker viewpoint with that of McGuinness (1989) after she completed an extensive review of the pertinent literature concerned with the use of stimulant drugs for ADHD children. McGuinness said simply: "The data consistently fail to support any benefits from stimulant medication" (p. 183). Interestingly, in a 1991 review, Whalen and Henker seemed to be closer to the McGuinness stance: "Despite the impressive track record established by stimulant therapies over the past two decades, this treatment has serious limitations. Not all children can be given these medications, nor do all who take them improve. In the majority who appear to benefit, the changes may be short-lived or may persist only as long as the drug regimen continues. It is also quite common to observe positive changes in only a subset of the major problem domains" (p. 135).

We are left in an equivocal position. It would appear that certain benefits are to be derived from the use of stimulant medications with children who have problems related to disinhibition and difficulties in focusing attention consistently. However, the magnitude of these benefits and their durability are, despite thousands of studies, still surprisingly poorly defined.

Having traversed the array of findings from the various chapters just presented, what commonalities emerge? What are some overall impressions?

The first matter we are stuck with is the amazing quantity of time, money, effort, and ingenuity already invested in trying to prove that psychoactive drugs really cure people of multiple symptoms, discomforts, and dysfunctions. More specifically, the aim has been to prove that chemical substances can promote cures by virtue of their direct (biological) action on brain functions. In general, the power of psychoactive drugs relative to placebo has been overstated. There has also been a show of public professional confidence in the research testing of the drugs that is unrealistic. In the preceding chapters, scrutiny of the research pertinent to a broad spectrum of psychoactive drugs relative to placebo has revealed inconsistencies, weaknesses in research designs, and some indications of total ineffectiveness:

- When sources of bias are minimized, the advantage of antidepressants over placebo practically disappears.
- Fluoxetine is no more therapeutic than other antidepressants.
- The most frequently prescribed anxiolytics do not seem to be effective beyond brief time intervals.
- Neuroleptics have a low base rate for alleviating schizophrenic symptoms and may conceivably attain levels of effectiveness at very low doses that can almost be regarded as active placebos.
- Lithium has shifted over time from being regarded as a magic bullet for manic symptoms to being thought of as rather ineffective.
- Drugs prescribed to treat depression, anxiety, and psychosis in children have proven to be entirely without therapeutic power beyond placebo.

It is true that Whalen and Henker see stimulant medications as helpful in the treatment of children diagnosed as ADHD. This is the one area of optimism that has emerged. Even in this instance, however, there are troubling questions and uncertainties.

Parenthetically, the extremely high relapse rates that occur when patients are taken off antidepressants, antipsychotics, or stimulant medications raise serious questions. What is the nature of the improvement produced by such drugs if their therapeutic effects are so temporary? Does this mean the underlying internal conditions that originally triggered the symptomatology are still present when the drugs are administered, but are simply masked by the transient brain changes the drugs initiate? The following quote highlights the doubt raised by the observed lack of permanence of antidepressant drug treatments (Hyman, 1995–1996):

> I'm sure most of us have worried about the data from the Pittsburgh (Kupfer et al., 1992) study. Twenty individuals had been maintained well for three years on imipramine and then rerandomized to imipramine or placebo, and 9 out of 11 on placebo relapsed rather rapidly. About 80% or 90% of those who stayed on active treatment stayed well. It's disturbing because having been well for three years, you certainly would expect that more than 10% to 20% would remain well. (p. 15)

This relatively rapid dissipation of antidepressant effects has been puzzling to those concerned with understanding how antidepressants affect the central nervous system (CNS). Why should the presumed alterations in amine levels be of such transient significance? No satisfactory explanations have emerged simply because the brain mechanisms involved in the antidepressant process are largely not yet understood. Hyman (1995–1996) indicates that researchers can only vaguely speculate that altering amine levels produces as yet poorly understood CNS adaptations. He notes:

> The simple monoamine hypothesis, that depression resulted from inadequate monoamine release, predicts . . . that monoamine turnover as measured by levels of monoamine metabolites be decreased in depressed subjects. Despite three decades of investigation, these predictions have not been borne out. . . . Overall, the concept of norepinephrine or serotonin "levels" in the brain is relatively meaningless. (p. 12)

A biologically phrased model of how depression can be modified or cured remains in a largely inchoate state.

FURTHER CONSIDERATIONS

The history of the enterprise directed at validating the psychoactive drugs has a "Greek tragedy" quality. Despite heroic efforts, it has been plagued by false assumptions and weak control procedures. The prime false assumption was that it is possible to eliminate psychologically disturbed behavior by means of agents that act directly in the brain and are relatively independent of the psychosocial context in which they are administered. An implicit underlying assumption was that the effects of psychosocial contexts (e.g., placebo expectations) are due less to direct brain changes than are those of the active drugs. We have examined this matter in some detail and demonstrated not only great overlap between active drugs and placebos in their therapeutic potentials but also that psychoactive drugs are highly influenced by what would conventionally be called nonbiological factors. For example, antipsychotics labeled as placebos can apparently lose a significant portion of their potency. Overall, the biological assumption resulted in treatment strategies that sought mightily to eliminate all placebo (psychosocial) factors and, in so doing, probably diminished an important source of treatment potency.

Perhaps more seriously, the basic research design adopted to test drug efficacy only pretended to control for experimenter bias because it used a double-blind paradigm with inactive placebos that were therefore distinguishable from the active drugs capable of arousing cues (body sensations) to signal they were pharmacologically active. It thus enabled both researchers and patient participants to identify fairly easily whether the ingested substance was a placebo or an active agent. This meant that all studies that had employed the double-blind design were suspect because, with rare exceptions, no effort was made to ascertain to what degree the double-blind had been penetrated. Thus, there was no way to determine whether the findings of any given study had been contaminated by bias and were not scientifically trustworthy.[3]

Defining the power of psychoactive drugs is particularly complex because two grossly different perspectives can be taken with respect to the pertinent published literature. One can accept the published findings at face value, except for reservations about gross and obvious defects in design, procedure, or analysis of data. However, one can also justifiably take the position that all the published results in this area are probably seriously flawed because of failures of the double-blind. Choosing the second alternative puts the investigator in the position of dismissing the bulk of the work in this area and declaring that we have almost no dependable knowledge about psychoactive drugs. This statement would be treated as absurd by those who have for many years worked so hard to put psychoactive drugs to the test. However, they would have to deal with the hard question how one can have faith in data that have not been adequately shielded from the bias of investigators who are almost invariably highly motivated to demonstrate that given drugs are successfully therapeutic. We see no quick or easy way to resolve this dilemma and favor maintaining an attitude of uneasy skepticism. The keynote is uncertainty, with the attached obligation to refrain from making overly confident statements about efficacy issues.

ERRONEOUS ASSUMPTIONS

Apropos of this matter of uncertainty, the following list is a compilation of assumptions, notions, and procedures current in the psychopharmacology literature that have directly or indirectly been shown in the preceding chapters to lack dependable and consistent scientific support:

1. The idea that the double-blind design for testing psychotropic drugs effectively eliminates researcher bias.
2. The assumption that the samples of patients evaluated in the typical drug trial are representative of the general clinical population to whom the treatment will be applied.
3. The practice of using an initial washout phase during drug trials, with the intention of eliminating placebo responders and therefore to minimize placebo effects.

---

[3] Carroll, Rounsaville, and Nich (1994) have actually presented research data demonstrating that the penetration of the double-blind results in biased ratings of patients' responses to drug versus placebo.

4. The assumption that any clear evidence has emerged that the therapeutic power of psychoactive drugs is linked to dose levels in any consistent fashion.
5. The belief that the therapeutic effects of psychoactive drugs are correlated consistently with their plasma levels.
6. The concept that psychotropic drugs produce effects that are more biological than placebo effects.
7. The confident belief that psychotropic drugs are much more therapeutic than placebos. This would be especially true with reference to the antidepressants and anxiolytic agents.
8. The practice of administering psychotropic drugs to children and adolescents to alleviate depression, anxiety, and psychosis.
9. The presumption that psychotropic drugs target specific symptom clusters that are empirically well defined and distinguishable.
10. The practice of testing psychotropic drugs by means of brief trials (e.g., 4–6 weeks) and assuming such brief evaluations will provide adequate information concerning long-term therapeutic potential.
11. The often promulgated idea that depressed patients can be better prevented from suicide by psychoactive drugs than by other therapeutic techniques.
12. The concept that severe depression (e.g., "endogenous") is better treated with antidepressants than with other therapeutic modes.
13. The comfortable self-serving conviction that the side effects of most psychoactive drugs are ephemeral and not of much consequence.
14. The notion that the placebo component of a response to a psychoactive drug can be adequately measured simply by inclusion of a matched placebo control. Since placebos are typically inactive, there is no way of ascertaining whether an enhanced placebo component is linked to the greater stimulation aroused by the active drug.
15. The idea that psychoactive drugs are routinely more effective than psychotherapy treatment or more helpful in preventing relapse.

This amounts to a litany of weighty problems that plague the psychopharmacological enterprise. As a matter of science, it is appropriate and important to raise these questions. However, what are the practical implications of our observations?

Are we suggesting that psychoactive drugs do not work? No, that is not our message. Although such drugs probably often do not work much better than active placebos, many troubled individuals likely have benefited from them. The degree of this benefit, as against no treatment, cannot be scientifically defined at this point in time. Also, the issue of how much of the benefit derives from the action of chemical substances (e.g., serotonin, norepinephrine, dopamine) targeted, in terms of theory, to specified CNS systems cannot currently be spelled out. However, in some conglomerate way, different factors unite to impart apparent therapeutic power to the act of an authority figure administering a psychoactive substance to troubled individuals. The complex of ingesting a substance that palpably induces "druglike" body experiences, in the context of personally feeling the need to change or improve, and the added element of receiving authoritative reassurance that now there is a good probability of changing—all seem to offer an opportunity for a therapeutic process to be set in motion. However, we know this only in a diffuse, uncertain fashion.

COPING WITH DESIGN DEFECTS

Earlier, we proposed that systematic studies be undertaken to determine the conditions that will optimize a psychoactive drug's various pathways to influencing the brain. For example, aside from inducing effects derived from selectively altering levels of monamines, other therapeutic brain responses should be fully mobilized that are linked to placebo power. How can we optimize the reassuring potency of the drug administrant, the appearance of the "pill," and the subjective experiences aroused by ingesting the drug? Incidentally, it is pertinent that Kirsch and Rosadino (1993) have shown that merely being aware that one is involved in a double-blind drug trial (with the potential one might receive a placebo rather than a "real" drug) is sufficient to create a skeptical set that can reduce the therapeutic effectiveness of a placebo.

A number of variables need to be considered when trying to decide whether a drug is the treatment of choice for psychological discomfort. Besides such factors as the availability of other treatment options, serious attention must be directed to the so-called side effects each drug will induce. The euphemistically labeled side effects can have such serious consequences as delirium, neurological damage, sexual dysfunction, memory loss, Parkinsonism, orthostatic hypotension, addiction, and even death (Dewan & Koss, 1989). Customarily, most side effects are dismissed as transient and unimportant. However, it is documented that they can cause real suffering, and little is factually known about their potential long-term consequences. We were unable to find any studies that actually measured, over extended follow-up periods, the probabilities that drug side effects like sexual dysfunction will largely dissipate. Obviously, an informed decision whether to take psychotropic drugs calls for fairly detailed and accurate knowledge concerning their impact on multiple body systems.

Troubling doubts have been repeatedly raised about the cogency of the typical double-blind design for evaluating the efficacies of psychoactive medications. Studies have shown that the double-blind is usually vulnerable to bias; that the often used initial washout to control placebo response is useless; and that the patients who participate are simply unrepresentative of the modal clinical population. What can be done to devise a more sensible design? First of all, inert placebos can no longer be justified and should be replaced by placebo substances that arouse body sensations mimicking the active drug being tested. This would close a big hole in the objectivity of the double-blind as it is now practiced. Another technique for attaining greater objectivity would be to introduce periodic inquiries of both patients and research staff concerning whether they have a greater-than-chance accurate awareness of who is receiving active drug versus placebos.

Hughes and Krahn (1985) developed a methodology for analyzing reports concerning the degree to which one has penetrated the double-blind. They outlined formal modes of analysis of the reports of patients concerning whether they believed they had received an active drug or a placebo or were uncertain. On the basis of such data, the patients would be assigned to 1 of 6 cells in a 2×3 table comparing actual drug group (placebo vs. active drug) and accuracy of drug identification (correct vs. incorrect vs. uncertain). Three forms of analysis are derived from the table. First, the patients' degree of blindness is computed by comparing the numbers who correctly and incorrectly identify their drug assignment. Second, the impact is ascertained of any failure to maintain blindness on the validity of the results. This calls for comparing the sizes of the drug effects (i.e., the difference in active drug and placebo among patients who correctly or incorrectly identify the drug they received and also those who are uncertain in this respect). It is assumed that if drug identification affected the validity of the results, then the drug effect should vary significantly among the three groups. Third, the size of the drug effect, with identification held constant, is computed by determining drug effects within specific groups (e.g., those definitely blind because they are truly "uncertain"). This analytical scheme seems promising and could be informative if routinely applied in drug trials. Should any analysis reveal serious penetration of the double-blind, one would expect the study to be declared invalid. This may be setting a difficult standard but there is little choice. Data contaminated by serious bias are worse than no data at all.

With respect to improving the basic drug trial design, an interesting idea was put forward by Suedfeld (1984). He proposes a new approach to measuring placebo effects that copes to some degree with the problem of how to conceal adequately from patients that they are receiving a placebo control substance. He devised a strategy that he refers to as the "Subtractive Placebo Procedure." His description is as follows:

It consists of administering an active, specific therapeutic procedure but introducing it with the orientation that it is inert with respect to the problem being treated. In other words, the client is led to expect less of an effect than the treatment is known to produce. The Subtractive Expectancy Procedure avoids the need to invent or find an inert technique. . . . (It) can be used to answer some questions that are currently moot . . . It is very difficult to identify . . . procedures that actually are inert, or to specify inert and active components . . . This is not a problem in the Subtractive Expectancy Procedure, since the treatment administered as a placebo is in reality an established active one. The ethical problem of randomly assigning some groups of clients to a condition in which they get no active treatment even though such treatments are available is also avoided, since in fact one such treatment is being administered to the placebo group. . . . Deception still occurs; but almost any effective placebo procedure has to use at least passive deception (allowing the client to believe something that the therapist thinks is untrue). (p. 162)

Suedfeld discusses potential problems related to the credibility of the Subtractive Placebo approach: "How does one explain to a client the use of a technique for which any active effect is specifically disclaimed? This may be relatively easy to do in a research setting. . . . Possible solutions of the credibility problem are to represent the procedure as an adjunct to or a preparation for actual treatment, or as an information-collecting device relevant to future or previous treatment" (p. 162). Actually, Suedfeld points out that the Subtractive Placebo Procedure is already widely used in the "balanced placebo design" often employed in the study of alcohol effects. In that balanced placebo design, the experimenter arranges various conditions in which subjects do or do not anticipate being given alcohol and in which they actually do or do not receive alcohol (relatively tasteless vodka, mixed in a tonic). The condition in which the subject anticipates only tonic but gets the vodka and tonic mixture is an analogue of the Subtractive Expectancy design. It should be recalled too that Guy (1967) employed an analogous approach when, as earlier described, he presented Thorazine® to subjects disguised as a placebo (and observed a decrease in the drug's potency).

A prime advantage of this approach to placebo control is that it avoids convincing subjects that an inert substance (producing few body sensations) is an active drug. But at the same time, it provides a measure of the power of expectancy when the effects of the active drug labeled as a placebo are compared with those of the active undisguised drug. To the degree that the placebo version is reduced in therapeutic power, the investigator can designate that reduction as an index of the contribution of placebo expectancy to the total "drug effect." We would assign high priority to retesting the efficacy of a number of the major psychotropic drugs within the context of this new placebo marker.

Researchers also must cope with the difficult problem of drug trial samples being unrepresentative of the modal clinical population. The biased selectivity of most drug trial samples stems from two factors. First, only those patients are chosen whose symptoms fall clearly into a defined *DSM* category and who manifest no significant signs of comorbidity. Second, about 25% to 30% of those patients who gain entrance to the drug trial usually drop out for a variety of reasons (e.g., unacceptable side effects, sudden improvement).[4] Actually, little is solidly known about the nature of the sampling selectively resulting from the dropout process. Probably not much can be done to eliminate this source of selectivity.

However, it is worth giving some thought to dealing with the comorbidity issue. Investigators could simply decide to admit into the drug trial patients who have comorbid symptoms—at least in the same proportion as they are represented in the general population with a given *DSM* cluster of symptoms. Thus, since comorbidity occurs in about 50% of patients with depression, 50% of the patients admitted to a trial of an antidepressant could have comorbid symptomatology. Of course, this would get into all sorts of complications, such as the upper limit of the number of comorbid diagnoses that would be acceptable in terms of maintaining the identity of the diagnostic category supposedly being appraised. But more perplexing would be that while an average level of improvement (drug versus placebo) could be computed, it would probably become apparent that the improvement was greater in the noncomorbid subsample than in the comorbid one. In fact, the overall average improvement in the mixed group would really no longer specify the response of a group with a *DSM* identity. It would, with its comorbid mixture, no longer represent a recognizable *DSM* entity.

The logic of these observations forces one to ask whether it might be more meaningful to conduct many drug trials outside the *DSM* paradigm. Reports in the literature have already shown a lack of therapeutic specificity (in *DSM* terms) for major classes of psychotropic drugs. Hudson and Pope (1990) offer data indicating that antidepressants may produce apparent significant improvement in the following: major depression, bulimia, panic disorder, obsessive-compulsive disorder, attention-deficit disorder with hyperactivity, cataplexy, migraine, and irritable bowel syndrome. Antipsychotics are widely used not only for schizophrenic disturbance but also manic-depressive symptomatology, poorly controlled

---

[4] There are also other incidental biases related to underrepresentation of various ethnic and socioeconomic groups.

aggressive outbursts, autism, and so forth. Hudson and Pope were so impressed with the diversity of symptoms that apparently respond to antidepressants that they conceptualized a larger underlying "disorder family" that simply does not match any existing *DSM* definition. Any observer of the current psychopharmacological literature quickly perceives that the *DSM* is no longer the sole major paradigm for treatment choices involving psychoactive drugs. Not only is any given individual drug often used across diverse, supposedly separate *DSM* categories, but also multiple different combinations of drugs are often prescribed for an individual patient.

What does such complexity and confusion imply for structuring the recruiting of patients for drug trials? Quite simply and boldly, it suggests that recruitment should no longer revolve primarily around the *DSM* axes. One need not be looking for psychotropic drugs that "cure" this or that *DSM* syndrome. Although it is unclear what new treatment categories should be substituted, one possibility comes to mind.[5] Perhaps, apropos of the comorbidity issue, research energy could be focused on ascertaining which of the psychotropic drugs are most effective over a broad versus narrow spectrum of symptomatology.[6] The focus would be on the range of therapeutic prowess rather than the power to ameliorate a defined *DSM* species. Patients would be classified primarily in terms of the total severity[7] of their symptoms before treatment was instituted. Other variations on this approach could involve studies dealing with whether the power of a given psychotropic drug to reduce total symptomatology was of short- or long-term duration; greater or lesser magnitude as a function of the placebo context (e.g., "authoritative reassurance" versus "friendly support"); and higher or lower in relation to gender, ethnic background, or educational level.

Those who would reject the notion of a drug trial paradigm not anchored in the *DSM* must in any case eventually confront themselves with

---

[5] This perspective does not mean that we completely reject the possibility of some *DSM*-related specificity (e.g., obsessive-compulsive response to clomipramine). However, the literature suggests few well-validated examples of such specificity.

[6] To classify patients in terms of overall disturbance rather than specific symptom categories makes sense, interestingly, in relation to a number of studies (Watson & Clark, 1984) that have examined the nature of happiness-unhappiness. When subjects are asked to report the gamut of discomforts or symptoms they are experiencing on a number of questionnaires, each designed to measure a specific parameter (e.g., depression, anxiety), substantial correlations among the specific forms of discomfort are reported. A major factor that emerges is one of general demoralization or vulnerability. Persons can be most meaningfully classified as to their degree of *overall* preoccupation with negative affectivity.

[7] Previous studies have found that the total degree of personality instability is predictive of extreme forms of response to various drugs. These findings are discussed in Chapter 1.

the need to redo most of the earlier *DSM*-based studies that are, because of their lack of genuine blindness, open to challenge. Until such repeat studies are carried out with tighter designs, uncertainty will prevail and undermine confidence in the psychotropic enterprise.

MARKETING STRATEGY BIASES

A major aim of this book has been to present a balanced analysis of the relative effectiveness of psychoactive drugs compared with alternative treatment approaches, including placebo. It is assumed that level of effectiveness (as determined by objective scientific research) should be the most important factor guiding the selection of treatments (of course, cost and potential side effects will also be weighed in making treatment decisions). There are a number of indications that treatment decisions are not always as tied to evidence as is commonly believed. The skewing of evidence as well as the perceptions of practitioners and patients are skillfully undertaken with surprising frequency. In recent years, *Consumer Reports* has published two articles detailing an array of methods that have the effect of manipulating prescribing practices so that they become detached from strict dependence on proof regarding the merits of the prescribed drugs ("Miracle Drugs or Media Drugs?" 1992; "Pushing Drugs to Doctors," 1992). The reports highlight (and document with research) several commonplace practices that bias treatment decisions. These practices directly affect researchers as well as clinicians and patients.

One concern relates to the influence that pharmaceutical companies may exert by being a major source of research grants. Aside from the possibility that favored researchers (i.e., those who produce results benefiting a particular company's products) are likely to receive more grants and profit financially, there are other more subtle ways to influence research findings. For example, pharmaceutical company influence has been suggested by A. Hillman and his colleagues at the University of Pennsylvania in a paper published in the *New England Journal of Medicine*. Their comments about such companies, reproduced in *Consumer Reports* ("Pushing Drugs to Doctors," 1992), indicated:

> They fund projects with a high likelihood of producing favorable results . . . They exclude products that may compare favorably with the sponsor's own. Sometimes, only favorable clinical data are released to investigators. . . . Negative studies may be terminated before they are ready for publication. . . . Corporate personnel may seek to control the content and use of the final report, including the decision to publish. (p. 93)

The importance of these maneuvers is highlighted by another piece of research cited by *Consumer Reports* ("Pushing Drugs to Doctors," 1992) showing that drug-company supported studies of new drugs are significantly more likely to favor the use of those drugs than are studies not receiving drug company funding. Similar conclusions were reached by Levy (1992) after analyzing several reviews of the medical literature in which new drugs (that were higher priced as a result of being protected by patent law) were compared with older ones. Invariably the newer drugs were reported to be more effective and to have fewer side effects. Again, drug company support proved to be linked to results favoring new drugs over the old. In fact, Levy could not locate a single case where research found a sponsoring company's medication to be less effective than a drug produced by a competing company. It was also noted that bias and statistical errors were frequent and they almost always favored the new medication. Relatedly, both an editorial in the *New England Journal of Medicine* (Relman, 1989) and a feature article in *The Wall Street Journal* (Chase, 1989) call attention to growing concerns about the contamination of clinical investigations by researchers having vested economic interests in drug-manufacturing companies.

Another unexpected potential source of bias can be found in peer-reviewed medical journals. Such journals are a well respected source of objective information in the eyes of the professional medical community. However, it is not unusual for these publications to produce "supplements" subsidized by pharmaceutical companies. These supplements (which are often based on drug-company-sponsored symposia) are appended to regular journal issues and printed in the same style as regular journal articles. As detailed by *Consumer Reports* ("Pushing Drugs to Doctors," 1992), supplements have been shown to lack balance and objectivity and are therefore not reliable sources of information about drug treatments or research.

Some also express alarm at the revelation that drug companies have hired ghostwriters to produce journal reviews and articles on clinical trials. These articles are then passed off as having been written by respected scientists who are paid a fee for the use of their names as authors (Levy, 1996). Professor Lois DeBakey who teaches ethics and medical writing at Baylor College of Medicine, labels the practice of ghostwriting of medical articles as "pernicious." She asks, "How far is it from ghostwriting to ghost data?" (Levy, 1996, p. 2A).

Physicians often prescribe drugs that were introduced after they completed their formal medical education. Thus, large numbers of prescriptions, perhaps the majority, are written for medications that the prescriber did not formally study in medical school (Leavitt, 1995). How then do physicians learn about many of the treatments they are prescribing? Two of the major ways are through advertisements in medical journals and continuing medical education (CME) lectures and courses. Each of these vehicles for imparting information has been found to be tainted.

Although advertisements represent a significant influence on prescribing practices (e.g., Avorn, Chen, & Hartley, 1982; Leavitt, 1995; Wilkes, Doblin, & Shapiro, 1992), studies have suggested they frequently present slanted or inaccurate data (e.g., Mehta, Sorofman, & Rowland, 1989; Stimson, 1977; Wilkes, Doblin, & Shapiro, 1992). For example, Wilkes et al., (1992) presented 109 full-page pharmaceutical advertisements drawn from 10 major medical journals to panels of three experts in the relevant clinical area. In 30% of cases, the panels disputed the ad's claim that the drug was the "drug of choice." Experts also judged that the headlines were misleading in 32% of the ads. Information on efficacy was judged not to be balanced by information on side effects and contraindications in 40% of the ads. Experts felt that physicians would prescribe improperly if they depended on the information provided in 44% of the ads. In general, the reviewing panels judged that 57% of advertisements had little or no educational value.

Pharmaceutical companies are a major source of funding for CME lectures and symposia (e.g., Leavitt, 1995; "Pushing Drugs to Doctors," 1992). Although even critics would agree that industry-supported educational presentations can be useful, there is reason to be wary. Frequently, companies exercise control over who will speak and mandate selection from lists of speakers known to favor the sponsor's products. In fact, *Consumer Reports* ("Pushing Drugs to Doctors," 1992) stated that experts were able to identify the specific drugs being promoted by simply hearing the names of the speakers. The article also cited a provocative study by Dr. Majorie Bowman that analyzed the content and outcome of two CME courses on the same topic, but sponsored by competing drug companies. As might be expected, the sponsoring company's drug was presented more favorably at each conference, with negative effects more often attributed to the competitor's product. A follow-up analysis of the prescribing patterns of those in attendance revealed that doctors favored the drugs produced by the company sponsoring the course they took.

Additional factors reduce the likelihood that treatment recommendations will be based purely on objective research. Included are the influences of pharmaceutical sales representatives: one for every 12 prescribing physicians in the United States (Leavitt, 1995). Sales representatives who obviously have a vested interest in the products they are touting, ply physicians with gifts, dinners, free samples, and objective-looking supplements to medical journals described earlier. In recent years, *Consumer Reports* conservatively estimated the annual promotional cost to the pharmaceutical industry to be about $5 billion ("Pushing Drugs to Doctors," 1992).

Drug companies have also actively attempted to influence the media through such activities as payment to journalists for producing favorable stories, the provision to the media of paid physician spokespersons who are presented as independent experts, and unacknowledged payment to celebrities for testimonial statements or interviews endorsing specific drugs ("Miracle Drugs or Media Drugs?" 1992). A newer marketing innovation has focused directly on the public in an attempt to get laypeople to request specific prescription drugs from physicians (Leavitt, 1995). These promotional efforts have been so successful that almost one third of prescriptions for new products are now the result of patient requests ("Miracle Drugs or Media Drugs?" 1992).

The bottom line is that scientific research is only one factor among many influencing treatment decisions. There is reason to believe that the impact of empirical results may be much diluted by competing forces that promote marketing interests while compromising the objective gathering and analysis of data.[8]

CONCLUSION

Having immersed ourselves in the diverse data in this book, we now confront the question of how properly to answer patients who ask quite directly what the probabilities are they can obtain significant therapeutic help from psychotropic drugs. What can one confidently say about the antidepressants or the anxiolytic agents or the so-called antipsychotics? We have debated possible answers at some length and have gradually perceived that confident rational statements are almost impossible to make. To begin with, we sorely lack dependable data as to the spontaneous rates of recovery for various forms of disturbance. How, then, do we know how much better any of the treatments are than no treatment? Actually, the data we possess concerning spontaneous recovery in such categories as unipolar depression and mania do not suggest that active drug treatments provide imposing advantages in recovery rates (e.g., Winokur & Tsuang, 1996). But beyond this matter, the drug trials dealing with the efficacies of psychoactive drugs are befuddled with poor research designs that allow an undefined and probably large amount of bias to intrude. Superimposed on this confused state of affairs are the twists and spins that drug companies

---

[8] There are ways to minimize the influence of possible biases resulting from drug-company-sponsored research. For example, it could be required that, before receiving approval, new drugs attain validation from a set of efficacy studies conducted by independent researchers. The research, possibly government funded, would have to be performed by scientists having no connections with pharmaceutical companies to ensure freedom from conflict of interest.

have managed to insinuate into the drug research establishment and its messages to practitioners and consumers.

In the end, we would have to say that at this moment no one is in a confident position to tell patients how effective psychoactive drugs truly are. Paradoxically, the only confident stance is one of uncertainty. The best way out of this uncertainty is to adopt better research designs that will filter out the possibilities of bias. On a more optimistic note, it is certainly conceivable that the combination of novel new drugs and more imaginative ways of enhancing placebo effects may eventually lead to demonstrably better treatments.

As for future research priorities, our reviews of the psychopharmacological literature have convinced us that several key questions deserve special attention in future research. There is immediate need to understand better how bias intrudes into current psychotropic drug testing and what can be done to remedy that bias. One of the first steps that should be taken is to develop active placebo analogues for the major psychotropic drugs and to ascertain the therapeutic power of these drugs when compared with the active analogues versus the passive placebos. Probably the active analogue will provide greater protection against bias and thereby reduce the level of therapeutic difference between drug and the placebo marker. Incidentally, as part of such efforts to expand knowledge of placebo contexts, we suggest investigations in which the efficacies of standard doses of psychotropic drugs would be systematically compared with drug doses so low as to approach the active placebo level and also with standard doses of drugs disguised as placebos (Subtractive Expectancy design). Both of these variations might provide new strategies for bolstering the failed conventional double-blind, inactive placebo design.

More studies are needed to clarify the extent to which comorbidity reduces psychotropic therapeutic power. Research samples should be recruited that match modal clinical populations. Only in this fashion will we get realistic rather than rarified estimates of what the drugs are capable of attaining therapeutically.

A third priority is to acquire detailed, long-term data concerning the side effects produced by major psychotropic agents. We propose not only cataloguing such side effects but also determining how much pain and discomfort they produce, how seriously they interfere with daily functioning, and, especially important, how long they persist. In addition, we need to learn more about what classes of side effects (e.g., pain, loss of function, interference with cognitive clarity) are particularly likely to counteract therapeutic processes.

A final prime issue is the impact of abrupt versus gradual withdrawal from a psychotropic drug on the probabilities of relapse. We have some information on this matter but need a good deal more in view of how many important tests of efficacy (e.g., involving lithium, antipsychotics) have been based on designs that compare individuals stabilized on a drug and then put on a placebo with those who are stabilized and not shifted. As earlier described, it is quite possible that the abruptness of the change (rather than the fact of change) determines whether removal from a drug causes recurrence of symptoms.

Numerous other questions would be interesting to address, but at this point we regard those just enumerated as the most cogent and profitable.

Finally, there is a dramatic contrast between the negative pictures we present concerning the efficacies of the major psychoactive drugs and the largely positive images predominating in public psychiatric expositions (e.g., psychiatric textbooks, recommendation to patients). How can such divergence exist? How can observers look at the same pool of data and arrive at such opposed perspectives?

This is not a rare occurrence. The history of medicine and other sectors of science are filled with examples of sharply different opinions about the meanings of observations and data collected. On the current medical scene, investigators continually find quite divergent evaluations of treatment modes and surgical procedures (Eisenberg, 1996). The history of psychiatry is populated with polarized ideas about how to cure various forms of psychopathology (Valenstein, 1986). Many variables mediate the divergent perspectives ranging from personal bias (e.g., self-aggrandizement, profit motive) to inertia and doctrinaire educational background.

What are the potential irrational sources of our differences with the standard positive view of psychoactive drugs held by biological psychiatry? Since all of the contributors to this volume are psychologists, one could ascribe the disagreements to turf or guild factors (psychological vs. biological). One cannot too easily dismiss such a possibility; it must be alertly entertained. Other observers may eventually conclude that we have not been wholly innocent of this form of bias. Further, psychologists have experienced a course of education quite different from that of most psychiatrists. They also do not have the same intimate clinical experiences with psychoactive drugs as do psychiatric practitioners.

We have tried to factor in these potential sources of bias. In the end, however, we can only appeal to the force of our intellectual arguments. In essence, the skepticism we recommend with reference to the psychoactive drugs is based on not only clear-cut deficiencies in the typical research design used to test such drugs but also the repeated evidence that when proper controls are introduced the differences in therapeutic power between the active drugs and placebos largely recede.

REFERENCES

Avorn, J., Chen, M., & Hartley, R. (1982). Scientific versus commercial sources of influence on the prescribing behavior of physicians. *American Journal of Medicine, 73,* 4–8.

Baldessarini, R. J., & Viguera, A. C. (1995). Neuroleptic withdrawal in schizophrenia patients. *Archives of General Psychiatry, 52,* 189–192.

Carroll, K. M., Rounsaville, B. J., & Nich, C. (1994). Blind man's bluff: Effectiveness and significance of psychotherapy and pharmacotherapy blinding procedures in a clinical trial. *Journal of Consulting and Clinical Psychology, 62,* 276–280.

Chase, M. (1989, January 26). Mixing science, stocks, raises question of bias in the testing of drugs. *Wall Street Journal,* pp. A1, A6.

Dewan, M. J., & Koss, M. (1989). The clinical impact of the side effects of psychotropic drugs. In S. Fisher & R. P. Greenberg (Eds.), *The limits of biological treatments for psychological distress* (pp. 189–234). Hillsdale, NJ: Erlbaum.

Eisenberg, L. (1996). What should doctors do in the face of negative evidence? *Journal of Nervous and Mental Disease, 184,* 103–105.

Fisher, S., & Greenberg, R. P. (1993). How sound is the double-blind design for evaluating psychotropic drugs? *Journal of Nervous and Mental Disease, 181,* 345–356.

Greenberg, R. P., Bornstein, R. F., Greenberg, M. D., & Fisher, S. (1992). A meta-analysis of antidepressant outcome under "blinder" conditions. *Journal of Consulting and Clinical Psychology, 60,* 664–669.

Guy, W. H. (1967). Placebo proneness: It's relationship to environmental influences and personality traits. *Dissertation Abstracts, 28*(5-B), 2137–2138.

Hudson, J. I., & Pope, H. G., Jr. (1990). Affective spectrum disorder: Does antidepressant response identify a family of disorders with a common pathophysiology? *American Journal of Psychiatry, 5,* 552–564.

Hughes, J. R., & Krahn, D. (1985). Blindness and the validity of the double blind procedure. *Journal of Clinical Pharmacology, 5,* 138–142.

Hyman, S. (1995–1996). How antidepressants might work. *Progress notes: American Society of Clinical Psychopharmacology, 6*(4), 11–15.

Kirk, S. A., & Kutchins, H. (1992). *The selling of DSM: The rhetoric of science in psychiatry.* New York: Aldine de Gruyter.

Kirsch, I., & Rosadino, M. J. (1993). Do double-blind studies with informed consent yield externally valid results? *Psychopharmacology, 110,* 437–442.

Krupnick, J. L., Sotsky, S. M., Simmins, S., Moyer, J., Elkin, I., Watkins, J., & Pilkonis, P. A. (1996). The role of the therapeutic alliance in psychotherapy and pharmacotherapy outcome: Findings in the National Institute of Mental Health Treatment of Depression Collaborative Research Program. *Journal of Consulting and Clinical Psychology, 64,* 532–539.

Kupfer, D. J., Frank, E., Perel, J. M., Cornes, C., Mallinger, A. G., Thase, M. E., McEachran, A. B., & Grochocinski, V. I. (1992). Five-year outcome for maintenance therapies in recurrent depression. *Archives of General Psychiatry, 49,* 769–773.

Leavitt, F. (1995). *Drugs & behavior.* Thousand Oaks, CA: Sage.

Levy, D. (1996, September 25). Ghostwriters a hidden resource for drug makers. *USA Today*, pp. 1A–2A.

Levy, G. (1992). Publication bias: Its implications for clinic pharmacology. *Clinical Pharmacology and Therapeutics, 52,* 115–119.

Lipman, R. S. (1989). Pharmacotherapy of the anxiety disorders. In S. Fisher & R. P. Greenberg (Eds.), *The limits of biological treatments for psychological distress: Comparisons with psychotherapy and placebo* (pp. 69–103). Hillsdale, NJ: Erlbaum.

McGuinness, D. (1989). Attention deficit disorder: The emperor's clothes, annual "pharm," and other fiction. In S. Fisher & R. P. Greenberg (Eds.), *The limits of biological treatments for psychological distress: Comparisons with psychotherapy and placebo* (pp. 151–187). Hillsdale, NJ: Erlbaum.

Mehta, K., Sorofman, B., & Rowland, C. (1989). Prescription drug advertising trends: A study of oral hypoglycemics. *Social Science and Medicine, 29,* 853–857.

Miracle drugs or media drugs? (1992, March). *Consumer Reports, 57,* 142–146.

Pellegrino, E. D. (1996). Clinical judgments, scientific data, and ethics: Antidepressant therapy in adolescents and children. *Journal of Nervous and Mental Disease, 184,* 106–108.

Pushing drugs to doctors. (1992, February). *Consumer Reports, 57,* 87–94.

Relman, A. S. (1989). Economic incentives in clinical investigation [Editorial]. *New England Journal of Medicine, 320,* 933–934.

Stimson, G. (1977). Do drug advertisements provide therapeutic information? *Journal of Medical Ethics, 3,* 7–13.

Suedfeld, P. (1984). The subtractive expectancy placebo procedure: A measure of non-specific factors in behavioural interventions. *Behavioral Research and Therapy, 22,* 159–164.

Thomson, R. (1982). Side effects and placebo amplification. *British Journal of Psychiatry, 140,* 64–68.

Valenstein, E. S. (1986). *Great and desperate cures.* New York: Basic Books.

Watson, D., & Clark, L. A. (1984). Negative affectivity: The disposition to experience aversive emotional states. *Psychological Bulletin, 96,* 465–490.

Whalen, C. K., & Henker, B. (1991). Therapies for hyperactive children: Comparisons, combinations, and compromises. *Journal of Consulting and Clinical Psychology, 59,* 126–137.

Wilkes, M., Doblin, B., & Shapiro, M. (1992). Pharmaceutical advertisements in leading medical journals: Experts' assessments. *Annals of Internal Medicine, 116,* 912–919.

Winokur, G., & Tsuang, M. T. (1996). *The natural history of mania, depression, and schizophrenia.* Washington, DC: American Psychiatric Press.

Author Index

Subject Index